Initiating and Sustaining the
CLINICAL NURSE LEADER ROLE

A PRACTICAL GUIDE

SECOND EDITION

Edited by

James L. Harris, DSN, APRN–BC, MBA, CNL, FAAN
Education and Practice Consultant
Nashville, Tennessee

Linda Roussel, DSN, RN, NEA–BC, CNL
University of Alabama Birmingham
School of Nursing
Birmingham, Alabama

Patricia L. Thomas, PhD, RN, FACHE, NEA-BC, ACNS-BC, CNL
Director, Nursing Practice & Research
Trinity Health
Livonia, Michigan

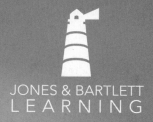

JONES & BARTLETT
LEARNING

World Headquarters
Jones & Bartlett Learning
5 Wall Street
Burlington, MA 01803
978-443-5000
info@jblearning.com
www.jblearning.com

Jones & Bartlett Learning books and products are available through most bookstores and online booksellers. To contact Jones & Bartlett Learning directly, call 800-832-0034, fax 978-443-8000, or visit our website, www.jblearning.com.

Substantial discounts on bulk quantities of Jones & Bartlett Learning publications are available to corporations, professional associations, and other qualified organizations. For details and specific discount information, contact the special sales department at Jones & Bartlett Learning via the above contact information or send an email to specialsales@jblearning.com.

Production Credits
Executive Publisher: William Brottmiller
Acquisitions Editor: Amanda Harvey
Editorial Assistant: Rebecca Myrick
Production Editor: Keith Henry
Senior Marketing Manager: Jennifer Stiles
V.P., Manufacturing and Inventory Control: Therese Connell
Composition: Paw Print Media
Cover Design: Kristin E. Parker
Cover and Title Page Images: (top) © Jasonash/ShutterStock, Inc.; (middle) © Eliks/ShutterStock, Inc.; (bottom) © VICTOR TORRES/ShutterStock, Inc.
Printing and Binding: Edwards Brothers Malloy
Cover Printing: Edwards Brothers Malloy

To order this product, use ISBN: 978-1-284-03288-8

Library of Congress Cataloging-in-Publication Data
Initiating and sustaining the clinical nurse leader role : a practical guide / [edited by] James L. Harris, Linda Roussel, and Patricia L. Thomas. — [2nd ed.]
   p. ; cm.
Includes bibliographical references and index.
ISBN 978-1-284-02656-6 (pbk.)
I. Harris, James L. (James Leonard), 1956– II. Roussel, Linda. III. Thomas, Patricia, 1961-
[DNLM: 1. Leadership. 2. Nurse Clinicians. 3. Interprofessional Relations. WY 128]
RT82.8
610.7306'92—dc23
                          2013013530

6048

Printed in the United States of America
17 16 15 14 13   10 9 8 7 6 5 4 3 2 1

Contents

Unit 1   Introduction

CHAPTER ONE

Introducing the Clinical Nurse Leader: Past,
Present, and Future 3

Joan M. Stanley

Unit 2   Academic, Clinical, and Community Partnerships

CHAPTER ELEVEN

CHAPTER TWELVE

CHAPTER THIRTEEN

CHAPTER FOURTEEN

Unit 4   Health Promotion and Disease Prevention: Essentials for the CNL

CHAPTER EIGHTEEN

CHAPTER NINETEEN

CHAPTER TWENTY

The Clinical Nurse Leader: Transforming Nursing Care in Acute Care, Ambulatory, and Long-Term Care Settings

Michelle A. Lucatorto, Evelyn Sommers, Larry Lemos, and Storm Morgan

Unit 5   Foundations for CNL Success

CHAPTER TWENTY-ONE

Creative and Meaningful Clinical Immersions

Patricia L. Thomas, James L. Harris, and Linda Roussel

Foreword

Doreen C. Harper

The evolution and practice base of the clinical nurse leader (CNL) role has made considerable progress since its inception and conceptualization in 2003 through a partnership between the American Association of Colleges of Nursing and practice leaders. This advanced nursing generalist is the first new role in nursing over the past 40 years that focuses on transforming care at the point of care—a role sorely needed in this nation's fragmented, complex, costly, and highly technical healthcare system. This second edition of *Initiating and Sustaining the Clinical Nurse Leader Role* expands the knowledge and evidence about the advanced nursing CNL role to work with nursing and interprofessional teams for the coordination of care, accountable processes of patient care and outcomes, and the mitigation of the triple threats of cost, quality, and access.

As dean at the University of Alabama at Birmingham, School of Nursing, I am pleased to have this opportunity to write the foreword for the second edition. My background in nursing education and workforce development, health policy, and advancement of interprofessional education has led me to conclude that the CNL can serve as the guardian of nursing care, helping to navigate patients and families through the healthcare maze driven by payers and policy. The Institute of Medicine's 2009 report *The Future of Nursing: Leading Change, Advancing Health* calls for nurses to practice to the full extent of their education and training and educating nurses for life-long learning. Advances in highly technical, specialized medical care and clinical services require nurses who are prepared at the graduate level with the requisite knowledge, skills, and competencies in care coordination, health systems operations, and evidence-based practice; quality and safety; teamwork; and communication, mentoring, and coaching to translate care and services across the continuum of care.

The CNL movement emerged from collaboration between academia and service in response to the growing need for a highly educated nurse at the point of patient care delivery. As an academic leader, I can attest to the critical role played by education–practice partnerships in strengthening nursing over the past 20 years. The CNL role emerged as a product of these academic–practice partnerships as practice leaders identified gaps in nursing and healthcare delivery, and through the role's relatively short life, CNLs have demonstrated their positive impact on improved patient clinical and financial outcomes.

In the next 10 years, I fully expect the demand for the CNL role to accelerate as health care unfolds within the landscape of healthcare reform and the Affordable Care Act of 2010. The need and demand for care coordination, continuity of care, and high-performance care teams will only increase in the future. As the authors explain and further develop the knowledge and competencies associated with the CNL role in this text, I remain convinced that CNLs are part of the solution to improving patient care quality and safety, reducing unnecessary medical errors, and managing excessive cost in our health system. The authors of this text have laid out a bold agenda for CNLs—an agenda that promotes their value in the transformation of clinical care redesign. The CNL role incorporates the clinical knowledge and competencies that guide the transformation of patient care while keeping the patient and family at the center of care. I look forward to the next 10 years as the CNL role continues to evolve. This role will create a brighter future for nursing, health care, and most importantly for the patients, families, and populations we serve.

Doreen C. Harper, PhD, RN, FAAN
Dean and Fay B. Ireland Endowed Chair in Nursing
The University of Alabama at Birmingham School of Nursing
Birmingham, Alabama

Acknowledgments

Great leaders are visionaries. Support, focus, and innovation are hallmarks of great leaders. Such qualities are the essence of the many individuals who envisioned a need for the clinical nurse leader (CNL) role, a nursing professional skilled in managing complex systems of care and elevating outcomes by making improvements at the point of care. CNLs return the locus of control for quality to its rightful place (Porter-O'Grady, Sinkus Clark, & Wiggins, 2010). My colleagues, Drs. Linda Roussel and Patricia (Tricia) Thomas, and I are unable to identify each of the individuals who continuously direct energies and purposeful insights as the CNL role evolves. We acknowledge the vision of Dr. Geraldine "Polly" Bednash and Dr. Joan Stanley of the American Association of Colleges of Nursing (AACN), who through dedication and tenacity engage nursing colleagues in thought and action as the CNL role develops and is implemented nationally. The efforts of the CNL Advisory Committee, the current president and past presidents of the AACN, the AACN membership and board, the AACN staff, and the Clinical Nurse Leader Association are recognized for their efforts and ongoing support of the CNL vision and the call to action to improve the health of all Americans. We acknowledged the Department of Veterans Affairs' (VA's) endorsement of the role and its spread throughout the VA system as both forward thinking and central to quality care for America's heroes. The VA's steadfast belief in CNLs has continued to contribute to quality care and the dissemination of measureable outcomes nationally. We would also like to acknowledge Gay Landstrom (SVP and CNO for Trinity Health) for her vision and commitment to the development of the CNL role within Trinity Health. Her contributions to cocreating curriculum and gaining support from the Trinity Health board allowed 38 CNLs scholarship and financial support to complete their CNL immersions. These CNLs are now demonstrating clinical, patient, and financial outcomes in four Michigan hospitals.

Linda, Tricia, and I would be remiss if we did not acknowledge the CNLs, CNL students, their clinical partners, and faculty who continue to keep this role and skill set at the point of care. By coordinating and planning interdisciplinary care, serving as a liaison to physicians, and facilitating quality improvement—including identification and dissemination of best practices, mentoring and coaching novice nurses, and communicating with patients and families—CNLs continue to address fragmented care and reduce health disparities.

James L. Harris
Linda Roussel
Tricia L. Thomas

Reference

Porter-O'Grady, T., Shinkus Clark, J., & Wiggins, M. S. (2010). The case for clinical nurse leaders: Guiding nursing practice into the 21st century. *Nurse Leader, 8*(1), 37–41.

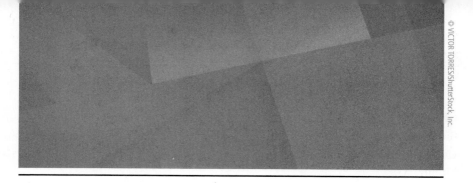

Chapter Contributors

Anna C. Alt-White, PhD, RN (Chapters 15, 16)
Department of Veterans Affairs
Office of Nursing Services
Washington, DC

Deborah Antai-Otong, MS, RN, CNS, NP, CS, FAAN (Chapter 6)
Veterans Integrated Systems Network
Arlington, TX

Laura Archbold, BSN, RN, MBA (Chapter 10)
Trinity Health
Livonia, MI

Alice E. Avolio, MS, RN, NE-BC (Chapters 5, 22)
Department of Veterans Affairs
Office of Nursing Services
Portland, OR

Michael R. Bleich, PhD, RN, NEA-BC, FAAN (Chapter 2)
Barnes Jewish College
Goldfarb School of Nursing
St. Louis, MO

Clista Clanton, MSLS (Chapter 14)
Biomedical Library
University of South Alabama
Mobile, AL

Greg Eagerton, DNP, RN, NEA-BC (Chapter 7)
VA Medical Center
Durham, NC

Alice J. Godfrey, MPH, RN, BC (Chapter 18)
University of South Alabama
College of Nursing
Mobile, AL

Larry Lemos, MSN, MHA, RN, GCNS-BC, NE-BC (Chapter 20)
VA Long Beach Health Care System
Long Beach, CA

Michelle A. Lucatorto, DNP, RN, FNCP-BC (Chapter 20)
Department of Veterans Affairs
Office of Nursing Services
Washington, DC

Margaret Moore-Nadler, DNP, RN (Chapter 19)
University of South Alabama
College of Nursing
Mobile, AL

Storm Morgan, MSN, MBA, RN (Chapter 20)
Department of Veterans Affairs
Office of Nursing Services
Washington, DC

Karen M. Ott, DNP, RN (Chapter 9)
Department of Veterans Affairs
Office of Nursing Services
Washington, DC

Beverly A. Priefer, PhD, RN (Chapters 15, 16)
Department of Veterans Affairs
Office of Nursing Services
Washington, DC

Carol Jefferson Ratcliffe, DNP, RN (Chapter 4)
Samford University School of Nursing
Birmingham, AL

Julia Stocker-Schneider, PhD, RN (Chapter 13)
University of Detroit Mercy
Detroit, MI

James M. Smith, PhD (Chapter 12)
Consultant
LaGrangeville, NY

Evelyn Sommers, MHSA (Chapter 20)
Department of Veterans Affairs
Office of Nursing Services
Washington, DC

Joan M. Stanley, PhD, RN, CRNP, FAAN (Chapter 1)
American Association of Colleges of Nursing
Washington, DC

Kathleen R. Stevens, EdD, MS, RN, ANEF, FAAN (Chapter 17)
Professor and Director
Academic Center for Evidence-Based Practice
University of Texas
Health Science Center at San Antonio
Improvement Science Research Network
San Antonio, TX

Melissa V. Taylor, PhD, RN (Chapters 15, 16)
VA Pittsburgh Health Care System
Pittsburgh, PA

Sandra E. Walters, DNP, RN (Chapter 3)
Consultant
Mt. Juliet, TN

Susan Wilkinson, MSN, RN, CNL (Chapter 8)
St. Vincent East
Birmingham, AL

Lonnie Williams, MSN, RN (Chapter 18)
Consultant
Nashville, TN

Marjory D. Williams, PhD, RN (Chapters 5, 22)
Department of Veterans Affairs
Office of Nursing Services
Washington, DC

Exemplar Contributors

Patricia Baker, MSN, RN-BC, CNL
South Texas Veterans Health Care System
San Antonio, TX

Miriam Bender, PhD, MSN, RN, CNL
University of San Diego/Sharp Healthcare System
San Diego, CA

Velinda J. Block, DNP, RN, NEA-BC
Chief Nurse Executive
University of Alabama Medical Center
Birmingham, AL

Barbara Bonnah, MSN, RN, CNL
Nursing Staff of 3 West, Medical Specialty Unit
Hunterdon Medical Center
Flemington, NJ

Laura Bozeman, MSN, RN, RNC-OB, CNL
Saint Joseph Mercy Hospital, Member of Trinity Health
Ann Arbor, MI

Kathy Carter, BSN, RN
University of Alabama Hospital
Birmingham, AL

Jennifer Densmore, BSN, RN
University of West Georgia
School of Nursing
WellStar Douglas Hospital
Douglasville, GA

Ann Eubanks, MSN, RN, CNL
Springhill Medical Center
Mobile, AL

Tina Fogel, PharmD
University of Alabama Hospital
Birmingham, AL

Madalyn Frank-Cooper, RN, MS, CNL
Winthrop University Hospital
Mineola, NY

Anita Girard, MSN, RN, CCRN, CNL
Nursing Quality Management Coordinator
Stanford Hospital & Clinics
Stanford, CA

Bridget Graham, MSN, RN-BC, CNL
Saint Mary's Health Care, Member of Trinity Health
Grand Rapids, MI

Deanne Guthrie, MCS
Systems Analyst
University of Alabama Medical Center
Birmingham, AL

Lauran Hardin, MSN, RN, CNL
Saint Mary's Health Care, Member of Trinity Health
Grand Rapids, MI

Mary Harnish, MSN, RN, CDE, CNL
Saint Mary's Health Care, Member of Trinity Health
Grand Rapids, MI

Kevin Hengeveld, MSN, RN, CNL
Saint Mary's Health Care, Member of Trinity Health
Grand Rapids, MI

Nancy Hilton, MN, RN
Chief Nurse Officer
St. Lucie Medical Center
Port St. Lucie, FL

Vicki Hogan, RN
Nursing Informatics
University of Alabama Medical Center
Birmingham, AL

Terri Johnson, MSN, RN
University of Alabama Hospital
Birmingham, AL

Lissy Joseph, MSN, RN
Michael E. DeBakey VA Medical Center
Houston, TX

Angela Jukkala, PhD, RN, CNE, CNL
University of Alabama
School of Nursing
Birmingham, AL

Jennifer Kareivis, MSN, RN, CNL
Nursing Staff of 3 West, Medical Specialty Unit
Hunterdon Medical Center
Flemington, NJ

Susan E. Koons, MSN, RN, CNL
Pine Rest Christian Mental Health Services
Grand Rapids, MI

Tracy Lofty, MSA, CAE, ACA
Director, Commission on Nurse Certification
American Association of Colleges of Nursing
Washington, DC

Sona H. Mahal, MSN, RN, PHN, CNL
University of California, San Francisco
Central Marin General Hospital
San Francisco, CA

Kristin Mast, MSN, RN, CNL, CNRN
Saint Mary's Health Care, Member of Trinity Health
Grand Rapids, MI

Mary E. Mathers, MSN, RN, CNL
South Texas Veterans Health Care System
San Antonio, TX

Lisa Mestas, MSN, RN, CORN
Assistant Administrator of Clinical Services
University of South Alabama Medical Center
Mobile, AL

Elizabeth A. Murphy, BScN, MSBA, RN, NEA-BC, FACHE
Vice President and Chief Nursing Officer
Saint Mary's Health Care, Member of Trinity Health
Grand Rapids, MI

Ann Nguyen, RN, WCC, MSN
University of San Francisco
San Francisco, CA

Kristen Noles, MSN, RN, CNL
Nurse Manager, ATCU/BDT
University of Alabama Medical Center
Birmingham, AL

Tommie Norris, DNS, RN
Director of MSN-CNL Program
University of Tennessee Health Science Center
Memphis, TN

Pamela Patterson, MSN, RN
University of Alabama Hospital
Birmingham, AL

Beverly Phillips, BSN, RN, CWOCN
Nursing Staff of 3 West, Medical Specialty Unit
Hunterdon Medical Center
Flemington, NJ

Leslie Phillips, MSN, RN, CNL
Saint Joseph Mercy Hospital, Member of Trinity Health
Ann Arbor, MI

Shea Polks, PharmD
Supervisor
Pharmacy Informatics
University of Alabama Medical Center
Birmingham, AL

Lisa Rasimowicz, RN, BSN, CIC
Infection Preventionist
Hunterdon Medical Center
Flemington, NJ

Shelia Cumbie Ross, MSN, RN, CNL
Stroke Coordinator
Mobile Infirmary
Mobile, AL

Kathy Roye-Horn, RN, CIC
Director of Infection Prevention
Hunterdon Medical Center
Flemington, NJ

Sunny Rutter, MSN, RN, CNL
University of San Francisco
Director, Emergency Department
San Francisco, CA

Sheri Salas, MSN, RN
Nurse Educator
University of South Alabama Medical Center
Mobile, AL

Marie San Pedro, MS, RN, CNL
New York Presbyterian Hospital Weill Cornell Center
New York, NY

Laurie Sayer, MSN, RN, RN-C, CNL
Saint Mary's Health Care, Member of Trinity Health
Grand Rapids, MI

Laurie A. Schwartz, MSN, RN, CEN, CNL
Saint Mary's Health Care, Member of Trinity Health
Grand Rapids, MI

Michelle Sheets, MSN, RN, CNL
Nursing Staff of 3 West, Medical Specialty Unit
Hunterdon Medical Center
Flemington, NJ

Barbara L. Summers, PhD, RN, NEA-BC, FAAN
Professor and Chair, Department of Nursing
Vice President and Chief Nursing Officer
Division Head, Nursing
University of Texas
MD Anderson Center
Houston, TX

Maureen Tait, MSN, RN, CNL
Saint Joseph Mercy Hospital, Member of Trinity Health
Ann Arbor, MI

Vidette Todaro-Franceschi, PhD, RN, FT
Hunter-Bellevue School of Nursing
New York, NY

Enna Edouard Trevathan, DNP, MSN, RN, MBA, CNL
University of San Francisco
Assistant Professor & Director of the Online RN/MSN Program
School of Nursing and Health Professions
San Francisco, CA

Elizabeth Triezenberg, MSN, RN, CNL, CNRN
Saint Mary's Health Care, Member of Trinity Health
Grand Rapids, MI

Tiffany Tscherne, BSN, RN (CNL Student)
University of South Alabama College of Nursing
Mobile, AL

Rebecca Valko, MSN, RN, CNL, CNRN
Saint Mary's Health Care, Member of Trinity Health
Grand Rapids, MI

Beth VanDam, MSN, RN-BC, CNL
Saint Mary's Health Care, Member of Trinity Health
Grand Rapids, MI

Sherry Webb, DNSc, NEA-BC, CNL
University of Tennessee, Memphis
Memphis, TN

Mary Lou Wesley, MSN, RN
Senior Vice President
Chief Nurse Executive
WellStar Health Systems
Marietta, GA

Donna Whitehead, BSN, RN (CNL student)
WellStar Health Systems
Marietta, GA
University of West Georgia, MSN-CNL Student
Carrollton, GA

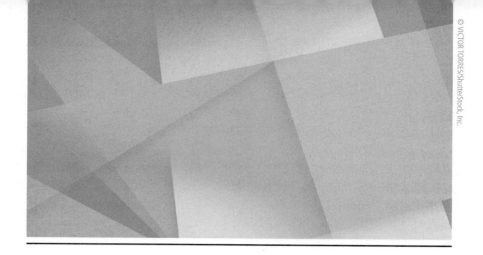

UNIT 1
Introduction

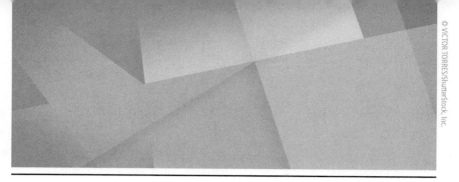

© VICTOR TORRES/ShutterStock, Inc.

ONE

Introducing the Clinical Nurse Leader: Past, Present, and Future

■ Joan M. Stanley

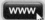 **Learning Objectives**
© Arenacreative/Dreamstime.com

- Discuss how the clinical nurse leader (CNL) contributes to care coordination within the evolving and constantly changing healthcare environment
- Describe the CNL role evolution—past, present, and future

Introduction

Health care is at a critical junction. Economic uncertainty, mushrooming costs, rapid growth in biomedical advances, workforce shortages, changing population demographics, and demands for better outcomes all call for new ways of delivering health care and educating future health professionals. Despite the many ways the profession has evolved over the past decade, nursing continues to be faced with unique challenges, including the fragmentation of care, retention of nurses in the profession, opportunities for

> "I have an almost complete disregard of precedent, and a faith in the possibility of something better. It irritates me to be told how things have always been done. I defy the tyranny of precedent. I go for anything new that might improve the past."
>
> Clara Barton

career advancement, utilization of nurses to the full scope of practice, and equipping clinicians with the knowledge and skills needed to address the competing demands of a complex healthcare system. Inter- and intraprofessional collaboration are key to meeting these challenges. Innovative partnering between the practice and education arenas is even more critical to address and sustain effective solutions for the long term. Within this environment, the American Association of Colleges of Nursing (AACN), in partnership with practice leaders, created the clinical nurse leader (CNL) role—the first new nursing role in over 40 years. The CNL is prepared to respond to today's challenges and readily adapt to meet the needs of the rapidly changing healthcare environment.

The Healthcare Environment

In 1999, the Institute of Medicine (IOM) released its landmark report, *To Err is Human: Building a Safer Health System*, which estimated that up to 98,000 Americans die each year as a result of medical errors (IOM, 1999). Subsequent estimates indicated that these numbers could be even higher (Leape & Berwick, 2005). The estimated national costs of preventable adverse events (medical errors resulting in injury) are in the billions. Medication-related errors and mistakes that do not result in actual harm are also extremely costly and have a significant impact on quality of care and healthcare outcomes. Over the past two decades, the IOM (2003) and others, including the American Hospital Association (AHA, 2002), The Joint Commission (2002), and the Robert Wood Johnson Foundation (Kimball & O'Neil, 2002), have all called on healthcare systems to refocus their efforts to reduce medical errors, improve patient safety, and reevaluate how future health professionals will be educated.

A report released by the U.S. Department of Labor in February 2012 reported that the growth in nursing jobs was the largest among all professions. The report projected that the number of employed nurses would increase from 2.74 million in 2010 to 3.45

million in 2020, an unprecedented increase of 26% (U.S. Department of Labor, 2012). Buerhaus and coauthors projected that the nursing shortage will increase to 260,000 nurses by 2025, twice the size of any previous shortage (Buerhaus, 2009). The nursing shortage will have dire consequences for quality of care and nursing outcomes if it is not addressed. Needleman and associates demonstrated that lower nurse staffing levels were associated with adverse patient outcomes, including higher rates of pneumonia, urinary tract infections, length of stay, and "failure to rescue" (Needleman et al., 2002). Aiken and colleagues (2002) found that low nurse-to-patient ratios were related to higher risk-adjusted 30-day mortality and "failure to rescue" rates. In addition, nurses practicing in settings with lower nurse-to-patient ratios were more likely to experience burnout and job dissatisfaction (Aiken et al., 2002).

In addition to the predictions of a long-lasting nursing shortage and the universal calls from outside nursing to change the way health professionals are educated and practice, several studies have demonstrated that nurses educated at baccalaureate or higher degree levels produce better patient outcomes, specifically reduced mortality and failure-to-rescue rates (Aiken et al., 2003; Estabrooks et al., 2005). In its report, *The Future of Nursing*, the Institute of Nursing called for 80% of the nursing workforce to hold a minimum of a baccalaureate degree by 2020 and recommended that all nurses be allowed to work to the full scope of their education in order to address and face the challenges of the country's healthcare system (Institute of Nursing, 2010).

Leading the Profession to a New Vision for Nursing Education

In direct response to the changing global demographics, the turmoil of the healthcare system, and the drastic shortage of nursing professionals, the AACN began a dialogue to examine and shape nursing education. For over a decade, this dialogue, which is participated in by a broad representation of stakeholders both inside and outside of the nursing profession, focused on the knowledge, skills, and competencies needed by professional nurses to address the demands of an evolving healthcare system. From this dialogue emerged a preferred vision of the future of nursing, as well as new models for nursing education. This vision encompasses all levels of nursing education, from the baccalaureate degree to the doctorate (Stanley, 2008). The CNL— prepared at the master's-degree level to practice in any healthcare setting, with a focus on quality improvement, interprofessional communication, evidence-based practice, and care coordination—is its linchpin.

In 1999, the AACN board of directors formed the Task Force on Education and Regulation for Professional Nursing Practice (TFER). The task force developed new education models, including a model for the "New Nurse" graduate, a clinician educated beyond the 4-year baccalaureate degree with a new license and legal scope of practice. After consultation with nurse executives, regulators, and other key stakeholders, the TFER determined that a new role was needed to differentiate professional nursing's scope of practice. At the same time, the National Council of State Boards of Nursing (NCSBN) indicated it was not possible to create a separate license for entry-level nurses educated at the associate and baccalaureate-degree levels unless the roles were well differentiated.

In 2002, in response to the recommendations from the TFER, the AACN board created TFER II, which was charged with examining what competencies were needed in the current and future healthcare system to improve patient care outcomes. A wide array of stakeholders, representing nursing education and practice, medicine, healthcare administration, pharmacology, public health, and others, were invited to provide input about what this "new nurse" role might look like. Their work resulted in the 2007 publication of the *White Paper on the Role of the Clinical Nurse Leader*. Prior to its publication, in addition to discussing the competencies needed for this new role, many discussions were held within AACN and with external groups about a possible name for the new role and the kind of education that would be needed to prepare someone to practice at this level.

The CNL Initiative Is Born

Since the early stages of the conception of the new role, the AACN board has remained committed to the implementation of the CNL and the involvement of both education and practice. In 2003, the Implementation Task Force (ITF), composed of representatives from both the education and practice arenas, was appointed to oversee the development of the new role. Modeling the importance of education–practice partnerships, the American Organization of Nurse Executives (AONE) was invited to appoint a representative to serve on the ITF. Another extremely important partner in this initiative was the Department of Veterans Affairs (DVA). Cathy Rick, chief nursing officer and an early stakeholder, has been a proponent of the CNL from its earliest stages, and the DVA has participated at all levels in collaborating on the design and implementation of the CNL role. This joint participation by education and practice has been a key factor in the success of the initiative. In January 2007, the ITF submitted its final report and recommendations to the AACN board. Tremendous strides had been made in moving the CNL initiative forward; however, continued support and leadership by AACN was critical to sustaining the early momentum and ensuring continued growth. Responding to the ITF's recommendation, in March 2007, the AACN board appointed the CNL steering committee, composed also of education and practice representatives, whose primary charge was to elevate the visibility and sustainability of the CNL role and support the measurement of the CNL's impact on patient care outcomes and costs.

Key Steps and Landmarks Along the Way

In October 2003, the AACN sent an open invitation to all deans of schools of nursing inviting them to participate in an exploratory meeting about the CNL role, which included exploring the implications and expectations for education programs and the transformation of care delivery models. The only requirement of participants was that they attend with at least one nurse leader from a practice institution. Over 280 individuals representing 100 potential partnerships attended this exploratory meeting. By March 2004, a request for proposals (RFP) was sent to all AACN member schools inviting schools and their practice partners to commit to implementing the CNL role, including the design of a master's-level CNL curriculum and integration of the CNL role within at least one unit in the practice setting. In June 2004, the ITF sponsored a CNL implementation conference for all education practice partners participating in the initiative. Representatives from 79 schools of nursing and 136 practice organizations participated with the goal of advancing the CNL movement.

By fall 2006, the number of partnerships had grown to 87, representing 93 schools of nursing and 191 healthcare practice settings. This number has continued to grow and now includes 98 schools and well over 200 practice settings, including a number of large healthcare systems. In a recent survey of the AACN member schools, 124 respondents indicated they had in place or were planning to institute a CNL program.

Numerous forums and conferences, including annual CNL conferences, have been held since the initial CNL implementation conference in June 2004. Over 400 faculty, deans, chief nursing officers, CNLs, students, healthcare administrators, and physicians attended the Fourth National CNL Summit, jointly sponsored by the AACN and the DVA, highlighting the success and continued growth of the

CNL initiative. The Fifth National CNL Summit occurred in January 2013 in New Orleans, Louisiana, and was widely attended by multiple stakeholders.

The CNL Association (CNLA), open to all CNLs and students, held its inaugural meeting during the First AACN–DVA National Summit in 2009. The CNLA has continued to grow its membership, supporting a regional conference annually and providing online education offerings, including a newly designed website.

Another landmark decision was the development of a CNL certification examination and designation. (*See "The CNL: Past, Present, and Future" at the end of this chapter, for more detail*). CNL certification provides a unique credential for graduates of the master's and post-master's CNL programs. The CNL Certification Examination was tested by 12 schools during the period from November 2006 to January 2007. The first regular administration of the CNL Certification Examination occurred in April and May 2007. Since that time, nearly 2,500 CNLs have been certified and may use the credential and title CNL. The Commission on Nurse Certification (CNC) was formed in 2007. An elected board and staff oversee all certification related activities and policies.

The AACN was also successful in trademarking the CNL title and the CNL Certification Examination in an effort to protect the integrity of this new designation. Only individuals who are successful in obtaining CNL certification may use the title CNL. In addition, the trademark symbol is to be used along with the CNL title, any reference to the title, or when citing the CNL Certification Examination.

The CNL Role

The CNL role was designed in collaboration with a broad array of stakeholders within the healthcare system. As the role emerged, it became evident that many leaders in practice had already identified the need for a nurse with these skill and knowledge sets. Similar roles were being developed and emerging on an ad hoc basis in settings across the country. Nurses were being recruited to fill these roles based on availability, clinical experiences, and self-selection. In many instances these nurses were completing classroom and clinical work without receiving academic credit or recognition of the advanced competencies being acquired. In addition, there was no standardization of the competencies and experiences required, and the utilization of these nurses varied from site to site. All of these factors prevented these CNL forerunners from moving from one care setting to another, discouraged the duplication of care models, and made it difficult to assess the impact these clinicians were having on care outcomes.

The patient care facilitator (PCF) role was designed by cardiovascular nursing staff in response to a challenge to describe the ideal unit staffing pattern. We piloted the PCF position, and it was so successful that we continued to implement the role across other areas and units. When the CNL role was first described we developed an academic practice partnership model and began to educate our PCFs to become CNLs.

Joan Shinkus Clark, DNP, RN, NEA-BC, CENP, FACHE, FAAN, Senior Vice President and System Chief Nurse Executive, Texas Health Resources

Assumptions About the CNL

Ten assumptions about the CNL were articulated early on by the AACN as role competencies were delineated and curricula designed. These assumptions included:

1. Practice is at the microsystem level.
2. Client care outcomes are the measure of quality practice.
3. Practice guidelines are based on evidence.
4. Client-centered practice is intra- and interdisciplinary.
5. Information will maximize self-care and client decision making.
6. Nursing assessment is the basis for theory and knowledge development.
7. Good fiscal stewardship is a condition of quality care.
8. Social justice is an essential nursing value.
9. Communication technology will facilitate the continuity and comprehensiveness of care.
10. The CNL must assume guardianship for the nursing profession (AACN, 2007).

The impact of the CNL has been even greater than expected. Nurses influence all of the critical metrics for our health system: quality and safety, patient experiences, finance, growth, employee engagement. The CNL plays a critical role in all of these.

MaryLou Wesley, MSN, RN, Senior VP & Chief Nurse Executive, WellStar Health System Inc., Marietta, GA

Key Components of the CNL Role

The CNL is seen as a leader in the healthcare delivery system—not just in the acute care setting, but in all settings in which health care is delivered. The implementation of the CNL role, however, varies across settings. The CNL is not an administrative or management role. The CNL assumes accountability for patient care trends and outcomes through the assimilation and application of evidence-based information to design, implement, and evaluate plans and processes of care. The CNL is a provider and manager of care at the point of care to individuals and cohorts of patients within a unit or healthcare setting. The CNL designs, implements, and evaluates patient care by coordinating, delegating, and supervising the care provided by the healthcare team, including licensed nurses, technicians, and other health professionals.

The defining aspects of CNL practice include:

- Leadership in the care of patients in and across all settings;
- Implementation of evidence-based practice in all healthcare settings for diverse and complex patients;
- Coordination of care;
- Lateral integration of care for a cohort of patients;
- Clinical decision making;
- Risk anticipation, specifically evaluating anticipated risks to patient safety with the aim of quality improvement and preventing medical errors;
- Participation in identification and collection of care outcomes;
- Accountability for evaluation and improvement of point-of-care outcomes;
- Mass customization of care;
- Interprofessional communication;
- Leveraging human, environmental, and material resources;
- Client and community advocacy;
- Education for individuals, families, groups, and other healthcare providers;
- Information management, including using information systems and technology at the point of care to improve healthcare outcomes;
- Oversight of care delivery and outcomes; and
- Team leadership and collaboration with other health professional team members (AANC, 2007).

An in-depth description of each of these practice components can be found in the AACN 2007 white paper, *The Role of the Clinical Nurse Leader* (AACN, 2007).

An expert panel representing CNL education, practice, and certification has been charged with the review and revision of the outcomes expected of all CNL graduates as currently delineated in the AACN 2007 white paper. This review and revision will be based on a 2011 job analysis conducted by CNC, a review of the CNL literature, and the lived experience of panel members. The process used to identify the new set of expected outcomes and competencies will be a national consensus-based process used previously to develop competencies for nurse practitioner and clinical nurse specialist competencies (Department of Health and Human Services, 2002).

> **The biggest impact the CNL has had in our healthcare system is how lateral integration and continuity of care has improved interdisciplinary communication and patient care outcomes.**
>
> Patricia Steingall, MS, RN, NE-BC, Chief Nursing Officer, VP Patient Care Services, Hunterdon Medical Center, NJ

Educating the CNL

As the CNL evolved, extensive dialogue occurred about the appropriate level of education to prepare someone with this unique set of competencies and to practice in this new role. Crosswalking the essential competencies for entry-level professional nurses (AACN, 1998) with those identified for the CNL (Stanley, 2008) clearly showed that the additional knowledge, skills, and experiences needed to practice in this new role could not be obtained within the confines of a 4-year baccalaureate nursing program. Based on this evaluation and input from multiple stakeholders, the decision was made by the AACN board that the educational preparation of the CNL should be at the graduate level, in a master's or post-master's degree program.

In fall 2007, 1,270 students were enrolled in 70 CNL programs, and in the 2006–2007 academic year, 265 students graduated from these CNL programs (Fang, Li, & Bednash, 2008). By fall 2011, these numbers increased to 2,817 students enrolled in 97 programs with 926 graduates in the 2010–2011 academic year (APRN Consensus, 2008). In addition, over 2,300 graduates of the CNL programs were certified by CNC by fall 2012.

After only 6 months of rolling out the CNLs on two pilot units, there were so many changes occurring in health care that I knew that nursing needed to take the lead in working with our physician colleagues in making these changes. These included pay for performance associated with core measures and the Hospital Consumer Assessment of Healthcare Providers and Systems Survey and decreasing hospital-acquired conditions. I quickly discovered that the new CNL role was the perfect fit to meet or exceed all of the goals for these new initiatives. The CNL now serves as the liaison between physicians, patients, families, and nursing staff.

Nancy Hilton, MN, RN, Chief Nursing Officer, HCA St. Lucie Medical Center, Port St. Lucie, FL

The CNL Curriculum Framework

Assumptions about CNL graduate education programs include:

1. The education program culminates in a master's degree or post-master's degree in nursing.
2. The CNL graduate is prepared as an advanced generalist with an emphasis on quality improvement and care coordination in any care setting.
3. The CNL graduate will be competent to provide care at the point of care.
4. The CNL graduate will be prepared in clinical leadership for practice throughout the healthcare delivery system.
5. The CNL graduate is eligible to matriculate to a practice- or research-focused doctoral program.
6. The CNL graduate is prepared with advanced nursing knowledge and skills but does not meet the criteria for advanced practice registered nursing (APRN) scope of practice (Institute of Nursing, 2010).
7. The CNL graduate is eligible to sit for the CNL Certification Examination.

The CNL curriculum framework encompasses three foci: nursing leadership, clinical outcomes management, and care environment management. Under each focus are major areas of emphasis, as shown in **Figure 1-1**. Ten threads that should be integrated throughout the curriculum in didactic and clinical experiences are also

Figure 1-1   CNL curriculum framework.

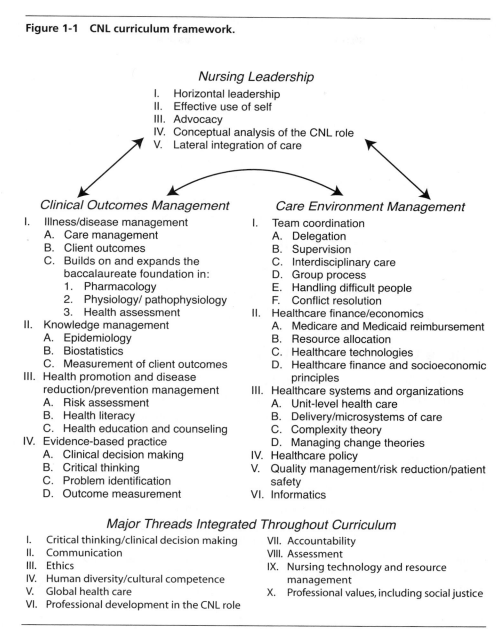

Nursing Leadership

I.   Horizontal leadership
II. Effective use of self
III. Advocacy
IV. Conceptual analysis of the CNL role
V.   Lateral integration of care

Clinical Outcomes Management

I.   Illness/disease management
  A. Care management
  B. Client outcomes
  C. Builds on and expands the baccalaureate foundation in:
    1. Pharmacology
    2. Physiology/ pathophysiology
    3. Health assessment
II. Knowledge management
  A. Epidemiology
  B. Biostatistics
  C. Measurement of client outcomes
III. Health promotion and disease reduction/prevention management
  A. Risk assessment
  B. Health literacy
  C. Health education and counseling
IV. Evidence-based practice
  A. Clinical decision making
  B. Critical thinking
  C. Problem identification
  D. Outcome measurement

Care Environment Management

I.   Team coordination
  A. Delegation
  B. Supervision
  C. Interdisciplinary care
  D. Group process
  E. Handling difficult people
  F. Conflict resolution
II. Healthcare finance/economics
  A. Medicare and Medicaid reimbursement
  B. Resource allocation
  C. Healthcare technologies
  D. Healthcare finance and socioeconomic principles
III. Healthcare systems and organizations
  A. Unit-level health care
  B. Delivery/microsystems of care
  C. Complexity theory
  D. Managing change theories
IV. Healthcare policy
V.   Quality management/risk reduction/patient safety
VI. Informatics

Major Threads Integrated Throughout Curriculum

I.   Critical thinking/clinical decision making
II.   Communication
III. Ethics
IV.   Human diversity/cultural competence
V.   Global health care
VI.   Professional development in the CNL role
VII. Accountability
VIII. Assessment
IX.   Nursing technology and resource management
X.   Professional values, including social justice

Source: AACN. (2007). *White paper on the role of the clinical nurse leader* (p. 32). Washington, DC: Author.

identified. The actual design of the curriculum rests with the faculty at the schools of nursing. However, the expectation is that the graduate will be prepared with the competencies delineated in the AACN *White Paper on the Role of the Clinical Nurse Leader*, as well as the required clinical experiences. The immersion experience is a critical component of the CNL curriculum. In addition to other clinical experiences integrated throughout the program, the immersion includes a minimum of 300 hours in practice in the CNL role with a designated clinical preceptor and a faculty partner. Many education programs partner with a clinical practice site and designate a single preceptor but also involve a variety of other individuals, including human resources personnel, financial officers, quality improvement personnel, patient safety officers, and nursing educators in the teaching of the CNL student.

CNL Curriculum Models

Five curriculum models for graduate CNL education programs have emerged. These five models are described in **Table 1-1**. The percentages of schools that have implemented each type of model are shown in **Figure 1-2**.

Where CNLs Are Practicing

The CNL competencies delineated in the AACN's *White Paper on the Role of the Clinical Nurse Leader* are meant to prepare nurses to practice as leaders in any healthcare setting. Stakeholders who were asked to review early documents describing the CNL

Table 1-1   CNL Curriculum Models

Model	Program Description
Model A	Program designed for BSN graduates
Model B	Program designed for BSN graduates; includes a post-BSN residency that awards master's credit toward the CNL degree
Model C	Program for individuals with a baccalaureate degree in another discipline; also known as a second-degree or generic master's
Model D	Program designed for ADN graduates; also known as an RN-MSN program
Model E	Post-master's certificate program

BSN, bachelor's of nursing science; AND, associate's degree in nursing; RN-MS, registered nurse with a master's of science in nursing

Figure 1-2 Percentage of schools offering CNL curriculum models (*n* = 99).

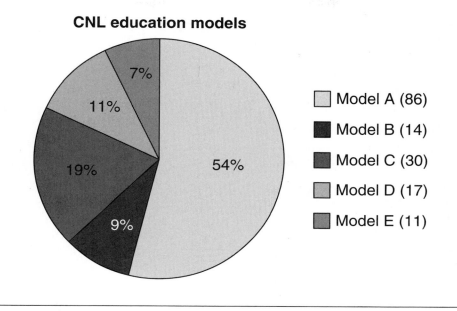

CNL education models

Model A (86)
Model B (14)
Model C (30)
Model D (17)
Model E (11)

Source: AACN CNL database 10/2012.

role and competencies unanimously stated that a nurse prepared with this set of competencies would be a valuable asset to their area of nursing practice or practice setting. The implementation of the CNL competencies, however, does vary across settings, and the CNL's day-to-day activities differ depending upon the setting, patient population, and care delivery model. To be most successful in any setting, however, the care delivery should be reshaped, and the CNL integrated into this revised model to fully use the unique skill and knowledge set brought to the point of care by this new nurse.

CNLs are practicing and making a significant impact in a variety of practice sites. A majority of the early graduates are practicing in acute care hospitals, where demands for improved outcomes and better ways of delivering care have been well documented. CNLs are also migrating to other employment settings including school health, long-term care, rehabilitation settings, outpatient clinics, home care, emergency departments, and state health departments. The employment settings for the early certified CNLs are displayed in **Table 1-2.**

Table 1-2   Employment Sites for Certified CNLs

CNL(r) Employment Settings (*N* = 535)

Acute care inpatient	304
Community/public health	11
Home health	6
School/university health	24
Nursing home/long-term care/subacute care	7
Hospice	1
Hospital outpatient	7
Outpatient clinic/or surgery center	22
Physician practice	2
Nurse-managed practice	2
School of nursing	89
Other	60

Source: CNC Certification Database, 3/09.

> I hope the CNL stays focused on the microsystem, either at the bedside or in an outpatient setting. We often move experienced nurses away from the point of care delivery and lose the effectiveness and impact.
>
> MaryLou Wesley, MSN, RN, Senior VP & Chief Nurse Executive, WellStar Health System, Inc., Marietta, GA

Impact of the CNL Role on Care Outcomes

As the number of CNLs in practice increases, the impact on patient care outcomes is becoming apparent. Although many of the reports on the impacts, costs, and benefits are anecdotal, outcomes are increasingly being reported in lay and professional publications and at professional conferences. Stanley and colleagues reported outcomes of care at three healthcare settings located in one state (Stanley et al., 2008). These outcomes included improvement in the Center for Medicare and Medicaid Services (CMS) core measures (e.g. pain management, acute myocardial infarction [MI], congestive heart failure [CHF], and pneumonia indicators), improved care coordination, improved physician–nurse collaboration, improved patient satisfaction, and decreased nurse turnover.

Gabuat and colleagues (2008) reported on a CNL pilot initiative that was conducted on a progressive care unit and medical/surgical unit at a for-profit hospital. Initially designed to be budget neutral, outcomes pre- and post-CNL implementation on these units also included decreased nursing turnover, increased patient and physician satisfaction, and improved core measures (acute MI, CHF, and pneumonia). Hartranft and colleagues reported significant patient safety improvements that included zero falls with injury and nosocomial infections and pressure ulcers, improved patient satisfaction, and 100% achievement of CMS core measures after implementation of the CNL role on several units (Hartranft, Garcia, & Adams, 2007). In addition, Hartranft notes that many of the outcomes achieved by the CNL are not captured in hard data.

> In the future, I see the CNL as the link between acute care and the outpatient settings, which is critically important with the current and impending changes in the healthcare environment.
>
> Patricia Steingall, MS, RN, NE-BC, Chief Nursing Officer, VP Patient Care Services, Hunterdon Medical Center, NJ

For that reason, the CNLs at this facility keep a daily journal of "saves" and qualitative accomplishments, for example identifying the need for early intervention and ability to stabilize a patient without moving to a higher level of care (a savings of approximately $1,150 per day just for the bed) (Stanley et al., 2008, p. 263). Other identified outcomes have been improvement in goal setting, greater engagement of staff nurses in projects, and improved nurse and physician satisfaction.

The DVA was involved in the early implementation of the CNL role, and the Veterans Health Administration is moving to fully implement the CNL role across all VA settings by the year 2016 (James Harris, verbal communication, March 6, 2009). One of the first VA settings where the CNL role was implemented was the Tennessee Valley Healthcare System (TVHS). AACN and TVHS collaborated on a pilot of an evaluation tool to capture clinical outcomes pre- and post-assignment of unit-based CNLs (Harris et al., 2006). Preliminary findings from this pilot were positive and encouraging, including decreased readmission rates for patients discharged with CHF, decreased length of stay for patients with CHF, increased discharge instructions for patients with CHF on an acute medical unit, and decreased patient falls

> The biggest impact the CNLs have had is in "just in time" training for the nursing staff. The CNLs have raised the level of nursing care on the units, including implementing evidence-based care processes, Core Measure compliance, and decreasing hospital-acquired conditions.
>
> Nancy Hilton, MN, RN, Chief Nursing Officer, HCA St. Lucie Medical Center, Port St. Lucie, FL

and surgical infection rates 30 days postoperative on an acute surgical unit. Since these early outcomes were reported, evaluation at TVHS of the outcomes on five care units (microsystems of care) have also been reported. Significant demonstrated outcomes included a 20% decrease in patients receiving a blood transfusion following total knee arthroplasty (TKA) on a surgical inpatient unit, a 28.6% increase in venous thromboembolism prophylaxis implementation for critically ill intubated patients, and an 8% increase in participation in a restorative dining program on a transitional care unit (Hix, McKeon, & Walters, 2009).

Other reported outcomes linked to CNL practice include an 18.2% decrease in critical care days and a 40% decrease in returns to the critical care unit netting $800,000 in savings over a 14-month period after a CNL implemented multidisciplinary rounds on long-term ventilator patients. Another CNL collaborated with a team of orthopedic surgeons and blood bank personnel to evaluate and then eliminate retransfusion of blood cells in TKA patients, which led to decreased opportunities for infection and netted an estimated $100,000 savings in time and equipment. At another facility, a CNL was able to decrease peripherally inserted central catheter (PICC) line infections from 179 blood stream infections (40 were related to the PICC line) to 0 infections, netting an estimated $500,000 savings over a 12-month period (Wiggins, 2008). These projects and their impact on patient safety and quality of care do not represent the entire impact that these 3 CNLs made in that particular setting. Rather, they represent 3 documented examples of the impact the CNL had in just 3 care settings. Increasingly, positive outcomes for quality of care and the related cost benefits are being reported in healthcare settings where the CNL role has been implemented. Although most of these examples are from acute care units, similar benefits and outcomes are being reported in a variety of other care settings.

Future of CNL Education and Role

Admittedly the CNL initiative is not the sole answer to the many issues that plague the healthcare delivery system; however it is one very promising strategy that is demonstrating a significant and sustained impact across settings. Calls for major changes in the way health care is delivered and the way health professionals are educated have prompted nursing education and practice, under the AACN's leadership, to develop a preferred vision for nursing education with the CNL at the center. The CNL, an advanced generalist with a focus on quality improvement and care coordination, is not a replacement for other nursing roles, such as the clinical nurse specialist, nurse practitioner, nurse manager, or the staff nurse. Rather the CNL is complementary to other nursing roles (Spross et al., 2004; Ott & Haase-Herrick, 2006) and works in tandem with these providers to deliver high quality, patient-centered nursing care. Healthcare leaders have identified the CNL as the future leader of quality improvement in the microsystem and at the point of care. The CNL initiative complements other quality improvement initiatives, such as those spearheaded by the Institute for Healthcare Improvement (IHI, 2013) and the Robert Wood Johnson Foundation's (RWJF's) Transforming Care at the Bedside (TCAB), which have greatly impacted the quality of care available in hospitals (RWJF, 2013). CNLs are taking a lead in these initiatives at multiple sites to implement quality improvement projects and improve patient safety. Partnering between education and practice has been identified as critical; collaboration and combining efforts are also crucial to making a lasting impact on enhancing care delivery.

The CNL initiative has grown considerably in the 9 years since the publication of the AACN "Working Paper," which is now the white paper, *The Role of the Clinical Nurse Leader.* The number of schools implementing CNL master's or post-master's

> In 10 years CNLs will be in every area of health care improving outcomes. The CNL has the expertise to provide insight and change as health care changes. As the lateral integrator and coordinator of care, I envision the CNL taking a leadership role in transitions of care, particularly from acute to post-acute care.
>
> Patricia Steingall, MS, RN, NE-BC, Chief Nursing Officer, VP Patient Care Services, Hunterdon Medical Center, NJ

> In the near future, the CNL will be the primary nurse interfacing with patients at critical junctures through the continuum of care. We are seeing a proliferation of roles like coaches and navigators to address smooth transitions for patients through the levels of care. Although these new roles may have functional worth for discreet tasks, we will still need someone (the CNL) who understands complexity and can help create systems and processes that promote seamless care, health, and well-being. The CNL will provide this leadership at all levels while staying patient focused in the day to day management of patients.
>
> Joan Shinkus Clark, DNP, RN, NEA-BC, CENP, FACHE, FAAN, Senior Vice President and System Chief Nurse Executive, Texas Health Resources, Dallas-Forth Worth, TX

programs has increased, and more schools are exploring the possibility of launching a CNL master's or post-master's program. For a number of schools, the CNL master's program represents the first graduate program offered at that institution. For others, the CNL master's program is a part of their evolution as advanced specialty nursing programs are transitioned to the doctor of nursing practice (DNP) degree. The number and type of healthcare institutions partnering with schools to implement the CNL also has expanded. Major healthcare systems across the country, including those providing acute and long-term care, are integrating the CNL into their care delivery models. As the impact of the CNL role on patient safety, quality care outcomes, care coordination, and cost benefits is more widely disseminated, it is anticipated that this expansion will occur exponentially. Particularly in this era of healthcare reform, cost containment, and changing reimbursement policies, the integration of the CNL into care delivery across settings offers a positive means of addressing these system-wide priorities.

The AACN remains steadfast in its support for the CNL initiative. However, to sustain the momentum and ensure that the CNL becomes embedded within the healthcare delivery infrastructure, ongoing networking and expansion of national and local partnerships are critical. Documentation and broad dissemination of the CNL's impact on patient safety, quality improvement, care coordination, transitions of care, and the related cost benefits across a variety of healthcare settings also will be vitally important to sustaining this movement and embracing the CNL as a catalyst for quality care.

I see the CNLs, working with other CNLs across settings, taking a leading role in overseeing care transitions from unit to unit and from acute care to home or other settings to decrease readmissions and improve other care outcomes. We are already working to implement this and have made significant changes in our Length of Stay (LOS) hospital wide and also our readmission rates. Introducing the CNL role at St. Lucie Medical Center is the most progressive and innovative strategy that I have implemented in my 17 years as a chief nursing officer. This will be my legacy to this hospital and nursing in general.

Nancy Hilton, MN, RN, Chief Nursing Officer, HCA St. Lucie Medical Center, Port St. Lucie, FL

References

AHA Commission on Workforce for Hospitals and Health Systems. (2002). *In our hands: How hospital leaders can build a thriving workforce.* Chicago, IL: American Hospital Association.

Aiken L. H., Clarke S. P., Cheung R. B., Sloane D. M., & Silber J. H. (2003). Educational levels of hospital nurses and surgical patient mortality. *Journal of the American Medical Association, 290*(12), 1617–1623.

Aiken, L. H., Clarke, S. P., Sloane D. M., Sochalski J., & Silber J. H. (2002). Hospital nurse staffing and patient mortality, nurse burnout, and job dissatisfaction. *Journal of the American Medical Association, 288*(16), 1987–1993.

American Association of Colleges of Nursing. (1998). *The essentials of baccalaureate education for professional nursing practice.* Washington, DC: Author.

American Association of Colleges of Nursing. (2007). *White paper on the role of the clinical nurse leader* (pp. 6–11). Washington, DC: Author. Retrieved from http://www.aacn.nche.edu/Publications/WhitePapers/ClinicalNurseLeader07.pdf

APRN Consensus Work Group & National Council of State Boards of Nursing APRN Advisory Committee. (2008). Consensus model for APRN regulation: Licensure, accreditation, certification & education. Retrieved from http://www.aacn.nche.edu/Education/pdf/APRN Report.pdf

Buerhaus, P. (2009). The recent surge in nurse employment: Causes and implications. *Health Affairs, 28*(4), 657–668.

Department of Health and Human Services, HRSA, BHP, DON. (2002). *Nurse practitioner primary care competencies in specialty areas: Adult, family, gerontological, pediatric, and women's health.* Washington, DC: Author.

Estabrooks, C. A., Midodzi, W. K., Cummings, G. C., Ricker, K. L., & Giovannetti, P. (2005). The impact of hospital nursing characteristics on 30-day mortality. *Nursing Research, 54*(2), 74–84.

Fang, D., Htut, A. M., & Bednash, G. D. (2008). *2007–2008 enrollment and graduations in baccalaureate and graduate programs in nursing.* Washington, DC: American Association of Colleges of Nursing.

Fang, D., Li, Y., & Bednash, G. D. (2012). *2010–2011 enrollment and graduations in baccalaureate and graduate programs in nursing.* Washington, DC: American Association of Colleges of Nursing.

Gabuat, J., Hilton, N., Kinnaird, L. S., & Sherman, R. O. (2008). Implementing the clinical nurse leader role in a for-profit environment. *Journal of Nursing Administration, 38*(6), 302–307.

Harris, J. L., Walters, S. E., Quinn, C., Stanley, J., & McGuinn, K. (2006). The clinical nurse leader role: A pilot evaluation by an early adopter. Retrieved from http://www.aacn.nche.edu/cnl /pdf/VAEvalSynopsis.pdf

Hartranft, S. R., Garcia, T., & Adams, N. (2007). Realizing the anticipated effects of the clinical nurse leader. *Journal of Nursing Administration, 37*(6), 261–263.

Hix, C., McKeon, L., & Walters, S. (2009). Clinical nurse leader impact on clinical microsystems outcomes. *Journal of Nursing Administration, 39*(2), 71–76.

Institute for Health Care Improvement. (2013). Home page. Retrieved from http://www.ihi.org/Pages /default.aspx

Institute of Medicine. (1999). *To err is human: Building a safer health system* (p. 1). Washington, DC: National Academy Press.

Institute of Medicine. (2003). *Health professions education: A bridge to quality.* Washington, DC: National Academies Press.

Institute of Nursing. (2010). *The future of nursing.* Washington, DC: National Academies of Science.

Joint Commission on Accreditation of Healthcare Organizations. (2002). *Health care at the crossroads, strategies for addressing the evolving nursing crisis.* Chicago, IL: Author.

Kimball, B., & O'Neil, E. (2002). *Health care's human crisis: The American nursing shortage.* Princeton, NJ: The Robert Wood Johnson Foundation.

Leape, L. L., & Berwick, D. M. (2005). Five years after to err is human. *Journal of the American Medical Association, 293*(19), 2384–2390.

Needleman, J., Buerhaus, P., Mattke, S., Stewart, M., & Zelevinsky, K. (2002). Nurse-staffing levels and the quality of care in hospitals. *New England Journal of Medicine, 346*(22), 1715–1722.

Ott, K. M., & Haase-Herrick, K. (2006). *Working statement comparing the clinical nurse leader and nurse manager roles: Similarities, differences and complementarities.* Washington, DC: AACN. Retrieved from http://www.aacn.nche.edu/cnl/pdf/roles3-06.pdf

Robert Wood Johnson Foundation. Transforming care at the bedside (TCAB) tool kit. Retrieved from http://www.rwjf.org/en/grants/national-program-offices/T/transforming-care-at-the -bedside.html

Spross, J. A., Hamric, A. B., Hall, G., Minarik, P. A., Sparacino, P. A., & Stanley, J. M. (2004). *Working statement comparing the clinical nurse leader and clinical nurse specialist roles: Similarities, differences and complementarities.* Washington, DC: AACN. Retrieved from http://www.aacn.nche.edu/CNL/pdf/CNLCNSComparisonTable.pdf

Stanley, J. M. (2008). AACN shaping a future vision for nursing education. In B. A. Moyer & R. A. Wittmann-Price (Eds.). *Nursing education: Foundations for practice excellence,* Philadelphia, PA.

Stanley, J. M., Gannon, J., Gabuat, J., Hartranft, S., Adams, N., Mayes, C., . . . Burch, D. (2008). The clinical nurse leader: A catalyst for improving quality and patient safety. *Journal of Nursing Management, 16*(5), 614–622.

U.S. Department of Labor, Bureau of Labor Statistics. (2012). Economic news release. Retrieved from http://www.bls.gov/news.release/ecopro.t06.htm

Wiggins, M. (2008, June 8). The clinical nurse leader demands in healthcare require new innovation. Presentation made to the Joint Commission-Nursing Advisory Council. Oakbrook, IL.

The CNL: Past, Present, and Future

Tracy Lofty
Director, Commission on Nurse Certification

The Commission on Nurse Certification (CNC), an autonomous arm of the American Association of Colleges of Nursing (AACN), is responsible for the administration of the Clinical Nurse Leader (CNL) Certification Program. CNL certification is awarded to individuals who meet the certification eligibility criteria (registered nurse [RN] licensure and graduation from a CNL education program) and who successfully complete a comprehensive exam.

The first official testing period of the CNL Certification Exam was launched in May 2007. By working with subject matter experts, key stakeholders, and a highly reputable testing agency, the AACN developed the exam blueprint based upon a model curriculum that was prepared by other subject matter experts and leading authorities. At that time, the CNL was a new role, and no formally trained CNLs were practicing. Therefore, the exam had to be developed based upon a very comprehensive model curriculum. Based upon feedback from examinees completing CNC's certification program evaluations, the model curriculum served as one of the resources for certification exam preparation.

By 2011, more than 1,500 individuals had earned the CNL credential. To maintain the quality of the exam and to adhere to certification accreditation standards, the board of commissioners (BOC) began to explore conducting a job analysis. What were the CNLs doing in practice—what were their specific tasks? More importantly, what common ground did all CNLs share? Did the AACN's model curriculum support the knowledge, skills, and abilities (KSAs) required of a novice CNL in practice?

The job analysis is a critical element of a valid certification exam. Knowing that CNLs were being employed in the role and that there were testimonies of positive outcomes linked to CNL practice, the BOC decided that it was an appropriate time to conduct a formal job analysis study. The greatest challenge and concern identified by the BOC related to conducting this study was identifying shared KSAs as CNLs were employed in a variety of settings.

In the spring of 2011, the CNC posted a call for volunteers to recruit CNLs to serve on the CNL Job Analysis Committee. In May 2011, 10 CNLs, along with CNC staff, met with the staff of the current testing agency, Schroeder Measurement Technologies, Inc. (SMT) to identify CNL tasks—specifically, knowledge, skills, and abilities of a novice, practicing CNL regardless of setting. This was an intense two-day meeting. Various publications related to the CNL role were reviewed prior to the meeting, and a list of more than 200 KSAs were considered to establish a CNL body of knowledge.

Discussion with the committee continued into the evening—clear evidence for just how passionate they were about the CNL role. Committee members could see the future of the CNL role and the critical importance of the work at hand. They believed that the CNL role was just at the cusp of being fully accepted and integrated; they viewed the CNL role as the most fundamental position in healthcare innovation. From their explanations, the CNC developed the brochure *Why Hire a CNL?*, which is currently posted on the AACN's website.

Following the meeting, SMT developed and emailed a survey based upon the KSAs to all CNLs. The survey would serve as the measuring tool to determine the significance of each KSA. Nearly 300 CNLs participated in the survey in the summer of 2011. By September 2011, SMT, along with the CNL Job Analysis Committee, completed the job analysis study, which was approved by the BOC in October 2011.

In April 2012, the CNC launched a completely new multiple choice exam based upon the job analysis study. During the first testing period of the new exam from April to May 2012, more than 300 individuals registered for the exam nationwide. This was a record number of examinees for any CNL testing period (four testing periods are offered throughout the year). This testing period also resulted in a 75% pass rate on the exam, an increase from the previous 2 years.

The CNL certification exam has evolved to reflect the practice of CNLs. The CNC offers a psychometrically sound exam with exam specifications based upon the job analysis study. The exam meets national standards that were determined by practicing CNLs. The past CNL certification exam reflected the curriculum; the present exam reflects the job analysis study. Although very similar to the past exam content outline, the exam blueprint now includes subdomains in advanced clinical assessment and ethics.

The job analysis was critical in the evolution of the CNL Certification Program. The job analysis study will undoubtedly impact the CNL curriculum and also provide an overview of CNL practice to those healthcare leaders who may still seek clarity on the role.

Following initial certification, CNLs, regardless of when they earned the CNL credential, must demonstrate continuous learning to maintain their credentials.

CNLs are required to renew once every 5 years, and the renewal criteria emphasizes enhancing competency.

What is the future of the CNL Certification Program? The BOC understands that the role continues to evolve and that the assessment must be relevant to practice. The CNC is committed to conducting a job analysis study every 5–7 years. However, exam items will be reviewed annually with new exam items developed and incorporated on a continual basis. The CNC will continue to collect feedback from examinees as well as from CNL faculty to maintain a quality certification program.

Go to www.aacn.nche.edu/CNL for information about the CNL Certification Program and the CNC.

TWO

The Clinical Nurse Leader: A Catalyst for Advancing Nursing

 Michael R. Bleich

www Learning Objectives
© Arenacreative/Dreamstime.com

- Identify the rationales for key messages and recommendations of the Institute of Medicine's report, *The Future of Nursing: Leading Change, Advancing Health*

> **Constant change is here to stay.**
>
> **Anonymous**

- Understand how the Institute of Medicine's key messages and recommendations relate to clinical nurse leader practice

Introduction

The clinical nurse leader (CNL) has the potential to be a powerful catalytic role that advances patient- and family-centered care in a rapidly fluid health-care system. Nursing is a relationship-based discipline, resplendent with intellectual, physical, and emotional demands, particularly at the point of care, where the art and science of nursing converge. Nursing is the sole health

Key Terms

Relationship based	Problem solving	Outcome based
Evidence based	Infrastructure	Point of service
Health leader		

CNL Roles

Leader	Advocate	Life-long learner
Educator	Manager	Decision maker
Lateral integrator	Risk anticipator	

CNL Professional Values

Accountability   Integrity   Advocacy   Collaboration

CNL Core Competencies

Communication   Delegation   Interpretation and analysis
Design/management/coordination of care   Critical thinking
Illness and disease management

discipline that embraces assessment, intervention, and evaluation skills by intentionally integrating individuals, families, and community. Nurses are hardwired to think through a clinical problem-solving lens that spans from human responses to health problems through to the care delivery systems where treatments are sought and to the community resources that support recovery. Further, nursing is the discipline that, arguably, best complements the work of physicians, whose contributions to the nature of disease, its diagnosis, and treatment serve a great public good. Nurses share knowledge of disease, fulfilling an adjunctive role in medicine. Through the decades, nursing science has evolved. Today's clinical nurse is holistic in focus—responding to the biophysical, psychosocial, and spiritual dimensions of human responses to health and illness—advanced through nursing science. Clinical nurses and scientists give more attention to the role of the family and environmental determinants of health. Nurses know that at the juncture of biological demise, individuals and families can be fulfilled in the dimension of psychosocial–spiritual well-being. This is the essence of nursing's contribution to healthcare and what it means to be a "clinical nurse" (Bleich, 2012).

When adding advanced leadership to the role of the clinical nurse, another catalytic dimension unfolds. Nurses have grown substantially as leaders for numerous reasons: advances in nursing science; the profound range of nursing's presence in all aspects of the healthcare system (e.g., acute care, long-term care, home care, school-based clinics, ambulatory, military, and correctional institutions); the increased fragmentation of the healthcare system, with nurses serving to bridge and navigate complexities; and the increased education and presence of nurses in venues that set policy. These factors all add to the credibility and demand for nurses in leadership roles and have contributed to the CNL role's emergence as a catalyst for advancing nursing.

From its inception, the CNL role was designed to link clinical care with process-based organizational improvements that are both evidence and outcome based in design. The CNL role was created to bring to the point of care an expert clinician with the ability to analyze caregiver interventions, linking care coordination efficiencies to a persistent focus on patient safety and patient- and family-centered outcomes. In this vision, the CNL would have the knowledge and skill to avoid costs and provide economic relief for the mutual benefit of the patient and family, the care team, and the organization. To illuminate the synergy between the clinical nurse role and leadership concepts, this chapter will review the key messages and recommendations of the Institute of Medicine's report, *The Future of Nursing: Leading Change, Advancing Health*, as they relate to the CNL.

The National Academies and the Institute of Medicine

The National Academy of Sciences advises the nation on science, engineering, and medicine through a charter granted to it by Congress in 1863 (The National Academies, 2013). The youngest of the three academies is the Institute of Medicine (IOM), established in 1970 to review matters pertaining to the health of the public and to shape policy through rigorous evidence-based work. The members of the IOM and those who are appointed to serve as its interdisciplinary advisers on various social issues are acclaimed in their respective fields. With their exclusive use of scientific data, followed by rigorous blinded external reviews, IOM studies are well regarded as valid and reliable and enjoy high public confidence in findings and recommendations.

Social issues involving nursing have been studied by the IOM, but until recently the discipline had not yet been comprehensively studied from the perspective of social policy. In 2009, the timing seemed appropriate, as the nation delved into crucial conversations about health care and the need for improved health policy, a debate that followed decades of gridlock. The key issues related to insurance coverage for Americans, access to care, and fragmented care between care delivery agencies. The issues of public health and disease prevention gained traction and increased attention as healthcare costs continued to skyrocket. As consumers of insurance, American industries were at risk, as both consumption and cost eroded their profitability in the global marketplace. Public awareness of the high cost of U.S. healthcare and its overall dismal outcomes surged.

During this debate, it became clear that despite its lag in clinical outcomes and its high costs of care, the United States continued to lead the world in medical advances, the use of high-cost technologies, and the advent of new therapies. This level of innovation increased the complexity of the health system, the knowledge needed to develop and execute these therapies, and the kinds of health personnel necessary to interpret and evaluate the impact on those with insurance coverage (Arrow et al., 2009). Nurses are central figures in this innovation implementation, and as the largest healthcare workforce (over 3 million strong) practicing across a wide range of settings, nurses must be at the center of any type of health reform.

With this in mind, the Robert Wood Johnson Foundation approached the IOM, and it was agreed that the first comprehensive review of nursing would be chartered in order to transform the nursing profession to fulfill the promise of a reformed healthcare system. Two years later, in October 2011, the report, entitled *The Future of Nursing: Leading Change, Advancing Health*, was issued (IOM, 2011). Its role in shaping the history of nursing remains to be fully determined, but all indicators point to it becoming the seminal blueprint for recasting the profession.

Findings and Recommendations

Led by Dr. Donna Shalala, 18 committee members convened to analyze and write the report, which was released on October 5, 2011. As a past secretary of health and human services and an IOM member, Dr. Shalala adeptly led the committee through a review of the dynamics of the health system; this contextual review is found in Part 1 of the report. Nursing is a central figure in the health system, but the discipline does not function in a vacuum, and the report addresses the issues of where and how nursing can best optimize its contributions in service to the public. This theme of public service resonates throughout the report, as it was not developed for nursing per se, but rather, for how nursing and nurses serve a larger public mission.

Key Messages

With intentional simplicity and boldness, the committee derived four key messages (presented in this section) and eight recommendations (presented in the next section) for its blueprint (IOM, 2011, p. 4). The key messages are as follows:

1. Nurses should practice to the full extent of their education and training.
2. Nurses should achieve higher levels of education and training through an improved education system that promotes seamless academic progression.
3. Nurses should be full partners, with physicians and other health professionals, in redesigning health care in the United States.
4. Effective workforce planning and policy making require better data collection and an improved information infrastructure. (IOM, 2011)

The First Message

The first message is based on the premise that nurses often have knowledge, skills, and abilities that are suppressed by institutional policies and practices, state nurse practice acts, and insurance practices; this at a time when human capital is critical to meet the health and illness needs of masses of individuals who cannot afford care. Along with other health disciplines, this message challenges unnecessary barriers that limit the practice capacity of health providers, including concerns for malpractice, negative imagery presented by the media, and social norms that misalign with actual practice. For instance, the public only recently became aware that there are nurses who can prescribe and treat common health problems, and many remain unaware that nurse scientists have made substantive contributions to the public's health and well-being. These factors delimit nursing's contributions and restrict the scope of practice.

The Second Message

The second message exhorts nurses to keep abreast of public expectations that health-care providers remain competent and confident in their abilities over the duration of a career through the acquisition of additional education. The scope of nursing (Message one) can expand, and with further education to drive added competencies, nurses are poised for greater influence in delivering care. Competency development should be driven by attention to rapidly changing societal demographics: the confluence of aging and increasingly diverse populations, socioeconomic variability, technological advances, and the explosion of scientific knowledge. A simple yet profound example of this is genomic mapping, which is transforming the basis of healthcare from rigid, protocol-driven knowledge to personalized knowledge that results in tailored treatment. Long-held traditions related to medication administration based on age and weight (past competency) are giving way to individualized dosing standards (new competency with decision-making ramifications).

Another factor worth considering with this message is that nursing demographics, too, are shifting in concert with societal aging. The nursing workforce needs to replace and expand the numbers and competencies of nurses with advanced degrees. Continuing education is one method to keep abreast of knowledge, but in a scientific era, formal education leading to graduate and doctoral degrees is critical within the discipline and the field of medicine. The IOM report notes the insufficient numbers of nurses who possess graduate-level development as a foundation for the number of leadership, academic, and scientific positions that are emerging, notably with the tipping point of nurses who hold these positions on the cusp of retirement.

The Third Message

With added scope and education, the third message calls for nurses to assume parity at decision-making tables where the nursing lens—with its holistic focus on individual, family, and communities, and with intimate knowledge of how clinical care is orchestrated and delivered—is a voice that legitimately resonates as healthcare reform unfolds. The dominant players at healthcare tables where policy and practice decisions are made have historically been physicians, administrators, insurers, and others; nursing's voice has been limited. Hassmiller (2012) and others call for nurses to assume greater roles, serving on healthcare boards where strategic decisions associated with clinical services, quality, and resource allocation are made. Many programs have developed to strengthen and engage nurses in functional system redesign. These efforts show promising results for nurse leadership, but are not yet scalable and exist only in organizations where leaders encourage nurse engagement. The third message embraces nurse input at micro, meso, and macro levels of system enhancement and redesign.

The Fourth Message

Finally, the fourth message suggests that an adequate workforce database is crucial for informed decision making. Today, there is a limited amount of standardized workforce data and infrastructure from which to make critical policy decisions. Supply and demand data are critical at all levels: local, regional, and national. For instance, nursing schools have ramped up enrollments to meet the demands associated with nurse shortages, but they have done so with little concrete data. This has sometimes produced an oversupply of graduates disappointed by their lack of employment opportunities (Mancino, 2011). In other cases, nurses have been turned away from schools because of capacity constraints, yet little concrete data is available about the attributes and motivations of these individuals related to their suitability for the discipline. Demand variables (that is, who and how much care will be needed in the future) are even more difficult to calculate. Knowledge of variables impacting demand could help with decisions about which segments of the health system to reconfigure, where to shift payments for services, and which competencies are needed in the workforce.

The focus on ensuring a competent workforce from which to base demands is a different conversation than ensuring that sufficient numbers exist. Further, there has been almost no national discussion that shows how various health disciplines intersect in their capacity to meet public needs.

Readers are encouraged to reflect on these messages and the specific recommendations that can be found in the full IOM report. Suffice it to say, this overview frames the importance of a nursing response to the public, and CNLs have an obligation to be aware of the findings, key messages, and recommendations found in the report.

The Clinical Nurse Leader: A Catalyst for Change, a Strategic Nursing Asset

The CNL is a special nursing role that fulfills the major recommendations found in the IOM *Future of Nursing* report. The following section highlights the contributions the CNL can make to the eight published recommendations. Giving special attention to clinical and leadership considerations in the CNL role will contribute to the successful implementation of the IOM recommendations and serve to motivate CNLs to take action.

Advanced Education and the CNL

Recommendations 4 (increasing the number of baccalaureate graduates) and 5 (doubling the number of doctoral-prepared nurses) in the IOM report clearly illustrate the need for a more educated workforce. Recommendation 4 is the pathway to gaining more nurses who are able to take on additional roles, such as the CNL. As such, CNL education directly contributes by preparing entry-level nurses or advancing nurses to the master's level. A partial listing of the fundamental aspects of the CNL role that align with the IOM report includes leadership in the care of the sick in and across all environments; the design and provision of health promotion and risk reduction services for diverse populations; population-appropriate health care for individuals, clinical groups/units, and communities; risk anticipation; mass customization of care; and team management and collaboration with other health professional team members (American Association of Colleges of Nursing, 2007). Specific competencies are acquired through CNL education that focus on health promotion, risk reduction, and disease prevention, critical aspects of health reform that nurses are uniquely prepared to carry out. Communication competencies are at an advanced level, consistent with functioning on an interprofessional team, drawing in evidence and serving in a patient/family advocacy role, when needed. Illness and disease management competencies link care delivery to internal and external care needs, notably with an aim toward risk management and quality of life outcomes that avoid rehospitalization. In the area of human diversity, graduate education as a CNL carries expectations for the nurse's ability to intersect with various cultures; ethnicities; and socioeconomic, linguistic, and religious and lifestyle variations, consistent with the IOM's notations on diversity. Finally, as the IOM calls for nurses to engage with health system redesign, competencies that include an understanding of healthcare systems that incorporates the ability to design and evaluate healthcare, using principles of quality improvement, systems knowledge, and policy development skills are acquired; this could be within a healthcare institution or extend beyond into political arenas as needed. Based on these acquired graduate-level competencies, the CNL is in a position to pursue doctoral-level education if that is a personal goal.

Nurses Leading and Diffusing Collaborative Improvement Efforts

As noted, the CNL acquires cognitive and experiential competence in leadership within the healthcare team and beyond. The emphasis on microsystem design as it affects care populations is within the purview of CNL responsibilities. The CNL contributes a unique and often missing function by linking the patient to meso- and macro-level integration of care. The CNL's ability to guide and lead care at the point of service is critical, but with a defined skill set and training that detects patterns and trends in care such that practice can be standardized for the sake of efficiency and effectiveness. While the goal is always individualization of care, the CNL assists other nurses and health team members coordinate care through personalized delivery and delivery system design that maximizes the impact of service delivery. IOM Recommendation 2 states that healthcare organizations should support and help nurses take the lead in developing and adopting innovative, patient-centered care models and further, engage nurses at the front lines to work with developers and manufacturers to benefit clinical information exchange and products that advance patient care. Critical to this recommendation is that the Centers for Medicare and Medicaid Services should support the development and evaluation of models of payment and care delivery that use nurses in expanded and leadership capacities to improve health outcomes and reduce costs while ensuring evidence-based best practices. CNLs, presented with this opportunity, have the skill set to impact new care models through design and evaluation competencies.

Ensuring an Adequate Workforce

Indirectly, CNLs have been and are currently playing a crucial role in the development of nurses. The IOM calls for nurses to engage in life-long learning and suggests that nurse residency programs (Recommendation 3) are one method of seamlessly progressing new nurses from academic programs into clinical practice settings. As the CNL role has evolved, organizations have reported that the CNL plays an indirect role in fostering the competency development of other nurses, particularly those who are new to nursing roles. Perhaps an unintended consequence, the CNL role is also creating an opportunity for the mid-careerist to return to school and advance as a nurse while remaining at the bedside in a nonmanagerial role. IOM Recommendation 6 calls for a commitment to life-long learning, and the CNL is a potential motivator by role modeling to peers a personal commitment to formal education, but also demonstrating to other nurses the outcomes of life-long learning through competent expanded practice.

The CNL as a Health Leader

With additional coverage, more Americans will have access to health services. The influx of additional covered lives will impact children and others across the life span.

Insurance coverage is not a panacea for ensuring access to care, however. Many Americans have no experience with the healthcare system, and institutional settings may create unintentional barriers to access by lacking sensitivity to cultures, ethnicities, socioeconomic groups, and the other multitude of variables that make seeking care comfortable and attainable. Rural and frontier citizens experience geospatial barriers to care, which must be bridged through the use of technology and relocation of existing urban-centric services.

As a health leader, the CNL can support the ideas that many diseases are preventable and that illness care is not the onset of the care delivery system. CNLs are currently aligned with acute care systems, but there is no reason this must or should be the case. CNLs have the competencies to lead care throughout the care continuum, and CNLs will bear the burden of demonstrating this through their own tenacity and willingness to give voice to the evolving role. In this way, the CNL will give credence to Recommendation 1, which calls for an expanded scope of nursing practice. The CNL has the potential to meet specific needs in acute, long-term, and transitional care, in addition to correctional nursing, public health, and other settings yet to unfold. Within nursing's reach in a reforming health system are opportunities to meet public needs consistent with IOM Recommendation 7, which calls for nurses to take responsibility for integrating leadership theory with business practices, including clinical practice.

While the CNL is not specifically addressed in the IOM report, it should be clear that the role was developing at the very juncture of the writing of the report, the passage of the Affordable Care Act, and there was insufficient evidence at that juncture for the role to be referenced in an evidenced-based report. That said, a close examination of the CNL founding principles, the competencies aligned with the role, and the key messages and recommendations found in the IOM report make clear the compatibility of the CNL role with public expectations for nursing now and in the next quarter century. The American public will benefit from an adequate supply of qualified nurses, such as reflected in the CNL role, who are competent to meet the projected demand for services in an informed manner (the essence of which is Recommendation 8).

Summary

- The CNL role is congruent with the seminal IOM report, *The Future of Nursing: Leading Change, Advancing Health.*
- An examination of the context of the IOM report frames how the CNL role aligns with the four messages and eight recommendations found in the report.

- In both direct and indirect ways, the CNL is poised to contribute substantively to the blueprint identified in the IOM report that will improve the health of the nation through leadership, system design, advanced competency attainment, and patient-centered clinical care.
- The unique perspective that nurses bring to the decision-making table is made explicit; the CNL must seize the opportunity to bridge individual care with a population- and evidence-based perspective.

`www` Reflection Questions
© Arenacreative/Dreamstime.com

1. How can the CNL respond to public needs in the era of healthcare reform?
2. How can the CNL influence change based on the IOM key messages and recommendations?

`www` Learning Activity
© Arenacreative/Dreamstime.com

- Identify one IOM recommendation and how the CNL can take action to meet it. Discuss the idea with classmates and generate an action list to share with state action coalition groups.

References

American Association of Colleges of Nursing. (2007). *White paper on the role of the clinical nurse leader*. Retrieved from http://www.aacn.nche.edu/publications/white-papers/cnl

Arrow, K., Auerbach, A., Bertko, J., Brownlee, S., Casalino, L. P., Cooper, J. . . . van de Ven, W. (2009). Toward a 21st-century healthcare system: Recommendations for healthcare reform. *Annals of Internal Medicine, 150(7)*, 493–495.

Bleich, M. R. (2012). Certification as an emerging force in competence development and attainment. *AHNA Beginnings, 32(1)*, 5. Retrieved from www.national-academies.org

Hassmiller, S. B. (2012). Professional development: Nurses on boards. *American Journal of Nursing, 112 (3)*, 61–66.

Institute of Medicine. (2011). *The future of nursing: Leading change, advancing health*. Washington, DC: The National Academies Press.

Mancino, D. J. (2011). Inaction is not an option. *Dean's Notes, 33*(2), 1–3.

The National Academies. (2013). Who we are. Retrieved from http://www.national-academies.org/about/whoweare/index.html

Developing a Clinical Nurse Leader Practice Model: An Interpretive Synthesis of the Literature

Miriam Bender

Objective

The Institute of Medicine's *Future of Nursing* report identifies the need for nurses to engage in innovative practice in order to meet higher healthcare quality standards. The purpose of this study was to clarify CNL practice components contributing to improved interprofessional collaborative patient care standards. The American Association of Colleges of Nursing CNL white paper defines CNL core competencies necessary for practice. The literature documents preliminary evidence of improved outcomes associated with CNL integration into clinical microsystems. However, the CNL role is not yet clearly defined in terms of the fundamental activities and responsibilities necessary to produce outcomes. Lack of practice clarity limits the ability to articulate, implement, and measure CNL-specific practice and outcomes.

Methods

An interpretive synthesis was conducted to integrate the extant CNL literature into a coherent understanding of CNL practice. A literature search was conducted in CINAHL, Pubmed, Dissertations and Theses, and Google, using the search term "Clinical Nurse Leader." Results were reviewed and included if they described any aspect of CNL practice *in action*. Thirty implementation reports, 8 qualitative/mixed methods studies, 3 quantitative studies, and 244 conference abstracts were included in the final synthesis. Grounded theory methodology was utilized to reanalyze primary CNL evidence and identify domains and components of CNL practice.

Results

CNL practice encompasses five domains: preparation for CNL practice; the structure of CNL practice; the core phenomenon of CNL practice, which is continuous leadership at the point of practice; outcomes of CNL practice; and acceptance. *Preparation for CNL practice* components include clear understanding of current care delivery deficits, strong leadership support, and an effective change management strategy. *Structure of CNL practice* components include microsystem care delivery redesign, competency-based CNL workflow, and accountability for a defined set of outcomes. *Continuous leadership at the point of practice* components include supporting staff engagement, source of constant communication/information, strengthening interprofessional relationships, team creation, and shifting focus from person to process. *Outcomes of CNL practice* components include improved care environment, improved care quality, and nursing brought to the forefront of healthcare redesign. *Acceptance* components include initial buy-in, exposure, and understanding.

Discussion

The CNL practice model proposes five domains that interact to produce the structure, function, and outcomes of CNL practice. The core phenomenon of CNL practice involves developing relationships across professions to promote and manage information exchange, shared decision making, and effective care processes. The model highlights the importance of a systematic approach to CNL development and implementation, including macro- and microsystem preparation, care delivery redesign, allowing CNLs to function to their full scope of practice, and allowing time for role acceptance. The extent to which each domain is adequately addressed influences the degree of CNL practice success.

Implications

This study advances understanding of the relatively new CNL role by synthesizing an empirically derived model for CNL development and practice. It clarifies CNL practice components and differentiates them from existing nursing roles and practices. The model can provide a guideline to organizations wanting to implement the CNL. It can also provide a basis for future research identifying quantifiable measures of CNL practice and CNL-specific influence on outcomes.

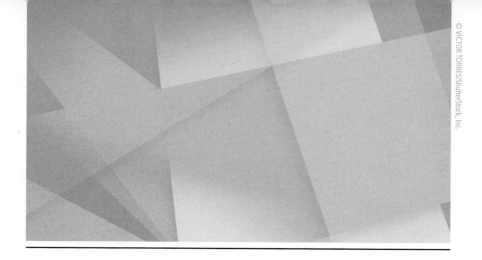

UNIT 2
Academic, Clinical, and Community Partnerships

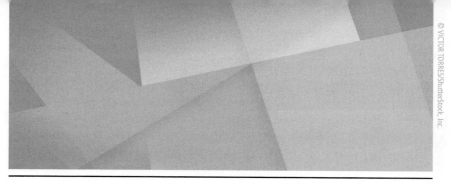

THREE

Building and Sustaining Academic, Clinical, and Community Partnerships

■ Sandra E. Walters

www Learning Objectives

- Define partnership
- Identify key components of a partnership
- Identify the significance of academic, clinical, and community partnerships in building and sustaining the clinical nurse leader role
- Describe the process for building a sustainable clinical nurse leader academic, clinical, and community partnership
- Discuss microsystems analysis and its importance in relation to academic, clinical, and community partnerships

> There is no peace among equals because equality doesn't exist in this universe. Either one prevails and the other follows, or both negotiate their differences and create a greater partnership.
>
> Harold J. Duarte-Bernhardt

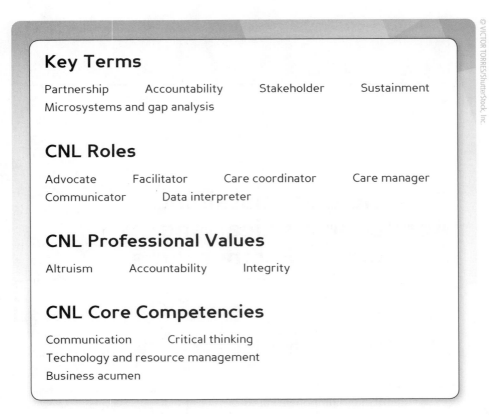

Key Terms

Partnership   Accountability   Stakeholder   Sustainment
Microsystems and gap analysis

CNL Roles

Advocate   Facilitator   Care coordinator   Care manager
Communicator   Data interpreter

CNL Professional Values

Altruism   Accountability   Integrity

CNL Core Competencies

Communication   Critical thinking
Technology and resource management
Business acumen

Introduction

A shortage of nurses in the United States focused the attention of clinicians, academicians, and communities on its causes, impacts, and possible solutions. The results of multiple studies have included recommendations for the development of partnerships between academic and clinical organizations. As early as 1998, the Pew Health Professions Commission called for the development of partnerships for the education of health professionals that would integrate the commitments of the care delivery systems with those of health education professionals and the needs of the communities served. In similar manner, a study by the Institute of Medicine (IOM, 2000) resulted in recommendations for increased collaboration between institutions as a means to enhance patient safety, and the Robert Wood Johnson Foundation called for new practice models to enhance education/

practice partnerships (Kimball & O'Neil, 2002). Additionally, the National League for Nursing (2003) called for nurse educators, students, consumers, and nursing service representatives to form partnerships that would dramatically reform learning and teaching and enhance the relationships between and among students, teachers, researchers, and clinicians.

Efforts to address the need to transform professional nursing care and nursing education led to the development of four separate task forces by the American Association of Colleges of Nursing (AACN). With the establishment of an implementation task force to launch the clinical nurse leader (CNL) role through education–practice partnerships, the AACN ushered in an educational model that could be responsive to the changing needs of the healthcare environment (AACN, 2007). The development of partnerships between educators, clinicians, and communities is an essential element to the successful implementation of the CNL role and forms the foundation for education and practice.

In 2010, the IOM, in its report, *The Future of Nursing: Leading Change, Advancing Health*, made recommendations that require collaborative actions by nurses, the government, healthcare institutions, and other stakeholders in nursing education in order to improve the delivery of high-quality, seamless care. The education of CNLs in an environment where clinicians, educators, patients, and other community agencies form partnerships to maximize care outcomes is critical to the success of the CNL role.

Definition of Partnership

The word *partnership* was derived in the 14th century from the Middle English use of the word *partner*. The original meaning designated joint heirs or part holders and was itself derived from the Anglo-French word *parcener*, which referred to a division or share (Merriam-Webster, Incorporated, n.d.). Terms that appear closely related to the concept of partnership include *partner, partnering, part, partnered, partial*, and *partition*. These words have also evolved from the word *partner* and are generally used to describe a relationship in which there is a division or sharing of some larger whole with joint rights or responsibilities. The term *partnership* is used in many ways, including to describe legal transactions as may be seen in a business, personal relationships that may express the state of committed bonding between two individuals, and even to describe individuals who engage in a specific activity together, such as dancing.

> Friendship is essen-
> tially a partnership.
>
> Aristotle

A partnership can be defined as an alliance or union between individuals or groups that is characterized by mutual cooperation and responsibility to achieve a specified goal (*American Heritage Dictionary*, 2007). Gallant, Beaulieu, and Carnevale (2002) and Hook (2006) focused on the context of the professional–patient relationship in partnerships. Their work established attributes for partnership such as shared decision making, relationships, professional competence, shared knowledge, autonomy, communication, participation, and shared power. Steinhart and Alsup (2001) identified trust, effective communications, shared values, monitoring programs, and long-term relationships as necessary to the formation of successful partnerships. In similar manner, the European Foundation for Quality Management (EFQM) model for health care includes partnership development as one of eight elements of quality improvement (Vallejo et al., 2006). Their content analysis included the following elements as part of the model:

- Requiring clearly identified mutual benefit;
- Consisting of shared goals;
- Being supported with expertise, resources, and knowledge;
- Delivering enhanced value to stakeholders by optimizing core competencies; and
- Building a sustainable relationship based on trust, respect, and openness. (Vallejo et al., 2006)

Creating Academic, Clinical, and Community Partnerships

Antecedents for the development of partnership within the CNL role must include recognition of unmet needs within the partner settings. In the education arena, unmet needs arise as the result of factors such as faculty vacancies, space constraints, limited equipment or supply resources, increased population diversity, and a lack of available practice models (Stanley, Hoiting, Burton, Harris & Norman, 2007; Stark, 2003).

In the clinical arena, unmet needs may result from increased complexity of the healthcare environment, the rapid advances in technology, an aging population, or licensure and certification requirements to maintain a well-educated professional workforce (Bartels, 2005; Bartels & Bednash, 2005; Zahner & Gredig, 2005). A review of hospital initiatives to support the education of nurses cited drivers for the formation of partnerships as including the need for mechanisms to help nurses balance work and education, mechanisms for delivery of continuing education, the need for increased levels of nurses with bachelor's (BSN) and master's (MSN) degrees, and pressures to decrease recruitment and retention costs (Cheung & Aiken, 2006).

In communities, in addition to their roles as employers and procurers of goods and services, clinical and education partners may be needed to produce additional benefits including being a source of volunteers, positively affecting productivity and safety, and acting as a source for health promotion. Concurrently, communities can contribute to health care through the provision of expertise as demonstrated by enterprises such as the auto industry, whose human factors engineering has been applied to health care (Kerfoot, Rapala, Ebright, & Rogers, 2006).

When unmet needs are recognized within academic, clinical, and community institutions, the evaluation of the suitability of partnership may then progress. The role of the CNL in the formation of partnerships at any level should begin with a needs assessment or gap analysis (see **Box 3-1**). This systematic collection of information will be necessary for setting goals, developing an implementation plan, allocating resources, and establishing success indicators.

In order for a partnership relationship to be formed, the essential attributes of trust, respect, openness, and shared values must be present within the proposed relationship. If any of these is absent, the partnership will fail to progress, and needs

Box 3-1   Facets of Gap Analysis

1. Determine the current state of the organization or microsystem in terms of available resources, performance, goals, values, knowledge, or internal and external constraints using performance data, stakeholder input, employee responses, or other sources.
2. Determine the desired or necessary state based on stakeholder input, benchmark data, community standards, or other comparison measures.
3. Analyze the gap between the current and desired states to identify problems, opportunities, strengths, weaknesses, or other concerns.
4. Prioritize needs and determine their importance to meeting organizational objectives, cost effectiveness, impact on stakeholders, or other goals.
5. Identify potential solutions and opportunities for improvements.

will continue to be unmet. If the essential attributes are present, however, the partnership will progress with the formulation of shared goals, establishment of communication strategies, and designation of shared resources and a monitoring program (Gallant et al., 2002).

The role of the CNL as a facilitator in the establishment of partnerships provides the opportunity to implement strategies to ensure the success of these initiatives. From the beginning, sharing of information with stakeholders throughout all involved organizations is crucial to successful implementation of partner initiatives. The clinical, academic, and community partnership is believed to result in empowerment, integration, collaboration, effectiveness, increased satisfaction, quality enhancements, innovation, learning, improvements, and higher quality services within the partnering institutions. When these results are realized, the positive outcomes form the basis for a sustained partnership. In the event that expected results are not achieved, reevaluation of the partnership will result in the need to reassert the essential attributes of the partnership and may also lead to continued unmet needs. **Figure 3-1** depicts a model of the partnership formation process.

Exemplars of Partnership

The University of Maryland

The University of Maryland found itself in need of additional faculty, clinical sites for student experiences, additional resources, and employment opportunities for new graduates to ensure the success of its academic program. At the same time, the University of Maryland Medical Center faced the challenges of an increased inpatient census, sicker patients, increased staff vacancies, and a need to provide opportunities for the continuing education of their nurses (University of Maryland Office of Communications, 2007). The two institutions initiated an exploration of each other's needs, assets, and individual visions. When a shared vision emerged, they began to develop a plan with priorities and starting points. Planning evolved to a commitment of resources, sharing of a nurse researcher, and participation of both institutions in research and grant applications. Outcomes from the partnership have included increased clinical experiences for students, increased faculty, integration of the nursing education program and hospital to provide mobile healthcare services to rural areas, and increased enrollment by staff nurses in continuing education initiatives. Data collection on

Figure 3-1   Partnership formation process.

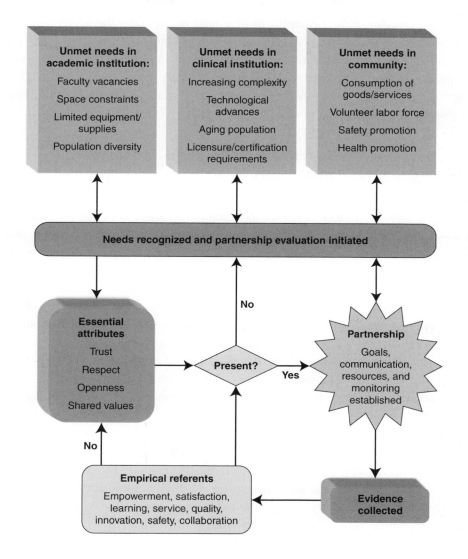

partnership outcomes has allowed formal evaluation of program results and has led to continued modifications and expansion of the program.

The exemplar of the University of Maryland incorporates the antecedent factors of identified needs at an educational and clinical institution and recognition of the need to initiate partnership evaluation. When the essential attributes of trust, respect, openness, and shared values were present, the partnership was formed. The partnership progresses with the formation of shared goals, communications, shared resources, and monitoring programs.

The Tennessee Valley Healthcare System and Vanderbilt University School of Nursing

In 2004, the Department of Veterans Affairs medical centers of the Tennessee Valley Healthcare System (TVHS) faced multiple challenges in the provision of patient care. Among these challenges was a fragmented care delivery system that often resulted in frustration for patients, their families, providers, and nurses when patients transitioned from one level of care to another within the system. Nurse managers recognized the need for enhanced multidisciplinary collaboration in the care delivery process but were often overwhelmed by the operating demands of the units and were unable to focus sufficient attention on clinical care issues. Staff nurses found themselves unable to meet the care needs of their patients as new equipment, advanced information technologies, increased patient acuity, and an aging patient population eroded the amount of time available for individual patients.

Concurrently, Vanderbilt University School of Nursing (VUSN) was facing the challenge presented by rapid technological advances—demands from employing institutions to produce highly skilled and educated nurse generalists who could direct the care of patient populations rather than diagnostic groups. An education focus group including hospitals, educators, and members of the community was formed to identify future nurse management needs. The result of the partnership between the TVHS and VUSN was the initiation of the CNL role, with the first CNLs graduating from VUSN in August 2005.

Community involvement and participation was evident in the implementation of the CNL role as VUSN customized its program to address the special needs of the United States Air Force Academy. Additionally, the TVHS, VUSN, the Veterans Affairs Office of Nursing Services, and the AACN collaborated to produce a video for national distribution explaining the CNL role. In 2006, the TVHS and VUSN began a pilot study for evaluation of empirical referents for successful implementation of the CNL role as developed in collaboration between the AACN and the Department of Veterans Affairs. The results indicated significant improvement in financial and satisfaction indicators (Hix, McKeon, & Walters, 2009); success of the clinical, academic, and community partnership was evidenced by joint participation of partners in scholarly publishing activities such as presentations at national conferences, mentorship activities for CNLs throughout the country, and even the joint celebration of special events and holidays. Effects of academic–clinical partnerships have been categorized as reaching multiple domains including economic, human capital, social capital, knowledge, and place (Davies & Bennett, 2008). While it may be difficult to make clear distinctions between domains, it may be beneficial to begin by examining how each institution impacts each domain and how a partnership may be used to bring about change.

Sustaining Partnerships

The lack of progress in changing the delivery of health care to match the complexity of patient needs has been attributed to a failure to recognize interdependencies (Wiggins, 2006). Partnerships offer organizations the opportunity to not only recognize interdependencies, but to embrace them as providing mechanisms for effecting positive changes. Examination of the elements of successful partnerships in the implementation of the CNL role has provided insights into strategies that offer the potential to sustain these relationships. Evaluation of partnership outcomes is often measured in terms of the impact on the clinical setting, the academic setting, and the outcomes of care delivered. It is also important to consider the impact one partnership will have on other academic–clinical partnerships, as many hospitals serve as clinical sites for multiple academic institutions (Glazer, Erikson, Mylott, Mulready-Shick, & Banister, 2011).

Contract negotiations for student placement in clinical settings present an opportunity to incorporate evidence-based practice outcomes such as review or development of practice guidelines. Nurse executives can influence course content through discussion of important clinical and administrative issues (Newhouse, 2007). Establishment of a joint academic service journal club may be used in a clinical setting to enhance staff awareness of evidence-based practice, promote leadership development, and enhance the learning environment of the organization (Duffy, Thompson, Hobbs, Niemeyer-Hackett, & Elpers, 2011).

> I have found no greater satisfaction than achieving success through honest dealing and strict adherence to the view that, for you to gain, those you deal with should gain as well.
>
> Alan Greenspan

For example, the partnership experience of leaders at the Hunterdon Medical Center and the College of New Jersey at Ewing led to recommendations for sustaining the partnership through frequent open dialogue, openness to learning, and close collaboration. Specific recommendations included that meetings be held on a monthly or other regular schedule and include the chief nursing officer, faculty, and other academic administrators, and that students and other practice stakeholders should meet and provide feedback regarding education or implementation matters (Rusch & Bakewell-Sachs, 2007).

The extent to which academic, clinical, and community partnerships can be maintained depends in part on the investment in efforts to understand the culture and values of the individual organizational participants. To this end, feedback between and among all stakeholders must be sought and given with the goal of continuously improving outcomes. Although activities such as curriculum development, orientation of students and faculty, and assessment and improvement of performance are critical to evaluation and implementation, it is equally important to maintain a focus on the relationships within the partnership. In this manner, celebrating success, recognizing achievements, and sharing the credit for what is accomplished are essential to the establishment of a common culture and keeping the spirit of the partnership alive.

Summary

- The formation of partnerships begins with recognition of unmet needs and challenges within and between academic, clinical, and community entities.
- The collection of data and stakeholder input form the basis for a gap analysis that can be used to initiate dialogue for negotiation of the partnership.
- A partnership can only move forward when trust, respect, shared values, and openness are present.
- In the implementation phase, partnership goals, communication strategies, resources, and monitoring mechanisms are determined.

- As the work of the partnership progresses, evidence is collected for use in outcome evaluation.
- Empirical referents as indicators of the results of the partnership are then evaluated, analyzed, and shared among partners and stakeholders.
- If essential attributes of the partnership remain in place, the process of goal revision and review of needs is undertaken as the partnership is sustained.
- As the partnership continues, activities such as publishing results of the work, joining to provide recognition to staff, and celebrating success become important to maintaining the relationship between organizations.

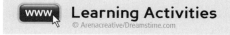

Reflection Questions
© Arenacreative/Dreamstime.com

1. The focus of this chapter is on establishing and maintaining partnerships between and among nursing organizations and the community. What, if any, changes would you expect in the partnership model if the partnerships were interprofessional, as might occur between a medical school and a hospital?
2. Formal relationships between institutions are not always possible or necessary. What types of informal collaborative initiatives could a CNL engage in with other healthcare institutions in the community? What types of indicators could be used as empirical referents?

Learning Activities
© Arenacreative/Dreamstime.com

1. Conduct a needs assessment of a microsystem in a healthcare facility. Use the gap analysis outline from Box 3-1 to guide your work.
2. Working with your CNL preceptor, identify how each partner benefits in an academic–clinical relationship.

References

American Association of Colleges of Nursing. (2007). White paper on the role of the clinical nurse leader. Retrieved from http://www.aacn.nche.edu/Publications/WhitePapers/Clinical NurseLeader.htm

American Heritage Dictionaries. (2007). *American heritage college dictionary* (4th ed.). Boston, MA: Houghton Mifflin.

Bartels, J. (2005). Educating nurses for the 21st century. *Nursing and Health Sciences, 7*(4), 221–225.

Bartels, J., & Bednash, G. (2005). Answering the call for quality nursing care and patient safety. *Nursing Administration Quarterly, 29*(1), 5–13.

Cheung, R., & Aiken, L. (2006). Hospital initiatives to support a better-educated workforce. *Journal of Nursing Administration, 36*(7/8), 357–362.

Davies, S. M., & Bennett, A. (2008). Understanding the economic and social effects of academic clinical partnerships. *Academic Medicine, 83*(6), 535–540.

Duffy, J. R., Thompson, D., Hobbs, T., Niemeyer-Hackett, N. L., & Elpers, S. (2011). Evidence-based nursing leadership. *Journal of Nursing Administration, 41*(10), 422–427.

Gallant, M. H., Beaulieu, M. C., & Carnevale, F. A. (2002). Partnership: An analysis of the concept within the nurse-client relationship. *Journal of Advanced Nursing, 40*(2), 149–157.

Glazer, G., Erikson, J. I., Mylott, L., Mulready-Shick, J., & Banister, G. (2011). Partnering and leadership: Core requirements for developing a dedicated education unit. *Journal of Nursing Administration, 41*(10), 401–406.

Hix, C., McKeon, L., & Walters, S. (2009). Clinical nurse leader impact on clinical microsystems outcomes. *Journal of Nursing Administration, 39*(2), 71–76.

Hook, M. L. (2006). Partnering with patients—a concept ready for action. *Journal of Advanced Nursing, 56*(2), 133–143.

Institute of Medicine. (2000). *To err is human: Building a safer health system.* Washington, DC: National Academies of Science.

Institute of Medicine. (2010). The future of nursing: Leading change, advancing health. Retrieved from http://www.iom.edu/Reports/2010/The-Future-of-Nursing-Leading-Change-Advancing -Health.aspx

Kerfoot, K. M., Rapala, K., Ebright, P., & Rogers, S. M. (2006). The power of collaboration with patient safety programs: Building safe passage for patients, nurses, and clinical nurses. *Journal of Nursing Administration, 36,* 582–588.

Kimball, B., & O'Neil, E. (2002). *Health care's human crisis: The American nursing shortage.* Princeton, NJ: Robert Wood Johnson Foundation.

Merriam-Webster, Incorporated. (n.d.). *Merriam-Webster online dictionary.* Retrieved from http:// www.merriam-webster.com

National League for Nursing Board of Governors. (2003). Position statement: Innovation in nursing education: A call to reform. Retrieved from http://www.nln.org/aboutnln/Position Statements/innovation.htm

Newhouse, R. P. (2007). Collaborative synergy. *Journal of Nursing Administration, 37,* 105–108.

Pew Health Professions Commission. (1998). *Recreating health professional practice for a new century: Fourth report of the Pew Health Professions Commission.* San Francisco, CA: Author. Retrieved from http://www.futurehealth.ucsf.edu/Public/Publications-and-Resources/Content .aspx?topic=Recreating_Health_Professional_Practice_for_a_New_Century

Rusch, L., & Bakewell-Sachs, S. (2007). The CNL: A gateway to better care? *Nursing Management,* 32–40.

Stanley, J. M., Hoiting, T., Burton, D., Harris, J., & Norman, L. (2007). Implementing innovation through education-practice partnerships. *Nursing Outlook, 55*(2), 67–73.

Stark, P. (2003). Clinical teaching and learning in the clinical setting: A qualitative study of the perceptions of students and teachers. *Medical Education, 37*(11), 975.

Steinhart, C. M., & Alsup, R. G. (2001, May). Partnerships in health care: Creating a strong value chain. *Physician Executive, 27,* 50–56. Available at http://findarticles.com/p/articles/mi _m0843/is_3_27/ai_75451945

University of Maryland School of Nursing, Office of Communications. (2007). *Nursing: Leadership, partnership, innovation* (pp. 1–30). Baltimore, MD: Author. Retrieved from http://nursing .umaryland.edu/sites/default/files/uploads/docs/publications/UM-NURSING-Sprg07.pdf

Vallejo, P., Saura, R. M., Sunol, R., Kazandjian, V., Urena, V., & Mauri, J. (2006). A proposed adaptation of the EFQM fundamental concepts of excellence to health care based on the PATH framework. *International Journal for Quality in Health Care, 18*(5), 327–335.

Wiggins, M. (2006). The partnership care delivery model. *Journal of Nursing Administration, 36*(7/8), 341–345.

Zahner, S., & Gredig, Q. (2005). Improving public health nursing education: Recommendations of local public health nurses. *Public Health Nursing, 22*(5), 445–450.

WellStar Health System— CNL on All Acute Care Units

Donna Whitehead
WellStar Health System, Marietta, GA
University of West Georgia, MSN-CNL Student

Senior nursing leaders at WellStar Health System (WHS) are dreaming of the day that there is a clinical nurse leader (CNL) on every inpatient unit. WHS supports the 12-bed hospital model for the delivery of patient care lead by CNLs in acute care.

WellStar Douglas Hospital is a 102-bed hospital with four acute care units. Currently there is one CNL working on the 16-bed postoperative unit. This CNL is paving the way for four additional CNL students to join her during their clinical immersion experience. By the end of fiscal year 2013, WellStar Douglas will have five CNLs leading the way to improve patient outcomes in acute care. WellStar Paulding will have one CNL functioning on the acute care unit.

WellStar Cobb Hospital will start its implementation journey of CNLs with four CNLs in spring 2013. Two CNLs are being placed on the stroke/neurological unit, and two are being placed on the renal failure unit.

WellStar Kennestone Hospital will have eight CNLs working on four of the acute care units. Senior nursing leaders have chosen units where they believe the CNLs will make the biggest impact on improving clinical outcomes for patients. Two CNLs will be on the stroke/neurological unit, two on the cardiac dysrhythmia unit, two on the renal/hemodialysis unit, and two on the medical unit.

WHS will be adding 23 additional CNLs to Cobb and Kennestone Hospitals in spring 2014, when the second cohort graduates from the University of West Georgia.

FOUR

Creating a Business Case for the Clinical Nurse Leader Role

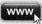 Carol Jefferson Ratcliffe

Learning Objectives

- Define the business case
- Identify the steps in developing a business case
- Discuss the importance of determining organizational/system readiness for the business case
- Identify and discuss the components of a business case
- Discuss how to quantify the economic value of the clinical nurse leader role within an organization/system
- Identify and discuss quality, safety, and financial outcomes of the business case

> To raise new questions, new possibilities, to regard old problems from a new angle, requires creative imagination and marks real advance in science.
>
> **Albert Einstein**

Key Terms

Strategic plan   Business case   Organizational/system readiness
Economic value   Measurable improvement

CNL Roles

Risk anticipator   Advocate   Delegator   Communicator
Data manager   Lateral integrator   Leader

CNL Professional Values

Advocacy   Accountability   Integrity
Ethics   Altruism

CNL Core Competencies

Communication   Risk anticipation   Critical thinking
Leadership   Resource management   Analysis
Information management

Introduction

The clinical nurse leader (CNL) role has catapulted into a unique vision in nursing. The CNL has the ability to see care delivery through a new set of lenses, and the role facilitates getting to the core of opportunity and sustaining change (Ratcliffe, 2010). Transforming care at the bedside through implementation of the CNL role can create the culture of safety opportunities discussed and recommended by the Institute of Medicine (IOM, 1999, 2001, 2004). Other landmark documents affirm that care delivery today will not sustain the complex health needs of most patients, and thus change is required (American Association of Colleges of Nurses [AACN], 2007; IOM, 2010). An innovative nurse leader who is prepared to mentor and who is focused on improving patient outcomes and staff, patient, and physician satisfaction, and who is dedicated to building partnerships and collaboration and integrating best practices is a catalyst for the CNL role's success.

Successful immersion of the CNL into the patient care model requires the development of a business case that shows measurable improvement with economic value. As nurse leaders, we rely on our financial acumen and clinical astuteness to know when a process change makes good clinical and business sense. The challenges of today's healthcare environment make it necessary for nurse leaders to prove that any additional staff or new roles have positive fiscal implications. Although many organizations have garnered multimillion dollar success, nurse executives have found that the CNL role is not immune to this process. Making a business case that is specific to a patient care area, population, or program with metrics that matter and measurable outcomes will provide the fiscal and clinical leverage needed to obtain support. It is not the number of metrics that are important. It is important to choose wisely and yield big. Remember, go after the low-hanging fruit.

Let the Innovation Begin

Planting the Seed

When developing a strategy on paper, it is crucial to initially begin to raise awareness, assess organizational readiness, and gain support for the concept (Moore, 2006). Part of this process is creating an education and communication plan. In the case of the CNL, the first step is to ensure that nurse leaders understand the role and how it differs from other traditional nursing positions and specialists, and to ensure that they can articulate the role's benefits. As an advocate, you should think in terms of an elevator speech, striving to be effective and to the point and crafting your message wisely.

Once nursing leadership understands the CNL role and how effective it is in improving patient care, you should begin to seek the support of other key stakeholders within the organization, including staff nurses, physicians, and executive leaders. Knowing the organizational culture is a must. Relationships and the ability to garner individual support will be very important. You do not need to have a complete financial analysis at this time, but you will need to know where opportunities exist and emphasize the success of others.

A Deeper Look Within

Suppose the nurse leaders in your organization have prioritized goals for the upcoming year and agreed that the CNL role immersion is one of the top priorities. Their knowledge of the role was enhanced by attending conferences, networking with others, and reading an array of literature. A deep dive followed. Choose a model that works best for the organization. In some instances, integrating a business and clinical methodology may prove useful.

The McKinsey 7-S Framework

The McKinsey 7-S framework was developed by Tom Peters, Robert Waterman, and Anthony Athos in the early 1980s. It can be used to assess and evaluate organizational effectiveness and determine how well an organization is positioned to achieve a strategy. The McKinsey 7-S framework, depicted in **Figure 4-1**, tests for strategic fit. It uses seven elements: (1) structure, (2) strategy, (3) staff, (4) systems, (5) style, (6) skills, and (7) subordinate goals (shared values). There is no hierarchy of the elements; rather all are interrelated and should be addressed during the assessment. These elements are further grouped into hard and soft elements. Hard elements are strategy, structure, and systems. They are easier to define and are influenced by management. Soft elements are shared values, skills, style, and staff. Soft elements are more difficult to define and are influenced more by the culture of the organization than by management (Ginter, Swayne, & Duncan, 2004; Waterman, Peters, & Phillips, 1980).

Here is a further breakdown of the seven elements of the model as they can be applied to the CNL role:

1. **Structure**—What organizational reporting structure will best support the initiative? Who will the CNL report to, the nurse manager or the director of nursing?
2. **Strategy**—Does implementation of the CNL role give the organization a competitive edge?
3. **Staff**—What additional skills and knowledge does the management team need to help ensure the CNL role immersion and its sustained success?
4. **Systems**—Are the systems in place to get the work accomplished? How will you spread the word about improved outcomes from across the organization?
5. **Style**—What is the style of the nursing leadership team?

Figure 4-1   McKinsey 7-S framework.

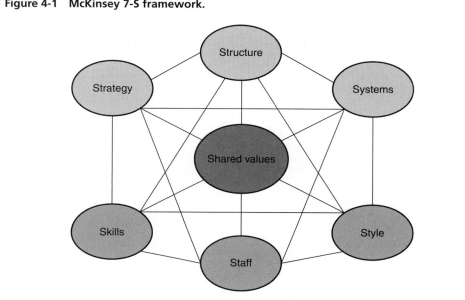

Source: Waterman, R. H., Peters, T. J., & Phillips, J. R. (1980, June). Structure is not organization. *Business Horizons*, 14–26.

6. **Skills**—Are there additional competency requirements of the staff to support the initiative?
7. **Shared values**—What is the organizational culture? Does the culture support the integration of the CNL role?

The Rosswurm–Larrabee Model

The Rosswurm–Larrabee model is an evidence-based model that is very easy for nurse leaders and staff-level employees to follow. Nurses who have been educated and understand the importance of synthesizing and applying the best evidence to an opportunity are using research to enhance patient care and cultivate knowledge to help make the right decisions about care. **Figure 4-2** depicts the components and flow of this evidence-based model and how it easily facilitates a thorough review of opportunities, comparison to the best evidence, action plan development, and sustainment of change.

Figure 4-2   Rosswurm–Larrabee model.

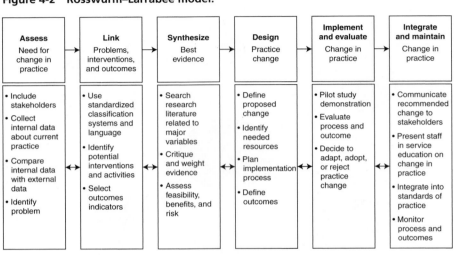

Source: Rosswurm, M. A., Larerabee, J. H. (1999). A model for change to evidence-based practice. *Journal of Nursing Scholarship, 31*(4). Reproduced with permission of Blackwell Publishing, Inc.

A Vision That Can Change the Future

A Solid Foundation

Nursing's foundation begins with leadership and a professional practice model that supports the mission and vision of nursing. Choose a model that is evidence based and measurable and that supports innovation and the emergence of new roles (Smith, Manfredi, Hagos, Drummond-Huth, & Moore, 2006). The practice model should be easy for the staff-level employee to understand, and it should facilitate and support an environment of high reliability, a commitment to life-long learning, collaboration and teamwork, satisfaction and service excellence, and improvement in patient outcomes.

An example of a practice model that fosters this desired atmosphere is the relationship-based care model. Koloroutis (2004) puts the patient and family at the center of the model. Fostering a strong relationship with other care providers and taking care of one's self creates what is necessary to care for the patient and his or her family. The relationship-based care model is built on the relationship with the patient and family, with other care providers, and with one's self. Positive relationships foster collaboration; the success of the CNL role is grounded in leadership, relationships and trust, implementation skills, coordination and lateral integration, and shared governance. The clinical partner(s) selected for role immersion must have a stable environment to include leadership and staffing.

The Strategy Behind the Strategy

In your role as the executive sponsor for the CNL role immersion, a solid business case is your platform. Prepare it as though it is the last opportunity to advocate your position in the negotiating process; be concise and strategically organized. The business case should cover who, what, and why with detail that helps to sell the idea. A highly successful business case is aligned with a strategic plan, supports innovation in practice, and builds on evidence that supports a culture of safety, quality, and service excellence (Simerson, 2011; Harris & Ott, 2008). The CNL role should support an existing strategy or strategies. Consumer expectations, market competitiveness, population health outcomes, and regulatory requirements have led nurse leaders to redesign and transform care using innovative delivery models (Rutherford, Lee, & Greiner 2004).

Highlighting how the CNL will help operationalize and sustain the desired outcome of an existing goal and the integration of concepts and transformation creates familiarity with the target audience. The business case for the CNL role immersion should be contained in a concise, strategically prepared document. The document should include, at a minimum, the following components:

- Cover page
- Table of contents
- Executive summary and recommendation
- CNL role highlights
- Background on the clinical nurse leader as a new and emergent role for nursing
- Role differentiation
  - How the CNL differs from the unit manager
  - How the CNL differs from the case manager
  - How the CNL differs from the clinical nurse specialist

- Implications for quality and safety
  - Pathways to excellence or magnet journey
    - Use innovative model for care delivery
    - Support the staff registered nurse
    - Foster teamwork
    - Improve relationships
  - Fostering of a high reliability organization
  - Performance and operational goals
  - Integration of care
  - Creation of systems
  - Selection of the CNL partner for implementation
  - Spreading success
- Business case objectives
  - Opportunity
  - Goals with measurable metrics and comparative baseline period
  - Expected outcomes and cost savings
- Quality investment and financial analysis overview
  - Detail expenses
    - Ongoing expenses
    - One-time expenses
  - Expected cost savings
  - Return on investment

Selecting Metrics That Matter

A crucial step in the planning phase for the CNL role is ensuring that the identified opportunities are prioritized. When beginning this process, one will likely have a list of projects that is many pages long. Choose metrics wisely. As the executive sponsor, one needs to serve as mentor and coach, provide resources, remove barriers, and manage workload by ensuring the CNL is not assigned to other projects. The CNL will be a hot commodity, and the CNL's expertise and organizational skills will be solicited by many across the organization.

Metrics must be measurable and produce the largest gain. It is best and less labor intensive when the information to support the metric is electronic and easily accessible. The CNL should spend the majority of time at the bedside working with staff and other team members, not manually collecting data. It supports role success when the CNL has been educated and can generate reports from applications. This access to data gives the CNL the ability to complete analysis in different ways and expedites receipt of information.

Keeping Your Finger on the Pulse

Operational controls, creation of a scorecard, and regularly scheduled meetings are crucial to the success of the CNL role immersion, attaining the established goals, and meeting the financial margin as expected (Ratcliffe, 2010). This level of detail clearly goes beyond a simple review of data. This structure provides key leader stakeholders, including the CNL(s), with a forum to review outcomes over time, manage using a scorecard, discuss what's working well, and what barriers exist. Empower the CNL to be candid during these meetings because the dialogue that occurs is invaluable. The group's membership should include, at a minimum, the nurse executive, CNL(s), and nurse leader(s) responsible for a unit or department with a CNL.

> **Some men look at things the way they are and ask why? I dream of things that are not and ask why not?**
>
> John F. Kennedy

This scheduled debriefing is prudent and enables the key stakeholders to really have a finger on the pulse of the CNL immersion. Corbett, Hurko, and Vallee (2012) describe how debriefings are important in determining the effectiveness of a plan. Scheduled debriefings eliminate surprises related to progress. One of the greatest challenges may be determining how to design reports for each metric. Agree upon this early in the process because these reports will be the visual for measuring success. Use scorecards and charts to communicate progress. As goals are met or major milestones are reached, celebrate, celebrate, and celebrate.

Immersion of the Clinical Nurse Leader Role on a Medical–Surgical Unit

In 2008, as vice president of patient care services and chief nursing officer of a medical–surgical unit, I recognized that the nursing landscape was changing. From the desire to create a new and innovative model for nursing care delivery that would enhance and improve care, the CNL role was born. Microsystem, macrosystem, lateral integrator, and risk anticipator were not terms routinely used by my organization's nurse leaders. However, after being educated about the CNL role by a clinical affiliate and a leading CNL educator and scholar, attending CNL conferences, and networking with other nurse leaders and CNLs, the nursing leadership team became zealous about the new concept. These learning opportunities and educational experiences sparked excitement and a commitment to undertake the steps to revise the nursing model of care and incorporate the CNL role.

A master's-prepared nurse at the bedside was a new concept in nursing at this time. Careful articulation of success stories, garnered from the Department of Veterans Affairs across the country and others, helped set the groundwork for acceptance and support by the organization's system chief operating officer, chief medical officer, and hospital president. The message was carefully crafted and focused on the CNL role highlights. A meeting was held with key system senior executive stakeholders to educate them about the role—how it differed from other traditional nursing roles, how it supported our existing organizational strategies, and how we could set the stage for rollout throughout our other system facilities. The time frame for implementation was approximately one and a half years. The length of the time frame was strategic, focused on finding dollars for the role and the right person to choose to be the organization's first CNL. A business case was required to add the new position. One of the charge nurses was so intrigued by the CNL concept and how it supported personal and professional goals that she enrolled in a CNL program.

Implementation

The critical phase of getting the organization ready for a change through CNL role implementation was only the first step. Implementing the role required deliberate, intentional strategies and tools. Developing an aim statement that was clear and meaningful was the next step.

Aim Statement

Our aim statement was articulated as follows: To implement a clinical nurse leader at the microsystem level who will have a positive impact on patient, associate, and stakeholder satisfaction, and who will demonstrate that good fiscal stewardship is a condition of quality care.

Elevator Speech

The CNL can be effective in various roles and departments across an organization. Some organizations are still determining how to define and implement this role. Buy-in is attained through effective communication.

The staff in our organization knew desired outcomes and assisted in CNL role immersion and creation of talking points. The elevator speech focused on the following role highlights with an explanation that resonated with staff and stakeholders:

- First new role introduced since the nurse practitioner role over 35 years ago
- Focus at the microsystem level and systems thinking
- Role enhances physician and nurse collaboration
- Master's-prepared nurse focused on quality, safety, and effective point of care delivery
- Role differs from the unit manager, the clinical nurse specialist, and the case manager
- Role achieves patient outcomes through lateral integration and coordination
- Role will assist in improving nursing-sensitive indicators by risk assessing patients with complex issues
- Role has a positive impact on patient, associate, and physician satisfaction (AACN, 2007)

Business Case Objectives
Nursing leadership had regularly scheduled meetings that included a review of nursing-sensitive measure results, patient satisfaction, and core measure compliance, to name a few. With opportunities identified, a nurse manager with a desire to implement the CNL role, and a dynamic and well-respected charge nurse a few months away from completing the CNL program, the organization was well positioned to implement the role.

Selected deliverables and the top opportunities and metrics were identified.

Table 4-1 describes the business case objectives, measurable metrics, and expected outcomes of the CNL immersion. All metrics were tracked monthly and reported quarterly for comparative purposes. Fiscal year 2010 was used as a baseline comparison to measure improvement.

Role Immersion
In preparation for the CNL role immersion, there were several strategies that were identified as important to the success of the role. The strategies included: (1) having a clear vision; (2) crafting the ideal CNL job description; (3) having the right person as the first CNL in the organization; (4) creating an orientation plan; (5) compensation

Table 4-1   Business Case Objectives with Expected Outcomes for the Medical Surgical Unit

Opportunity	Measurable Metric	Outcome
Quality/Cost/People		
1. Oversee processes to ensure the completion/ follow-through on core measure opportunities a. Evaluate the process and educate associates. b. Focus on nursing sensitive measures, surgical care improvement process (SCIP), and stroke with all core measures added over time. These units are the designated areas for stroke patients as part of our new protocol.	1. Obtain improvement fiscal year (FY) over fiscal year and attain compliance at the "top decile" with nurse-influenced core measures on the CNL unit.	1. Increase in core measure compliance
2. Integrate findings from the catheter-acquired urinary tract infections (CAUTI) research study conducted by graduate nursing students.	2. Decreased urine nosocomial infection markers (NIMs) as measured through CareFusion, using the average of Q3 FY2009 through Q2 FY2010 through May as the baseline. Cost for urine NIMs calculated using the FY 2009 data from CareFusion.	2. Decrease the urine NIMs rate by 25%. Total cost avoidance is $33,110.00.
3. Improve the average time a patient is discharged by 1 hour.	3. Average discharge time for the unit as measured by the electronic patient tracking board, using the period from February 2009 through June 23, 2009 as a baseline.	3. Improve the throughput of patients who need to be admitted.

Table 4-1   Business Case Objectives with Expected Outcomes for the Medical Surgical Unit (continued)

Opportunity	Measurable Metric	Outcome
Service/People		
4. Enhance collaboration between associates and physicians. a. Develop physician preference cards.	Measure nurse–physician collaboration on the nurse satisfaction survey tool, using the survey conducted in June 2010 as the baseline.	Increase in nurse–physician collaboration.
	a. Reported increases in physician satisfaction, using the most current physician satisfaction data as the baseline for comparison if a formal survey is conducted during FY 2011.	a. Increase in physician satisfaction.
b. Assess need for revision to processes in patient care that will increase patient satisfaction with nursing and communication related to medications.	b. Increase in patient satisfaction with nursing, communication with nursing, communication related to medications as measured by the patient satisfaction survey tool.	b. Increase in patient satisfaction with nursing, communication with nursing, and communication related to medications.
People		
5. Decrease incremental overtime and shift overage.	5. Decrease incremental overage by 50% using April and May 2010 as baseline.	5. $16,951

Total Savings/Cost Avoidance	**$50,061**

and the reporting structure; (6) regularly scheduled debriefings; (7) review of progress; (8) ensuring the CNL was not overextended; and (9) cultural acceptance and support for the role. Close attention to the structure of the CNL orientation was necessary and included time with a number of stakeholders. A decision was made to have the CNL report to the director of nursing and have a dotted line to the nurse manager. This structure was chosen to ensure that the CNL was not used to replace the bedside nurse in staffing and to keep the focus on the initiatives.

Although the first chosen CNL was a current employee and had been for 16 years, it was important that the CNL attend new nurse orientation. This approach ensured that the CNL was knowledgeable and had an overview of all practice revisions. As the current chair of the Staff Development Council, the CNL's insightfulness and attention to detail spearheaded changes to the orientation structure and content. Following completion of a 6-week orientation, the CNL's initial time was spent observing processes, performing searches for evidence-based and best practice literature, reviewing and collecting data, and developing tools. It was very important that the CNL was seen as a resource for the patient care team and not someone who would tell staff nurses how to provide patient care or complete assigned staff tasks.

CNL Sustainability and Success

The CNL role immersion on the medical–surgical unit was very successful. This innovative model was embraced and added value to the delivery of care. The role supported the staff registered nurse and the physician, fostered teamwork, and improved patient outcomes and relationships. The CNL identified cost savings and cost avoidances that would evidence fiscal responsibility and a high reliability organization. Measurable metrics were established for the CNL at the beginning of fiscal year 2010. Monthly meetings followed to review attainment of goals and progress made, provide feedback, and remove any barriers or obstacles that might inhibit goal attainment. The fiscal savings exceeded $3.5 million by putting the CNL role in place.

Specifically, the CNL initiated a variety of activities that contributed to the $3.5 million savings, including these examples:

- Through risk assessment, the CNL identified 176 core measure patients and 56 readmissions over a 12-month period of time. Interventions were implemented by the CNL with patients, families, nursing associates, and/ or physicians to ensure core measure guidelines were implemented. The readmissions were assessed for trends, including discharge location, and integrated into the hospital's readmission reduction program. There were only four instances over a 12-month period when the core measure compliance was not at 100%. Three of these instances occurred when the CNL was not working, and there was no documentation of congestive heart failure history on the fourth patient. The CNL prevented the occurrence of several hospital-acquired conditions (nurse-sensitive measures): catheter-associated urinary tract infections (18), urinary tract infections (3), pressure ulcers (36), and falls (33). All of these interventions were calculated as avoidance of adverse outcomes using the assumption that if the CNL had not intervened, there was a high probability that each would have occurred. The average cost to care for each occurrence was used in the calculation of the avoidance of the hospital-acquired conditions and totaled $3,475,944.

- There was a 33.33% decrease in infection rates with a savings of $43,037, as compared to a goal of 25% and a savings of $33,110. This included a 54.17% decrease in catheter-acquired urinary tract infections (CAUTIs).
- The average time to discharge a patient once an order was written decreased by 1 hour and 15 minutes. Identifying a dollar value for this improvement was not possible due to an increase in surgical volume and census, which limited the ability to determine if CNL role implementation improved the average number of admissions to the unit. However, an improvement in patient satisfaction related to the discharge process was evident. Staff nurses focused on ways to expedite patients' discharge.
- There was a 1% increase in nurse–physician collaboration identified through the nurse satisfaction survey. Communication about medications improved 7% overall and increased from 61.8% to 66.38%. The patient care unit also received "5 star status" by attaining the 90th percentile ranking in patient satisfaction three out of the four quarters studied. This was the first time the unit had achieved this ranking.
- An 8% ($3,253) decrease in incremental overtime was achieved, as compared to the goal of 50% ($16,951).

The success of CNL role immersion was achieved through careful planning and engagement but also because of the commitment and contributions of the CNL to create positive change and organizational history. The CNL understood the goals and mastered collaboration and a team approach to transforming care at the bedside.

The gains at the unit level were implemented housewide to reduce urine infections. The CNL collaborated with the clinical pharmacist, the surgical care improvement process outcomes manager, and the chief of anesthesia to develop a Lovenox (enoxaparin) protocol for surgical patients with epidurals.

In addition to the improvements seen in patient and physician satisfaction, there was marked improvement in associate satisfaction on this medical–surgical unit when comparing 2009 scores to 2011. The associate loyalty score improved from 84% to 96% and was higher than the overall hospital score of 87%. The work environment score improved from 70% to 84%. The equipment, tools, and resources score improved from 60% to 81% and was higher than the hospital's score of 74%. The spirit of cooperation score improved from 79% to 88%, which was equal to the hospital's score for this measure.

Since the initial role immersion, the CNL role has been expanded to four additional patient care units with two more units planned in the upcoming year. The role has either been implemented or there is planned implementation in other system hospitals. The CNL is regarded as an expert and is the epitome of advancing nursing practice.

Summary

- The chief nurse executive must have a clear vision for how the CNL will be immersed in the care delivery model and be prepared to demonstrate the economic value of the CNL role.
- Key stakeholders must be educated about the CNL role and how it supports the mission and goals of the organization. An elevator speech that articulates the key message is paramount when implementing the role.
- The success of the first CNL in an organization facilitates ongoing success of role immersion. Creating an orientation program that facilitates the success of the role is essential for sustainability.
- Performing a business and clinical organizational readiness assessment prior to role immersion is necessary. Being prepared to answer questions, remove barriers, and determine the reporting structure for the CNL role is also critical to success and sustainability.
- Selecting metrics that add value to patient care is important to the success of the CNL role immersion.

- Establishing regularly scheduled meetings with key stakeholders to review progress and discuss opportunities and barriers also is required.
- Communicating success on a regular basis to key stakeholders provides much needed input and feedback.
- Focusing on metrics and improving care at the bedside promotes the CNL role.

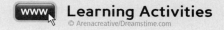

Reflection Questions

© Arenacreative/Dreamstime.com

1. Describe how you envision the role of the CNL in your organization.
2. Do you have a nursing strategic plan? Has the CNL role been included in your plan?
3. Identify where you would implement the CNL role and the opportunities. Would the culture in this microsystem support role immersion?

Learning Activities

© Arenacreative/Dreamstime.com

1. Perform an organizational readiness assessment for the CNL role. Do you have the foundation to support role implementation? Do you have the support of key stakeholders? If the answer to either question is no, what do you need to do to remove barriers prior to implementation?
2. Once you have identified the appropriate microsystem for role immersion, create a list of metrics, how success will be measured, and the expected outcome. Select initiatives that will improve care and processes and yield the greatest economic value.

References

American Association of Colleges of Nursing (AACN). (2007, February). *White paper on the role of the clinical nurse leader*. Retrieved from www.aacn.nche.edu/publications/white-papers/cnl

Corbett, N., Hurko, P., & Vallee, J. T. (2012). Debriefing as a strategic tool for performance improvement. *Journal of Obstetric, Gynecologic, & Neonatal Nursing, 41*(4), 572–579. doi: 10.1111/j.1552-6909.2012.01374.x

Ginter, P. M., Swyane, L. E., & Duncan, W. J. (2004). *Strategic management of health care organizations* (4th ed.). Malden, MA: Blackwell Publishing.

Harris, J. L., & Ott, K. (2008, August). Building the business case for the clinical nurse leader role. *Nurse Leader, 6*(4), 25–28.

Institute of Medicine (IOM). (1999). *To err is human: Building a safer health system.* Washington, DC: National Academies Press.

Institute of Medicine (IOM). (2001). *Crossing the quality chasm.* Washington, DC: National Academies Press.

Institute of Medicine (IOM). (2004*). Keeping patients safe: Transforming the work environment of nurses.* Washington, DC: National Academies Press.

Institute of Medicine (IOM). (2010). *The future of nursing: Leading change, advancing health.* Washington, DC: National Academies Press.

Koloroutis, M. (2004). Professional nursing practice. *Relationship based care: A model for transforming practice* (pp. 117–158). Minneapolis, MN: Creottative Healthcare Management, Inc.

Moore, R. (2006). Take seven successful steps to align your organization. *Plant Engineering, 25,* 33–34.

Ratcliffe, C. J. (2010). Getting to the core of opportunity: Using operational levels of control to improve and sustain compliance. In J. Harris, L. Roussel, S. Walters, & C. Dearman (Eds.), *Project planning and management: A guide for CNLs, DNPs, and nurse executives* (pp. 270–278). Sudbury, MA: Jones & Bartlett Learning.

Rutherford, P., Lee B., & Greiner A. (2004). *Transforming care at the bedside.* IHI Innovation Series white paper. Boston, MA: Institute for Healthcare Improvement. Retrieved from www.IHI.org

Simerson, B. K. (2011). *Strategic planning: A practical guide to strategy formulation and execution.* Santa Barbara, CA: Praeger.

Smith, S. L., Manfredi, T., Hagos, O., Drummond-Huth, B., & Moore, P. D. (2006). Application of the clinical nurse leader role in an acute care delivery model. *Journal of Nursing Administration, 36*(1), 29–33.

Waterman, R. H., Peters, T. J., & Phillips, J. R. (1980, June). Structure is not organization. *Business Horizons, 23*(3), 14–26.

An Innovative Approach to Implementation of the Clinical Nurse Leader at the Macrosystem Level, The University of Alabama at Birmingham Hospital

Kristen Noles and Velinda J. Block

Background Information

In response to the growing concern over patient safety, quality, and healthcare outcomes, the CNL role was created. One of the assumptions of the role is that the CNL practices at the microsystem level. As nurse leaders across the country seek ways to transform processes that will improve patient safety and quality care, it is essential not to limit the CNL skill set to the microsystem.

Aim

The purpose of this presentation is to describe how, at the macrosystem level, the CNL skill set was utilized at a 1,157-bed, magnet-designated, academic medical center.

Methods

The chief nursing officer (CNO) and CNL worked together to transform a passive model of shared governance into a functioning framework, supporting further integration into the organizational culture. The functioning of a sacred group was challenged, opening minds to the possibilities found in a true shared governance model. This new model, the nursing practice congress (NPC), empowers staff to use their knowledge about practice and determine the best course of action. Decisions rely on evidence-based practice, and all members are given the resources they need to find relevant information. The model provides a formal forum to openly share and evaluate current clinical practice, gain new knowledge, and work collaboratively with other members of the healthcare team; in this model systematic review and evaluation of work processes can be examined to evaluate and improve established practices and outcomes. The CNL skill set has been instrumental in establishing, mentoring, and supporting staff involved in this transformational process.

Outcome Data

After the first 2 years of existence at the organizational level, 36 issues were presented to the NPC, resulting in the formation of 29 work teams and 19 hospital-wide clinical practice changes. These results of these changes included (1) improvement in patient safety and quality, (2) standardization of practice, and (3) increased collaboration among a variety of disciplines.

Conclusion

As nurse leaders across the country seek ways to use the CNL skill set, it is essential that they remain open to the endless possibilities for the role within their organizations.

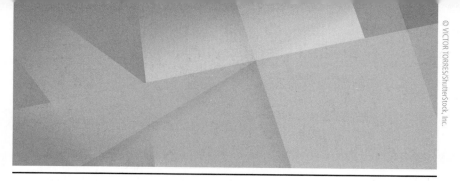

FIVE

Spreading the CNL Initiative: An Interprofessional Microsystem Approach

■ Alice E. Avolio and Marjory D. Williams

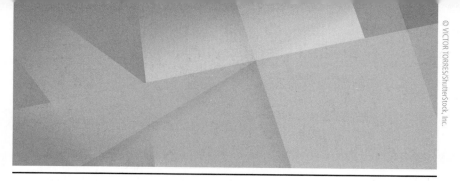

www **Learning Objectives**
© Arenacreative/Dreamstime.com

- Define microsystems within a collaborative practice model
- Identify the requisite steps, activities, and milestones associated with spreading the clinical nurse leader initiative within a healthcare system
- Discuss activities and methods to include in a communication plan that supports spreading the clinical nurse leader initiative
- Identify budget considerations and provide a sample budget plan that covers the lifecycle of the spread initiative
- Describe outcomes of a clinical nurse leader spread initiative within a healthcare system

> Initiative is doing the right thing without being told.
>
> Victor Hugo

77

Key Terms

Microsystems

Communication plan

Value

Interprofessional collaborative practice

Project and budget lifecycle

Measureable outcomes

CNL Roles

Communication

Risk anticipation

Member of profession

Leadership

Design and implementation

Evidence-based practice

CNL Professional Values

Collaboration

Advocacy

Accountability

CNL Core Competencies

Communication

Data interpretation and analysis

Resource management

Delegation

Introduction

Successful implementation and sustainment of the clinical nurse leader (CNL) role is best served by a strategic approach that creates opportunities and anticipates and addresses barriers and challenges. This chapter describes the components of a strategic approach to supporting implementation across a large national healthcare system, using the Veteran's Health Administration (VHA) as an example. Significant key components and instances of specific

> **Time is neutral and does not change things. With courage and initiatives, leaders change things.**
>
> **Jesse Jackson**

activities that can be included in the development, implementation, and evaluation of a strategic CNL spread initiative are described.

Background

In 2010, the Office of Nursing Services (ONS) of the VHA launched its CNL spread plan, a set of strategic initiatives designed to provide support for full implementation of the CNL role at all points of care across the system over a 5-year period (ONS, 2010). The plan, when first released, defined the scope, project lifecycle, activity descriptions, per annum costs, and markers of success. This portfolio of multiyear activities was specifically designed to:

- Overcome barriers to implementing and sustaining the CNL role
- Employ and fully integrate the CNL role into the patient care model
- Objectively embed quality, safety, and efficiency into patient care delivery
- Enhance collaborative partnerships with affiliating schools of nursing and interprofessional teams (ONS, 2010)

The impetus for the implementation of the CNL spread plan was difficulty encountered in attaining the goal of full implementation across the national VHA system. Multiple barriers existed, including budget constraints, geographic inconsistencies in understanding of and experience with the role, and lack of dedicated ongoing consultative support for facilities during implementation of the role. The multiyear spread plan was designed to address identified barriers while significantly enhancing care delivery and clinical processes at the microsystem level (ONS, 2010). Inclusion of the CNL role in current and future staffing plans and formation of valuable partnerships were considered fundamental to advancing the adoption and integration of the CNL role within VHA and the healthcare community.

The remainder of this chapter describes the component activities of the VHA's spread plan and outlines key activities and focus areas for consultative support. Priority concerns for communication and resource impact and examples of evaluation measures at the system, organization, and microsystem levels are identified. Chapter content incorporates insights gained from consultative activities and engagement with stakeholders at all levels. The significance of the multiple activities of the CNL spread plan in supporting CNL role implementation and sustainment are highlighted, as is the clear focus on the interprofessional team at the level of the microsystem.

Component Activities of the VHA's CNL Spread Plan

This section describes the component activities of the VHA's CNL spread plan. The activities included:

- Creating the Management Guidance Team
- Establishing the CNL Implementation and Evaluation Consultative Service
- Organizing the Academy for the Improvement of Microsystems
- Developing and implementing the CNL Transition-to-Practice Curriculum
- Partnering in identifying and establishing funding support for VHA employees pursuing requirements to become CNLs

As a beginning activity, a diverse group of stakeholders convened for an all day deep dive exercise to explore a systems redesign approach to the CNL role at the microsystem level across the organization (Harris, 2011). Theoretical underpinnings of the CNL spread plan and the vision of a CNL in every facility across the system by 2016 were reviewed. Barriers were identified, elements of a sound business case were delineated, marketing strategies were proposed, and measures of spread were discussed. The organization of the first Academy for the Improvement of Microsystems (AIM) was developed, as were mechanisms for integrating the multiple component activities of the CNL spread plan. The Management Advisory Group was created to consider feedback from various spread plan activities, make decisions about implementation of the CNL role, and conduct periodic monitoring and oversight during the proposed 5 years of the spread plan. The value of national leadership support was fully acknowledged. Following the deep dive exercise, the expectation that the CNL role would be included in current and future nurse staffing plans was communicated to all medical center directors.

A second activity of the VHA CNL spread plan was establishing the CNL Implementation and Evaluation Service to provide consultation and assistance to VHA medical centers, academic affiliates offering a CNL curriculum, and individual CNL students and preceptors. More specifically, the services included fostering clinical and academic partnerships, readying environments for CNL role implementation and sustainment, developing CNL preceptors, guiding the development and future analysis of metrics related to the impact of the CNL role, collaborating with other activities in the spread plan, disseminating findings, and submitting progress reports (ONS, 2010).

Core activities of the CNL Implementation and Evaluation Service were assessing system needs, establishing measures of success, and remaining responsive to the needs of stakeholders; these activities evolved over the lifecycle of the CNL spread plan. A system-level gap analysis conducted in April 2012 sought input from facility nurse executives to guide the development of consultative activities and products. Consultative site visits individualized to the needs of the requesting facility provided the opportunity to share effective strategies and practice and to create supportive networks across the system. Virtual consultative support was enhanced through access to resource tool kits developed to address common needs, promote standardization of role implementation, and disseminate effective practices. A virtual national community of CNL practice grew around shared online workspace and monthly CNL live meetings that offered CNLs and microsystem stakeholders the opportunity to discuss issues and share approaches. Dissemination of CNL activities and outcomes was supported through a virtual manuscript development workshop that provided step-by-step training and access to writing coaches. Examples of several of these core activities are included in the exemplars at the end of this chapter.

A third activity in the CNL spread plan involved collaboration between ONS and the MidWest Mountain Veterans Engineering Resource Center (VERC) to create the Academy for the Improvement of Microsystems (AIM). The goal of the AIM collaborative was to foster the development of the CNL role through an interprofessional approach emphasizing systems redesign and flow improvement (ONS, 2010). The vision and actionable goals for the AIM collaborative were created during the deep dive exercise using systems redesign principles and processes. AIM engaged cohorts of point-of-care teams from VHA medical centers to participate in guided learning sessions and activities focused on continuous improvement at the microsystem level. Cohort CNL team members were also provided the opportunity to complete a field-based analytics course to emphasize the importance of analytics-driven decisions for value, quality, access, and satisfaction.

A fourth activity in the CNL spread plan was the development and implementation of a 6-month transition-to-practice program and curriculum intended for new CNLs. This transition-to-practice program involved facilitation and mentoring by a facility-based preceptor or CNL mentor during the guided experience. The program was designed to enhance CNL knowledge, skills, and abilities in coordinating care, applying evidence-based practices, delivering care in a professional nursing practice environment, improving processes, demonstrating transformational leadership, and translating informatics and analytics data into practice.

A fifth activity in the CNL spread plan was the creation of a pilot scholarship program modeled after the VHA National Education for Employees Program (VANEEP) that would offer the necessary financial support to allow CNL students to complete their academic program. The pilot scholarship program offered salary replacement dollars to CNL students to complete the 400 hours of clinical practice immersion, the final requirement of the CNL academic curriculum.

Key Activities and Focus Areas for Consultative Support of CNL Role Implementation

Several consultative activities and focus areas emerged as pivotal to supporting CNL role implementation across the national system. Of paramount importance was the development and validation of a shared vision and conceptualization of the role. Even with the strong and well-represented national vision of the ONS, individual facilities and geographic regions often struggled with establishing a shared local vision among the diverse stakeholders at the facility level. Other critical focus areas for consultative support included identifying key stakeholders at the local level, employing a sound business case, creating capacity to support facility plans for CNL role implementation, leveraging stakeholder support in resource-constrained environments, and creating a community of practice networks and virtual resource repositories for sharing successes and innovations.

Developing/Validating a Shared Vision and Conceptualization of the CNL Role

The importance of approaching CNL implementation by first developing and validating a shared vision and understanding of the CNL role within the context of an organization cannot be overemphasized. This applies regardless of the level of consideration, whether that is across an entire national healthcare delivery system, a single organization, or an individual point-of-care microsystem. Failure to establish a common vision and understanding at the beginning of the journey can lead to misunderstandings and inconsistent expectations that threaten implementation efforts and may be difficult to overcome if initial attempts are unsuccessful (Moore & Leahy, 2012; Vestal, 2011). A particularly problematic barrier identified by nursing leadership in the VHA system was a history of failure in implementing the CNL role (ONS, 2010).

Development of a shared vision and understanding of the CNL role includes a set of activities that provide a strong foundation for initial success, growth, and sustainability (Scott & Mensik, 2010). These activities engage key stakeholders in viewing the role within the context of the organization, projecting and defining reasonable expectations and meaningful outcomes, and formulating an initial idea of the characteristics, role description, and competencies of an effective CNL.

Effective strategies for approaching a shared vision and understanding include clear articulation of the origin of the CNL role and the relationship of that origin to the challenges facing the organization. Some organizational leaders tend to start with looking at how nursing resources can correct issues in the organization, which is very likely to lead to role implementation that does not take advantage of the multiple domains of CNL practice and the potential influence of the role on microsystem practice, process, and outcomes. Concurrent with articulation of the origin of the CNL role, clarification of the role as a point-of-care generalist is an equally important foundational strategy. **Table 5-1** outlines key factors that led to the development of the CNL role that help to illustrate and emphasize a focus on practice at the level of the microsystem.

Clarification of the CNL role as a point-of-care generalist with a practice focus on the microsystem is an important early step in implementation. This step is the foundation for establishing and communicating expectations, as well as delineating evaluation measures. Although the terms *microsystem* and *interprofessional practice* are becoming part of the common language of health care, it remains important to

Table 5-1   Key Factors That Led to the Development of the CNL Role

Despite identification of quality and safety issues in healthcare delivery systems and implementation of structures to improve quality and safety, progress has been slow (Patrician et al., 2012) and improvement activities are often disconnected from the point of care (Reid & Dennison, 2011).

The complexity of healthcare needs, knowledge, delivery, and delivery systems continues to increase (Newhouse & Spring, 2010), yet the care environment remains fragmented and task oriented (Bender, Connelly, Glaser, & Brown, 2012; Stavrianopolis, 2012).

Interprofessional teamwork and collaboration have been identified as the foundation of safe, effective care (Bender et al., 2012; Buxton, Chandler-Altendor, & Puente, 2012; Herbert, 2005; Norsen, Oplanden, & Quinn, 1995), but the healthcare workforce remains inadequately prepared in the arena of interprofessional practice (Newhouse & Spring, 2010; Patrician et al., 2012; Wagner, Liston, & Miller, 2011).

clarify the definition of these concepts when approaching CNL role implementation. **Table 5-2** provides descriptive definitions. **Table 5-3** provides additional key points for articulating the importance of the microsystem focus.

Identifying Key Stakeholders

For the vision and understanding to be truly shared it is imperative that key stakeholders are identified and included as early as possible in the journey (Dearman & Davis, 2011). Failure is often due to paying inadequate attention to stakeholder groups and/or individuals who have not bought in and who introduce barriers that were not anticipated and adequately addressed in the early approach to role implementation (Harris & Roussel, 2011). Questions to guide stakeholder identification

Table 5-2 Descriptive Definitions of Healthcare Microsystem and Interprofessional Practice

A microsystem is a "small group of people who work together on a regular basis to provide care to discrete subpopulations including the patients. It has clinical and business aims, linked processes, shared information environment and produces performance outcomes. They evolve over time and are (often) embedded in larger systems/organizations" (The Dartmouth Institute, 2011).

Interprofessional practice is characterized by "coordinated and cohesive linkages between disciplines resulting in reciprocal interactions that overlap disciplinary boundaries, generating new common methods, knowledge, or perspectives" (Newhouse & Spring, 2010).

Table 5-3 Key Points About the Importance of a Microsystem Focus

The microsystem is the environment within which the interface with the patient actually occurs

The microsystem is the environment where culture and practice patterns directly impact patient outcomes

The microsystem is the environment where pride in work either flourishes or flounders

The microsystem is the environment where teams that include nurses create conditions of excellence, test changes in healthcare delivery, translate discovery into patient-centered care, provide safe and efficient care, support individuals to reach their potential, and roll up their sleeves and do the work

Shinn, J. K., & Ott, K. M. (2010). *The clinical nurse leader: Excellence at the microsystems level* [PowerPoint slides]. Retrieved from the VHA–ONS shared drive include the following: Who will this impact? How will this impact them? Who might be impacted unintentionally? Who are key stakeholders who can influence other stakeholder groups? How can we stage stakeholder engagement to maximize support and minimize barriers?

Employing the Business Case

Once a common understanding and shared vision have been defined, a solid and meaningful business case can help to consolidate stakeholder engagement and more specifically delineate expectations. Employing the business case can help address important questions such as the following: What can CNL implementation accomplish? What do we anticipate CNL role implementation will actually accomplish? Where in the organization do we most need what we anticipate will be accomplished? What factors maximize the ability to achieve anticipated/desired accomplishments? **Table 5-4** identifies ways that the CNL role adds value to the organization at the microsystem level. Value statements are an important component of the business case and provide a framework for presenting anticipated CNL accomplishments to diverse stakeholders (Bleich, 2011).

Creating Capacity

A common challenge facing many organizations in the early phase of CNL role implementation is the lack of a local CNL recruitment base. When an organization decides to move forward with CNL role implementation an important early issue is where to find the nurses to fill the role. The two options are recruiting external candidates and developing current employees into the role. Both options offer excellent opportunities

Table 5-4 How the CNL Role Adds Value to the Microsystem

- The role is incorporated into the care delivery model.
- The role embeds an advanced skill set in the microsystem at the point of care.
- The role assesses and addresses issues in real time and within context of microsystem reality.
- The role observes and evaluates patterns impacting practice and outcomes.
- The role partners with the nurse manager.
- The role supports direct care staff.
- The role influences point-of-care culture.

but also require thoughtful approaches to anticipate and avoid common pitfalls. As noted earlier, one of the activities in developing and validating a shared vision is formulating an initial idea of the characteristics, role description, and competencies of an effective CNL (Moore & Leahy, 2012). This activity is important to both external recruitment and selection of CNLs and to the development of current employees into the CNL role. Equally important to both approaches is a strong partnership with academic affiliates offering the CNL curriculum (Walters, 2011).

Many facilities across the VHA system identified the CNL role as a workforce development opportunity, recognizing the value of providing an opportunity to further develop strong nurse clinicians who wanted to remain at the point of care. Consultative services assisted facilities in identifying and establishing the key structures, processes, relationships, and resources that would be needed to support employee development into the CNL role. Successful approaches and lessons learned were shared, and important connections across facilities and with academic partners were facilitated. Virtual support was provided by experienced CNLs and CNL preceptors in those areas without current CNL capacity. Questions that helped guide the approach of "grow your own CNL" included the following: What do we need to have in place to do this? What do we currently have in place to support this? What do we need to obtain/develop to be able to do this? What are the stages of this process? What is the time frame for each stage and the overall process? What are alternative options?

Leveraging Stakeholders

Even if the decision to implement the CNL role is supported by leadership, nurse staffing resources may be limited. The resource environment may be further constrained by competition across stakeholder groups, and the challenge of actually creating the role without additional resources may generate new resistance within nursing (Moore & Leahy, 2012). An important issue to explore when resources are a problem is where the organization has buy-in and how it can use it to influence resistance. Anticipating resource competition may reveal opportunities for CNL role implementation to address unmet needs through transformation of care delivery models or approaches. Once barriers are identified, knowing where they are and who the organization can partner with to address them can be the basis of a strategic approach to strengthening organizational support of CNL role implementation.

Another issue to pursue is where resource deals can be made. This issue may identify opportunities for innovation and transformational change as resources are renegotiated and realigned to the point of care.

One strategic approach to leveraging stakeholders is a stratified staged marketing plan in which the nature and timing of information are designed to target specific stakeholder groups at key times in the sequence of activities supporting CNL role implementation. Influential stakeholders may help address resistance among other groups if they come on board first. The same set of stakeholders might conversely solidify barriers if the approach is to try to bring every group on board at the same time in the same way.

There are several examples in the VHA of the value of collaborative partnerships in leveraging support for CNL role implementation across programs. The AIM collaborative is one example. The mission of the VERC structures in the VHA is to "integrate the **principles of systems engineering** into the fabric of healthcare delivery" and to promote continuous improvement and lean system design through development of microsystem process and culture (VERC, 2012). Although the focus of the VERC mission is not specifically on the CNL role, the CNL in the microsystem provides an opportunity for the VERC to give tools for influencing microsystem processes to CNLs within the context of a team. Conversely, exposing microsystem teams without CNLs to teams with CNLs in the same cohort strengthens knowledge about the CNL role and helps teams value having a clinical team member with the particular focus and skill set of a CNL in the interprofessional microsystem environment.

Partnerships across clinical and evidence-based practice programs provide opportunities to keep the CNL role in the discussion of innovative and transformational models of care delivery and to engage in resource realignment considerations or proposals for small tests or pilot projects. These activities build evidence for a business case, increase organizational knowledge, and influence value and culture. Partnering with evidence-based practice program activities exposes CNLs and microsystem teams to consideration of practice change that is based on the best available evidence, clinical expertise, and patient preference. Workshops for teams including CNLs support development of CNL competencies in the area of facilitating microsystem evidence-based practice. **Table 5-5** includes examples of how the CNL can influence the microsystem.

Table 5-5   How the CNL Influences the Microsystem

- Patient outcomes in assigned microsystem
- Safety, effectiveness, timeliness, efficiency, quality, and the degree to which we are client centered
- Variations in clinical outcomes
- Critical evaluation and mitigation of risk
- Patterns of need and tailoring of interventions
- Evidence-based practice as way of practice
  - ▲ Uses evidence-based practice to facilitate, coordinate, and provide care
  - ▲ Engages other nurses in evidence-based practice to affect patient outcomes
- Quality and safety as everyday function
  - ▲ Redesigns practices, improves flow, coordinates processes
- Practice and practice change driven by outcomes
- Fosters interprofessional team environment
- Partners to create learning and problem-solving communities

Creating Communities of Practice

A primary consideration of activities designed to spread CNL implementation in a healthcare system is the scale of the overall effort. In a national system, such as the VHA, the ability to engage stakeholders across the diverse components of the system is a daunting challenge. Virtual communities of CNL practice provide a vehicle for increasing connections and communication that support adaptive change (Harris & Roussel, 2011) and build organizational knowledge across geographic boundaries. Rather than employing a prescriptive top-down framework for implementation, virtual communities of practice foster diverse relationships and promote action driven from the point of care (Harris & Roussel, 2011).

The VHA CNL Practice SharePoint site was created to provide ready access to information about the CNL role, VHA initiatives, and CNL practice across the VHA. This repository of resources includes a wide variety of tools that support CNL role implementation. Shared workspace is provided for special groups such as new CNLs participating in the Transition-to-Practice Program and CNLs who are participating in a manuscript writing workshop. While the CNL Practice SharePoint site was primarily created for practicing CNLs and CNL students, information and tools on this site are useful to other stakeholders as well. **Figure 5-1** is a screen shot of the VHA's CNL SharePoint site menu.

Figure 5-1   Menu of information, tools, and resources available on the VHA CNL SharePoint Site.

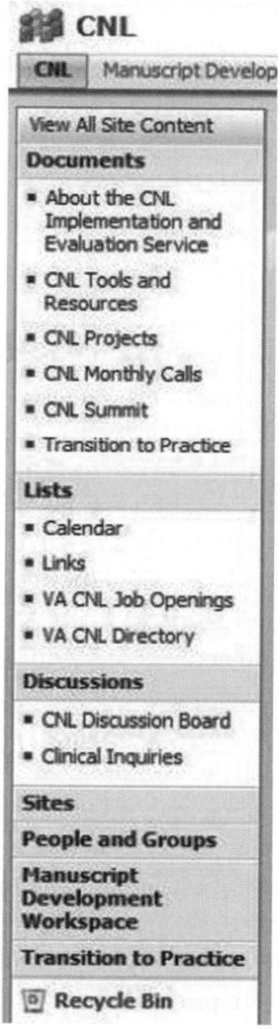

CNL

| CNL | Manuscript Develop |

View All Site Content

Documents
- About the CNL Implementation and Evaluation Service
- CNL Tools and Resources
- CNL Projects
- CNL Monthly Calls
- CNL Summit
- Transition to Practice

Lists
- Calendar
- Links
- VA CNL Job Openings
- VA CNL Directory

Discussions
- CNL Discussion Board
- Clinical Inquiries

Sites

People and Groups

Manuscript Development Workspace

Transition to Practice

Recycle Bin

The AIM collaborative provides another CNL online community. Cohorts of point-of-care teams from geographically dispersed facilities learn and work together using live or real-time Blackboard online learning technology. Faculty provides instruction in systems redesign and continuous improvement, emphasizing lean principles at the point of care. Teams have access to systems redesign coaches, faculty consultants, and a national network of subject matter experts. Team members who complete projects that meet specific requirements are eligible to take an exam to achieve Yellow Belt certification. Descriptions of team projects are available to other teams to promote dissemination of practices that reduce waste, improve throughput, and enhance quality care delivery.

Priority Concerns About Communication and Resource Impact

Communication is foundational to the success of any large-scale system change. Change in complex adaptive systems is effected through connections and networks that promote the exchange and flow of information (Crowell, 2011). Attention should be given to how communication occurs, what needs to be communicated, which stakeholders need to be part of which communications, and strategies for addressing barriers to communication (Harris & Roussel, 2011). In a multifacility national healthcare system, consideration should also be given to variable patterns of communication that may exist. A key element of the communication plan is identification of what works best and how the effectiveness of communication will be validated. Development and validation of a shared vision requires effective communication channels within and across system divisions. The success of marketing strategies is dependent on the timing and sequence of information delivery. Sustainable partnerships and supportive networks are not possible without continuous attention to appropriate and effective communication patterns.

Table 5-6 illustrates strategies employed to address communication among several internal stakeholders to support CNL implementation across the VHA system. A comprehensive communication plan identifies communication needs for both internal and external stakeholders.

Budget considerations are critical to the success of change initiatives. Projection of the economic impact of a proposed change includes consideration of fiscal barriers at all levels within the organization. Obvious dimensions of the economic impact of implementing the CNL role across a national healthcare system include costs associated with CNL salaries and training. Considerations for the cost of the necessary infrastructure to support this major change initiative include additional salary, technology, and community-building expenses. Equally important to the projection of anticipated costs is planning to address the impact of stakeholder

Table 5-6   Sample Internal Communication Plan to Support CNL Implementation Across a National System

Stakeholder Group	Communication Methods	Frequency
System and facility leadership	Leadership meetings/ briefings	As indicated by issues
	Strategic planning meetings	Annual reports
	Nurse executive conference calls	Monthly
	Nursing shared governance meetings	Monthly
	Elevator speeches	Impromptu opportunities
Interprofessional point-of-care teams	Discipline-specific conferences	Annual
	Informational webinars	Quarterly
	Grand rounds	Monthly
	Poster sessions	Semiannual
	Webpages	Ongoing
Practicing CNLs and CNL students	Conference calls	Monthly
	SharePoint community of practice	Ongoing
	National conferences	Annual; semiannual

disincentives related to resource competition that may occur over the lifecycle of the initiative. Strategies for addressing potential roadblocks to required resource alignments are also important components of budgetary planning. **Table 5-7** outlines examples of component costs of the VHA CNL spread plan and illustrates the projected economic impact over the lifecycle of the initiative.

Outcomes of a CNL Spread Initiative

A strategic approach to the implementation of the CNL role across a national healthcare system must include a framework for evaluating desired outcomes. The vision of the VHA's ONS set the primary objective for the CNL spread plan as having a CNL in every point of care across the system within 5 years. In addition to the primary

Table 5-7 Sample Budget Plan to Support CNL Implementation Across a National System

CNL spread plan Activity	Project Component Costs				
	YEAR 1	**YEAR 2**	**YEAR 3**	**YEAR 4**	**YEAR 5**
Academy for Improvement of Microsystems (faculty, coordination, technology, licensing, Yellow Belt [YB] certification, face-to-face meetings)	Salaries Start-up Travel	Salaries Virtual licensing YB testing	Salaries Virtual licensing YB testing	Salaries Virtual licensing YB testing	Salaries Virtual licensing YB testing
Implementation and Evaluation Consulting Service (Consulting team staff, site visits)	Salaries Travel	Salaries Travel	Salaries Travel	Salaries Travel	Salaries Travel
Transition-to-Practice Program (Curriculum development, pilot, 0.2 FTEE offset per participant and preceptor)	Start –up Travel FTEE offset	FTEE offset	FTEE offset	FTEE offset	FTEE offset
Organizational Level (at which cost impacts)	National	National and facility	National and facility	National and facility	National and facility

Note: FTEE = Full Time Equivalent Employee

objective, additional outcomes, milestones, and measures of success were embedded in the evaluation framework. Additional measures pertained to the effectiveness of spread plan components, growth and development of academic and interprofessional partnerships, workforce development, work environment enhancement, and improvements in microsystem performance. This included changes in patterns of microsystem practice, degree of transformational change, sustainability of change, return on investment, and generation of new knowledge.

Strategic action plans identified and tracked progress of component activities and the achievement of milestones. Measures for the AIM collaborative included the number of facilities and microsystem teams completing the training and the number of point-of-care staff achieving Yellow Belt certification. Measures for the Implementation and Evaluation Consultative Service included number of site visits and degree of success meeting facility needs. Outcomes of helping facilities address barriers to CNL implementation are reflected by increased numbers of certified CNLs and new patterns of growth in areas with a history of failure. Measures of the Transition-to-Practice Program include not only the number of new CNLs successfully completing the curriculum, but also the indicators of successful transition to effective practice. This is evidenced through the ability of the new CNL to influence microsystem patterns and practices through leadership and the specific domains of CNL practice.

Ideally, organizational indicators of performance will improve as practicing CNLs begin to impact and influence practices and processes leading to enhanced communication and throughput, competent and consistent high-quality care, reduction of risk for adverse events and hospital-acquired conditions, greater engagement of patients in care, and more efficient and cost-effective care practices. Indicators of healthcare transformation may emerge from more collaborative, innovative, and evidence-based care teams, and the spread of innovation may accelerate due to increased connections and energy across practice networks.

It is important to map out anticipated and desired outcomes to validate success and justify time and expenditure. It is equally important to remain open to unanticipated outcomes that emerge from diverse and novel connections. Healthcare transformation is not about doing the same thing better, but rather about being open to doing things in new ways, ways that have never been thought about or imagined.

As the VHA's CNL spread plan moves forward over its expected lifecycle, lessons will be learned and knowledge will be built. It is important to move forward in a manner that has sufficient fluidity and adaptability to embrace iterations of change as the innovation feeds its own evolution. Observation tells us that certain characteristics are commonly seen in successful CNL programs and that successful programs have common strengths. **Table 5-8** describes keys to successful CNL implementation and sustainability. **Table 5-9** identifies CNL program strengths.

Table 5-8   Keys to Successful CNL Implementation and Sustainability

Leadership that is engaged, understands, shares vision and expectations, and supports the CNL role

Microsystem staff that are knowledgeable, see the value of the role, and are willing to engage with the CNL in creating a safe environment characterized by patient-centered, high-quality, efficient, outcomes-focused, data-driven care

Interdisciplinary team members who actively partner with the CNL in lateral integration and effective communication

Advanced practice nurses who actively partner with the CNL and assist with role differentiation

Academic partners who are engaged with facility staff and leadership, and who help build knowledge about the CNL role and provide support for CNL students and preceptors

A strategic, thoughtful approach to implementing the CNL role in the organization that:

> Targets microsystems that would benefit most from role implementation

> Identifies and develops suitable candidates for the CNL role

> Prepares the clinical environment for role success

> Establishes and evaluates measures of success that are important to the organization

Table 5-9   CNL Program Strengths

CNL role implementation has maintained the integrity of the microsystem focus.

The CNL and nurse manager are true partners.

CNL role activities are primarily driven by microsystem needs.

CNL roles are strategically viewed from a systems perspective as critical to microsystem performance.

The CNL program represents a workforce development initiative.

Summary

- A CNL spread initiative for a major national healthcare system such as the VHA is composed of multiple activities designed to support implementation of the role and to reduce barriers to role implementation.
- The focus of a CNL spread initiative should be on (1) helping facilities establish the infrastructure to support CNL role implementation and practice, (2) providing point-of-care teams with the knowledge and skills to influence practice through system redesign and continuous improvement leadership, and (3) supporting the transition of new CNLs to effective practice at the point of care in the system.

- Establishing and validating a shared vision across stakeholders is key to the success of CNL spread and assists an organization in engaging key stakeholders in viewing the role within the context of the organization, projecting and defining reasonable expectations and meaningful outcomes, and formulating an initial idea of the characteristics, role description, and competencies of an effective CNL.
- Consultative strategies to support CNL implementation include creating capacity, leveraging stakeholders, and creating communities of CNL practice.
- A well thought out communication plan helps to identify information needs and communication patterns, as well as potential barriers to effective communication. Adoption and spread of adaptive innovation across a national system is affected by the nature of exchanges, connections, and networks.
- Projection of budget considerations is key to success. Costs of a CNL initiative need to be evaluated within the context of a framework that identifies objectives, milestones, and measures of success.

www Reflection Questions

© Arenacreative/Dreamstime.com

1. Review the individual components of the CNL spread plan described in the chapter summary. Which of the elements could your system or facility support?
2. What strategies does your facility or system have in place to develop mentors?
3. Does your facility have a shared vision of the CNL role? If not, what strategies could you employ to build or create a shared vision?

www Learning Activities

© Arenacreative/Dreamstime.com

1. Identify key stakeholders in your organization and map out a communication plan that addresses the needs of each of them. Think about what each stakeholder needs to know, when they need to know it, how they are best informed, and what barriers you should anticipate.
2. Think about how an organization might use a business plan to relate the economic impact of CNL implementation to a return on investment.

References

Bender, M., Connelly, C. D., Glaser, D., & Brown, C. (2012). Clinical nurse leader impact on microsystem care quality. *Nursing Research, 61*(5), 326–332.

Bleich, M. R. (2011). Measuring the value of projects within organizations. In J. L. Harris, L. Roussel, S. E. Walters, & C. Dearman (Eds.), *Project planning and management.* Burlington, MA: Jones & Bartlett Learning.

Buxton, J. A., Chandler-Altendorf, A., & Puente, A. E. (2012). A novel collaborative practice model for treatment of mental illness in indigent and uninsured patients. *American Journal of Health-System Pharmacology, 69,* 1054–1062.

Crowell, D. (2011). *Complexity leadership: Nursing's role in healthcare delivery.* Philadelphia, PA: F. A. Davis Company.

The Dartmouth Institute. (2011). Background. Retrieved from http://www.clinicalmicrosystem .org/about/background/

Dearman, C., & Davis, D. (2011). Planning a project for implementation. In J. L. Harris, L. Roussel, S. Walters, & C. Dearman (Eds.), *Project planning and management* (pp. 51–63). Burlington, MA: Jones & Bartlett Learning.

Harris, J. L. (2011, August 11). Chicago Deep Dive. Meeting minutes. Retrieved from personal files on VHA shared drive.

Harris, J. L., & Roussel, L. (2011). From project planning to program management. In J. L. Harris, L. Roussel, S. Walters, & C. Dearman (Eds.), *Project planning and management* (pp. 1–18). Burlington, MA: Jones & Bartlett Learning.

Herbert, C. P. (2005). Changing the culture: Interprofessional education for collaborative patient-centered practice in Canada. *Journal of Interprofessional Care, 19* (Suppl. 1), 1–4.

Moore, L. W., & Leahy, C. (2012). Implementing the new clinical nurse leader role while gleaning insights from the past. *Journal of Professional Nursing, 28*(3), 139–146.

Newhouse, R. P., & Spring, B. (2010). Interdisciplinary evidence-based practice: Moving from silos to synergy. *Nursing Outlook, 58*(6), 309–317.

Norsen, L., Oplanden, J., & Quinn, J. (1995). Practice model: Collaborative practice. *Critical Care Nursing Clinics of North America, 7*(1), 43–52.

Office of Nursing Services, Veteran's Health Administration. (2010). CNL spread plan. Retrieved from the VHA ONS shared drive.

Patrician, P. A., Dolansky, M., Estrada, C., Brennan, C., Miltner, R., Newsom, J., . . . Moore, S. (2012). Interprofessional education in action. *Nursing Clinics of North America, 47*(3), 236–241.

Reid, K. B., & Dennison, P. (2011). The clinical nurse leader (CNL): Point-of-care safety clinician. *The Online Journal of Issues in Nursing, 16*(3), 1–11. Retrieved from http://www.nursingworld .org/MainMenuCategories/ANAMarketplace/ANAPeriodicals/OJIN/TableofContents /Vol-16-2011/No3-Sept-2011/Clinical-Nurse-Leader-and-Safety.html

Scott, K., & Mensik, J. S. (2010). Creating conditions for breakthrough clinical performance. *Nurse Leader, 8*(4), 48–52.

Shinn, J. K., & Ott, K. M. (2010). *The clinical nurse leader: Excellence at the microsystems level* [Powerpoint slides]. Retrieved from VHA ONS shared drive.

Stavrianopoulos, T. (2012). The clinical nurse leader. *Health Science Journal, 6*(3), 392–401.

Vestal, K. (2011). Why transformational change often fails. *Nurse Leader, 9*(5), 22–24.

Veterans Engineering Resources Center. (2012). Homepage. Retrieved from http://www.newengland.va.gov/verc/

Wagner, J., Liston, B., & Miller, J. (2011). Developing interprofessional communication skills. *Teaching and Learning in Nursing, 6*(3), 97–101.

Walters, S. E. (2011). Foundations of project planning and program management. In J. L. Harris, L. Roussel, S. E. Walters, & C. Dearman (Eds.), *Project planning and management*. Burlington, MA: Jones & Bartlett Learning.

Pain and Complex Care

Lauran Hardin and Rebecca Valko

DL is a 36-year-old man with a devastating and rare neurological syndrome. In spite of being wheelchair bound, he maintains as much independence as possible with a service dog, high-end wheelchair, and a strong spirit.

The illness started to take his body in pieces—a Harrington rod, a colostomy, a urostomy, and a feeding tube were all necessary procedures in the last few years.

DL has had the same primary care physician (PCP) for many years, but as his physical status declined and he developed more complications, he added an array of specialists to his team, including urologists, gastroenterologists, hospitalists, pain physicians, and neurologists.

His admissions to the hospital escalated from once a year to six admissions within 3 months' time. Using the skills of systems analysis, CNLs looked at the root cause of these admissions to see if the outcomes of his care could be improved.

Several factors were identified, including fragmentation among the medical providers causing divergent plans of care, complex medical illness without framing it in the context of prognosis, fragmentation among the outpatient providers, lack of communication of plans of care between settings and electronic medical records (EMRs), and lack of a proactive intervention plan to anticipate and react early to problems.

CNLs led a cross-continuum conference of interdisciplinary providers, inviting everyone to come together to creatively see if we could improve outcomes in his care. A complex care plan was created and shared across systems and EMRs to coordinate his care. Evidence-based stoplight tools were engaged with the patient, his family, and the home care and PCP staff to teach everyone how to anticipate the development of complications and intervene before his medical condition required hospitalization.

Creating a web of support among his providers with a clear plan resulted in DL being able to manage his condition at home, with his family and his dog by his side and no hospitalizations or emergency room visits for more than a year.

Lateral Integration/Team Manager

■ Rebecca Valko

CNLs often work with the entire team so that discharges go smoothly. Here is an example scenario:

A complicated patient (complex psychosocial dynamics) with multiple specialists was being discharged to hospice. I **coordinated** the palliative care team and the attending physician to make rounds at the same time so that a final plan could be put in place. Proper antibiotic selection needed to be addressed. I called the infectious disease specialist, and she consulted via phone with the attending physician. The expensive antibiotic Zyvox (linezolid) was selected. I **respectfully challenged** the attending physician about the necessity of using this expensive antibiotic. We collaborated with the pharmacist, and an appropriate, much less expensive antibiotic was selected. The palliative care team was able to complete the pain plan with written prescriptions, the attending physician was able to complete the transfer paperwork, and final logistics were completed with the case manager and hospice liaison. In my role as CNL, I **collaborated** with six interdisciplinary **team** members **efficiently** in 2 hours to facilitate a discharge that could have taken several hours.

Innovation/Collaboration

■ Rebecca Valko and Lauran Hardin

Patients with gastroparesis comprise a highly complex patient population that is at high risk for readmissions and emergency room visits. Root cause analysis showed that most patients were not following a gastroparesis diet. Literature review showed that diet modification is essential to controlling this disease. Through **evidenced-based practice** and **collaboration** with the dieticians from the hospital and the diabetes center, we created an **innovative** gastroparesis diet guideline. This easy to read and informative patient education tool has been well received by patients and providers. A patient even told me that he kept it on his refrigerator! This was just the first step of an interdisciplinary complex care plan approach that decreased readmissions and the lengths of stays for this challenging patient population.

Quality, Core Indicators, and Vaccine Rates

■ Rebecca Valko

Vaccination rates for influenza and **pneumococcus** were a challenge on my acuity-adaptable/cardiac/medical/renal floor. I **educated** the staff several times regarding the importance and value of vaccinations for hospital patients. Even though we had improved since the implementation of the CNL role on the unit, the vaccination rates were still not meeting standards. With the **mentoring** of staff to assist in audits and a **process** change whereby vaccines were given at admission, not at discharge, our unit vaccination rates are now between 95% and 98%. The CNL must look at process steps that make it easier for the staff to do the right thing.

A Practice Innovation to Reduce Unit-Acquired Ear Pressure Ulcers on a Medical Specialty Unit

■ Beverly Phillips, Jennifer Kareivis, Michelle Sheets, and the nursing staff of 3 West
Medical Specialty Unit, Hunterdon Medical Center, Flemington, New Jersey

Background

An increase in unit-acquired pressure ulcers on a medical specialty unit was found to be device related, specifically to methods of oxygen delivery. The firm oxygen tubing and elastic strap from the facemask/tent were identified as factors contributing to ear pressure ulcers for patients unable to communicate needs, including stating pain/discomfort related to oxygen via nasal cannula or facemask/tent. Prior attempts to reduce ear pressure ulcers with alternative means failed. Data were presented by Certified Wound and Ostomy Care Nurse (CWOCN) at a unit meeting. The CNLs championed solving this problem.

Aim

To prevent device-related ear pressure ulcers in patients wearing oxygen cannula or facemask/tent.

Methods/Programs/Practices

Nasal oxygen cannula was changed to softer tubing for any patients requiring supplementation. The CWOCN designed an alternative to the facemask/tent strap, replacing it with a soft trach strap. The Braden scale sensory perception subscale identified patients at risk, with scores of 3 or below indicating that the patient might be unable to feel/communicate discomfort related to oxygen devices. Staff were educated and given visible protocol sheets and prepared supplies. The CNLs facilitated communication and education about the protocol. The CWOCN was the resource person/data collector. If the patient required facemask/tent and had a Braden scale sensory perception score of 3 or below the strap was replaced per protocol. Ear skin assessment was done every shift. Changes were reported to the CWOCN.

Outcome Data

In 2010, preintervention, nine patients developed ear pressure ulcers. Postintervention, one patient in 2011 had an ear pressure ulcer related to oxygen face mask/face tent. Unit-acquired ear pressure ulcers were reduced by 100% related to the oxygen tubing.

Conclusion

Collaboration between the CWOCN and CNLs led to a practice innovation that decreased unit-acquired ear pressure ulcers. The CNLs were integral in educating staff, improving quality care, and identifying patients at risk.

Clinical Nurse Leader and Infection Prevention Collaboration Leading to Decreased Hospital-Acquired Vancomycin-Resistant *Enterococcus* on a Medical Specialty Unit

Jennifer Kareivis, Barbara Bonnah, Michelle Sheets, Kathy Roye-Horn, and Lisa Rasimowicz
Hunterdon Medical Center, Flemington, NJ

Background

At Hunterdon Medical Center (HMC), the efficacy of the CNL is based on measurable indicators unique to each unit's population, as formulated by the chief nursing officer. Healthcare-acquired infections are one of the indicators. A 48-bed medical specialty unit, 3 West, screens all patients on admission for methicillin-resistant *Staphylococcus aureus* (MRSA) and vancomycin-resistant *Enterococcus* (VRE) to identify community-acquired cases.

Aim

To illustrate the correlation between the collaboration of CNLs and the infection prevention (IP) department and the decrease in hospital-acquired (HA) VRE at HMC.

Methods

In February 2010, an increase in the rate of HA VRE was noted. The CNLs collaborated with the IP department to decrease infection rates on the unit. A committee was formed to improve the rates of HA VRE. Staff nurses, housekeeping, patient care assistants, the IP department, unit management, and the CNLs on 3 West were included on the team. Observations were conducted to evaluate compliance with hand hygiene, use and cleaning of equipment, and wearing of personal protective equipment in isolation rooms. If a patient was positive for HA VRE, a review of his or her record was conducted. The CNL and IP department assessed if there was proximity to a patient with a known positive VRE, if the patient was on telemetry, or if the patient was utilizing a commode during his or her stay. An educational program was developed for the nursing staff, informing them of the increased rate of HA VRE and data from observations. The education focused on hand hygiene before/after patient contact and wiping of equipment before/after patient use.

Results/Conclusion

The overall rate of HA VRE decreased on the 3 West medical specialty unit from February 2010 to September 2010. The CNL cannot effect changes, such as decreasing HA VRE, without collaboration with other departments such as the IP department.

SIX

Effective Communication and Team Collaboration

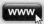 Deborah Antai-Otong

Learning Objectives
© Arenacreative/Dreamstime.com

- Explore the concept of effective use of self as related to written and verbal communication, interpersonal relations, diversity, ethical principles, and professional nursing
- Discuss the management of the healthcare environment using the concepts of delegation and supervision, interdisciplinary care coordination, group dynamics, and conflict resolution
- Describe a variety of communication tools, strategies, and methods such as appreciative inquiry, relationship-based care, crucial conversations, and confrontation

> The way we feel about ourselves is often communicated in the way we treat others.
>
> **Anonymous**

Key Terms

Appreciative inquiry   Assertiveness   Coalition and team building
Communication   Conflict   Crucial conversations
Essential qualities   Group dynamics   Organizational trust
Lean six sigma team

CNL Roles

Clinician   Client advocate   Educator   Information manager
Life-long learner   Member of a profession   Outcome manager
Team manager

CNL Professional Values

Accountability   Altruism   Empathy   Genuineness
Human dignity   Integrity

CNL Core Competencies

Critical thinking   Design/manage/coordinate care
Communicate information and healthcare technologies
Manage illness and disease   Human dignity   Ethics
Provider and manager of care   Healthcare systems and policy
Nursing technology and resources   Therapeutic use of self

Introduction

The novice clinical nurse leader (CNL) has vast opportunities to implement evidence-based care across the healthcare continuum. The success of this role delineation is based on effective communication skills and interpersonal relations that advance patient-centered care. Successful deployment also requires a basic understanding of human interactions, communication, problem-solving skills, conflict management, and coalition or team coordination.

The quality of all relationships stems from effective communication and concern for and appreciation of the rights of others. Effective communication is the matrix of nursing and a critical tool for the CNL, regardless of practice setting or role. This is particularly significant in an era of vast technological advances and substantial reliance on nonverbal communication interactions, such as social media, email, iPhones, and iPads with various applications (apps), such as Siri, a voice-activated app used to send messages, make calls, and set reminders. Other social media include informational blogs, Facebook, and Twitter, which are used to convey, analyze, interpret, and transmit messages.

The emergence of digital communication continues to reduce face-to-face nurse–patient interactions, as electronic devices and electronic communication become the norm. As more and more consumers use electronic devices and social media to access and share healthcare information and interface with the CNL, it is imperative to develop creative and innovative use of these social forums to advance the quality of nurse–patient relationships and provide health care in real time. While the explosion of digital communication is direct and cost saving, allowing consumers and nurses to generate healthcare information and feedback in real time, such may delay the natural progression and development of therapeutic nurse–client encounters. Furthermore, technological advances challenge healthcare providers with new ethical, confidentiality, and professional issues, including blurring nurse–patient boundaries (Ginory, Sabatier, & Eth, 2012; Moubarak, Guiot, Benhamou, Benhamou, & Hariri, 2011).

Apart from ethical, confidentiality, and professional issues associated with the explosion of technological advances, the CNL must be prepared to address changing demographics, such as a younger consumer who has come of age using social media as a primary source of communication. As a result of primary communication through social media and other digital technologies, younger consumers are unlikely to have developed interpersonal skills that enable them to effectively express feelings and opinions, manage and cope with criticism, and form meaningful relationships. Recognition of this potential communication barrier enables the CNL to use face-to-face interactions and other technologies to model effective interpersonal skills and educate younger consumers and families about healthcare issues. In comparison, some older adults with age-related and sensory deficits, psychological loss, and physiological change may require ample time to engage in discussions, express their feelings, and describe complex coexisting medical and psychiatric conditions. Working with all age groups provides a venue to discuss technological advances, such as telehealth, informational blogs, cell phones, and the Internet to access health care. Considerations in addressing age-related communication styles are critical to the CNL and must be mediated by developing person-centered approaches that are unhurried and involve appreciation of inept interpersonal skills and a willingness to address the needs and uniqueness of individuals across the life span.

The novice CNL is challenged to balance advantages and disadvantages and design innovative communication processes that facilitate and sustain quality interpersonal relationships. Healthy human interactions provide a venue for the CNL to form quality interpersonal relationships through effective verbal and nonverbal communication skills that address and resolve the needs of consumers, implement evidence-based interventions, and develop and improve across the healthcare continuum.

This chapter focuses on the effective use of self within vast social forums as related to effective communication, interpersonal relations, ethical principles, and professional values. The initial discussion centers on essential qualities possessed by the CNL—the foundation of communication, interpersonal relationships, and professional values. Later discussion integrates these principles into leadership skills and management of healthcare environments through delegation, supervision, interdisciplinary coordination of care, team collaboration, group dynamics, and conflict management.

Essential Qualities of the Clinical Nurse Leader

Regardless of where CNLs enter healthcare systems, they must possess certain essential qualities or competencies that enable them to quickly establish mean-ingful relationships; work effectively as a leader, team member, and team leader; and broker health care across the care continuum. Essential qualities are shaped by age, culture, gender, language, spiritual and religious beliefs, ethnicity, and educational and socioeconomic factors. These factors must be considered when conversing with internal and external consumers to ensure verbal and nonverbal communication is appropriately and accurately transmitted and received.

Essential qualities or core competencies are the building blocks of effective communication and interpersonal relationships. Essential qualities are therapeutic use of self, genuineness, warmth, empathy, acceptance, maturity, and self-awareness (Antai-Otong, 2008). Each quality promotes respect and person-centeredness, embraces strengths and positive attributes, maintains human dignity, displays care and acceptance, and sustains healthy interpersonal relations.

Therapeutic Use of Self

Therapeutic use of self is a core quality of nursing. It engenders trust and acceptance and a willingness to share personal experiences. Sharing personal feelings helps the nurse glean insight into another person's experience. This interactive process requires active listening skills, such as attentiveness and patience, congruent verbal and nonverbal communication, and mutual respect. It allows the CNL to impart support, reassurance, and health education, and to gather important data to ensure appropriate decision making.

Genuineness

Genuineness is the second quality; it refers to honesty and authenticity and infers openness and lack of defensiveness. Genuineness and openness must be prudent, tactful, discreet, and appropriate. Genuineness is communicated verbally with comments like this, "This must be a difficult time for you. How can I assist?" Nonverbal communication occurs with a handshake; embrace, when appropriate; active listening; eye contact; and open body language, such as unfolded or uncrossed legs. It is imperative that verbal and nonverbal communication are congruent when displaying genuineness.

Warmth

Warmth is the third quality. It is often associated with empathy, patience, kindness, and concern for others. It may be expressed with a smile, handshake, or eye contact. Warmth and genuineness often occur simultaneously and are core elements of therapeutic use of self, quality interpersonal relations, high consumer confidence and satisfaction, and positive healthcare outcomes. A lack of warmth is perceived as "cold and aloof" and noncaring. It is likely to generate distrust, anger, resentment, poor treatment outcomes, and low consumer satisfaction.

Empathy

Empathy is the fourth essential quality. It is the capacity to identify with or vicariously experience another's situation, feelings, and motives without them becoming part of the self. Its usefulness lies in helping the CNL "walk a mile in someone's shoes" and understand the meaning of another's anger, sadness, joy, grief, and other strong emotions. Empathy enables the CNL to use objective approaches to evaluate and resolve highly emotionally charged situations. It is the antithesis of pity, which infers one takes on the feelings and motives of others as one's own. Pity is counterproductive because it reduces objectivity and makes it difficult to separate one's feelings from others. It often leads to "rescuing" behaviors, blurred boundaries, and inappropriate relationships.

Acceptance

Acceptance is the fifth essential quality. It refers to favorable reception, belief in or approval of others, and value of differences. The extent of acceptance arises from the individual's values, beliefs, maturity, nonjudgmental attitude or tolerance, and self-awareness. Rapid societal and demographic changes, particularly in race, age, ethnicity, gender, religious beliefs, and health practices necessitate greater value and appreciation and acceptance of diversity and different views and attitudes. Inherent to acceptance is respect and maintenance of human dignity and integrity. An example is when the CNL encounters an emotionally charged situation in which a patient, family, or colleague is shouting. Although this behavior is unacceptable, the nurse must respond in an accepting manner using assertive and calming verbal and nonverbal communication to convey concern and willingness to help, quickly assess the problem, and work with the individual to resolve it in a timely manner. For example, the nurse might say, "I understand you are pretty upset because your prescription has not been filled, but is difficult to help if you are shouting. Let me check with pharmacy to see what has happened. I will be back in a few minutes." This approach involves therapeutic use of self, genuineness, warmth and caring, and acceptance, yet it is firm and calming.

Maturity

Maturity is the sixth essential quality. Maturity extends beyond chronological age and entails the ease with which an individual forms trust and meaningful relationships; displays empathy and warmth; and utilizes sound judgment, decision making, and problem-solving skills. Essential attributes of maturity include confidence in self and others, recognition of personal strengths and vulnerabilities, assertiveness, and overall respect for self and others. Individuals who lack these mature attributes tend to blame others for their mistakes, are argumentative and defensive, fail to see positives in others, and use manipulative behaviors to meet personal and professional needs. Distrust and strong negative emotions in others are often engendered, and difficulty in forming trust and healthy interpersonal relations is commonplace.

Self-Awareness

Self-awareness is the seventh essential quality. It is governed by mature behaviors and involves acknowledging and understanding personal strengths and attributes and shortcomings and vulnerabilities. Recognizing personal strengths and areas that require improvement helps the CNL appreciate these qualities in others. It promotes an objective portrait of how one fits into society within individual, group, and organizational domains. It is imperative to understand oneself to form meaningful relationships, recognize and value personal and professional values, and negotiate with others.

A lack of self-awareness often results in defensiveness, personalization of negative or constructive feedback, and unwillingness to listen to others and negotiate differences. The likely results are poor interpersonal relations, miscommunication, low consumer satisfaction, and poor outcomes.

The complexity of working with individuals, groups, and systems requires the CNL to acquire the essential qualities aforementioned. The successful CNL promotes self through effective communication skills, maintains personal balance, establishes coalitions across the healthcare continuum, and advances the values and mission of the organization. Predictably, distrust; impatience; failure to establish meaningful relationships, display empathy, warmth, and genuineness; and immature behaviors result in hostile work relationships, conflict, exhausted resources, and poor treatment outcomes.

As the novice CNL begins to understand self and use essential qualities to work with others individually, in groups, and in organizations, personal and professional values will direct how individuals are treated, individual accountability, and the use of sound judgment and decision making based on personal integrity and ethical principles. The following section describes these concepts and the impact on the CNL role.

Professional Values

The novice CNL brings a repertoire of personal and professional values and beliefs based on innate attributes, knowledge, educational preparation, socioeconomic factors, and clinical expertise that either synchronizes or diverges with organizational expectations, values, and beliefs. Divergence in values between staff and the organization often results in conflict and miscommunication and may negatively impact the successful deployment of the CNL role.

Professional values are individual and organizational expectations and ideas that direct social and environmental responsibilities, accountability, and proficiency. These values influence decision making, cultural communication, judgment, daily routines, and practices. The principles also underlie organizational policies, mission, decision making, culture, and receptiveness to internal and external consumers and healthcare delivery (Lloyd, Wise, Weeramanthri, & Nugus, 2009). Even more importantly, successful health-promoting programs are responsive to local communities and structures, cultural values, and communication and welcome community involvement and leadership in the organization (Barnett & Kendall, 2011).

Professional values that facilitate successful transition into the CNL role include altruism, accountability, integrity, and ethical principles. Professional and personal values govern how individuals:

- Communicate
- Form interpersonal relations
- Respond to and manage conflicts
- Provide health care
- Respond to failure
- View differences in others, including ethnicity and culture
- Cope with stress
- Accept success
- Display empathy and concern for others

Altruism

Altruism is the practice or display of unselfish concern for or devotion to the welfare of others without regard to personal reward or benefits (Yalom & Leszcz, 2005). True altruism is innate and occurs as a natural part of interactions with others. It is a character trait that is easily recognized and valued by others. The foundation of altruism is openness, empathy, genuineness, and sensitivity to the needs of others (Watson, 1988).

Accountability

Accountability and responsibility are interrelated. Responsible people account for what they do and how they perform. Effectively working with others or individually, and completion of tasks that achieve expected outcomes are common. Accountability and responsibility generate trust when a person commits to achieving the expected outcome. Trust is built on predictable behavior associated with keeping promises and being accountable, even when expectations are not achieved. Being accountable is a reliable way to build and sustain organizational trust and a crucial leadership skill. Leadership skills are discussed later in this chapter.

Integrity

Integrity, similar to other professional values, is a critical component of accountability and altruism that guides ethical decision making. It infers that an individual consistently maintains and exhibits high character (i.e., follows societal and cultural norms, expectations, and professional standards). Strong integrity is directed by ethical principles and moral character. It also fosters trust, respect, personal confidence, and self-esteem.

Ethical Principles

Ethical principles and integrity are interrelated and comprise a moral framework in which the CNL directs practice. From a professional perspective, this includes a code of ethics outlining how to act in accordance with the highest standards and mission of the profession, conscience, and the organization. Principles of professional practice include integrity, honesty, truthfulness, and adherence to obligation to safeguard public trust. Ethical principles also include developing and maintaining professional knowledge and competencies to ensure performance and demonstrate concerns about the well-being of others, adhering to all applicable federal, state, and local laws and regulations; cultivating and valuing cultural diversity and pluralistic values; and treating all people with dignity and respect.

As the CNL role is deployed, costs must be justified by healthcare organizations. The novice CNL must seek employment prepared to lead with a vision guided by essential qualities, proficient communication skills, professional values, and a willingness to learn. Understanding of the mission, values, and expectations of the organization is essential and must be demonstrated by results of external surveys, such as The Joint Commission, care delivery models, safety history, clinical outcomes, and consumer and staff satisfaction. The CNL must secure early wins and establish coalitions that produce organizational adjustments to environmental and political demands (Watkins, 2003). Most successful organizations value leadership as an asset and a sustainable competitive advantage. This advantage opens the door for the CNL, a natural leader, to be developed as a future leader. The following section discusses how the beginning CNL can move from a novice to expert leader.

Building Leadership Skills

Leadership is an integral part of nursing. The CNL has an advantage over some nurses because leadership in this role is expected and encouraged. High-performing leaders make an impact on the success of the organization. High-performing leaders are expert communicators, coalition builders, culturally sensitive, and proficient in technological advances. The transition from novice to expert leader occurs over time and facilitates leadership development.

The evolution of expert leadership skills requires confidence, a vision, and belief in self as a leader and contributor to the organization's values and mission. Normally, initial leadership roles generate tremendous anxiety and uncertainty. The CNL must employ effective communication and critical thinking skills, celebrate early successes, and nurture personal attributes to manage anxiety, uncertainties, and fears through constructive appraisal of self and others. High-functioning leaders use these building blocks to motivate individuals, groups, and systems toward a common goal. A positive, realistic, and confident attitude coupled with core competencies in management and leadership predicts success. Core competencies include organizational trust, communication, problem solving and decision making, cultural sensitivity, and coalition building.

Organizational Trust

Organizational trust is earned based on proven accountability, credibility, personal integrity, effective communication skills, the ability to work with others, and the ability to implement strategies with positive results. Trust is the heart of healthy relationships and effective communication. Trust is not immediately granted to the beginning CNL. According to Barker (1992), organizational trust is not inherent and must be earned and nurtured through all encounters and situations. Organizational trust is rooted in role theory.

Role theory posits that members of the organization assume responsibilities and roles within the system (Biddle, 1986). Role expectations of a leader vary from specific (such as an organization in which the leader defines personal style) to broader perspectives (for example, where roles are determined by organizational expectations held both by the individual and by other people). The novice CNL must understand roles and expectations within organizations, including goals, actions, and outcomes, as well as performance and proficiency. This is necessary in given situations or encounters. Trust arises from predictable behaviors based on actual or expected role performance. A substantial proportion of organizational trust is nurtured through observable, daily social interactions of individuals carrying out roles.

Building trust involves an array of basic principles and behaviors. The CNL must exhibit confidence and patience, employ effective communication skills, and validate expected technical proficiency as part of role development. Technical proficiency skills, such as data management and computer literacy, are critical competencies for the CNL. In addition, the CNL must:

- Demonstrate knowledge and clinical competency about the subject matter
- Ask appropriate questions and seek advice from mentor(s)
- Keep promises, establish realistic and measurable outcomes, and meet deadlines
- Seek to understand others' positions
- Employ assertive communication skills
- Exhibit consistency and reliability
- Express genuine interest and enthusiasm about the subject matter
- Accept others' feelings and ideas (this does not mean agreeing)
- Encourage active participation in decision making
- Provide ongoing feedback using an assertive and constructive approach
- Recognize and celebrate strengths and successes
- Recognize vulnerabilities
- Be accountable for failures and vulnerabilities and learn from these experiences
- Effectively manage crucial conversations to communicate and build relationships

Crucial conversations refer to spontaneous or unplanned interactions created by strong emotions, opposing opinions, and high stakes situations (Patterson, Grenny, McMillan, & Switzler, 2011). During crucial conversations, the CNL often feels vulnerable and unprepared to respond appropriately. Effective management of crucial conversations depends on the nature of the situation and preparation prior to the encounter. Examples of crucial conversations include speaking to a colleague who smells of alcohol or confronting a team member who consistently fails to complete an assignment or dealing with an in-law who continuously interferes with child rearing. Professional responses to these situations often parallel responses to personal situations.

Patterson and colleagues assert that what really matters during these interactions is the ability to speak openly and candidly about difficult or emotionally "charged issues," getting things done and at the same time forming and maintaining meaningful relationships. Perfecting this communication skill requires practice and expertise in one's personal and professional life. Assertive communication is the basis of this approach, which generally requires recognition and effectively managing physiological stress responses through deep breathing or other stress reduction exercises and maintaining cognitive or intellectual responses to highly charged situations. Such an approach enables the CNL to speak and express views persuasively while mitigating defensiveness and anger in others (Patterson et al., 2011).

Every encounter and situation, whether positive or negative, is an opportunity to learn and grow. Growth occurs with time and is based on understanding the roles and expectations of nurse leaders. Growing evidence implicates strong leadership skills are necessary to work effectively with others, advance the mission and values of the organization, and facilitate positive outcomes. A great example of this concept is crucial conversations.

Early successes require the CNL to identify and resolve organizational barriers inherent in roles and implementation of evidence-based practice. Important barriers include a lack of time, inadequate resources, a lack of nursing autonomy and empowerment, and cultural factors. Growing evidence demonstrates significant correlations between these barriers and practice, knowledge, and attitudes associated with evidence-based practice. Solutions to overcome these barriers include learning opportunities, mentoring, culture and relationship building, and cost-effective outcomes (Hauck, Winsett, & Kuric, 2012; Melnyk, Fineout-Overholt, Gallagher-Ford, & Kaplan, 2012).

A qualitative study that focused primarily on performance of the nurse consultant's role in relation to transformational leadership theory concluded that participants ($n = 4$) lacked considerable technical competencies, cognitive and interpersonal skills, and risk taking (McIntosh & Tolson, 2009). As a result of early findings from the study, leadership implemented several approaches to facilitate transformational leadership skills and processes, including developing a vision for designated services, acting as mentors and champions, and using assertive communication and interpersonal skills to advance complex change initiatives. Emphasis was placed on organizational support and educational opportunities to develop effective communication and interpersonal skills that facilitated role development and competencies to attain outcomes (McIntosh & Tolson, 2009).

Organizational trust is also guided by the unique contributions of the CNL, particularly leading research-driven activities and practice. Integration of research into clinical nursing practice is pivotal to the delivery of high-quality health care (Cummings, Hutchinson, Scott, Norton, & Estabrooks, 2012; Kajermo et al., 2008). The CNL must incorporate research findings into practice. To do so, the CNL must make practice more research transparent, providing necessary leadership, enlisting staff participation at all levels within the organization, establishing a research agenda, and implementing evidenced-based practice to improve outcomes. Although the CNL, along with other staff, is sometimes not provided ample time to lead research-driven research activities and may lack the motivation to review studies and apply findings to practice, it is critical to consider these initiatives to promote organizational trust and improve outcomes (Chummun & Tiran, 2008). Conclusions from the transformational leadership study indicate that successful organizational trust requires effective communication and interpersonal skills, confidence and patience, and clinical competencies to lead and participate in complex situations and encounters.

High-performing leaders clearly understand the significance of purpose, vision, and alignment to revitalizing an organization. Leaders must discern what drives organizational success and expectations. What are an organization's expectations about health care, internal and external consumers, quality, and safety? Are providers expected to develop and implement evidence-based interventions and clinical outcomes? What healthcare models are in place to address and manage complex patient problems and ensure appropriate monitoring, tracking, and trending of quality improvement activities? Does the organization embrace evidence-based practice? If not, why? By answering these questions the CNL can generate ideas and develop a niche within the organization that is consistent with its mission, values, and expectations. How can this knowledge guide the CNL to lead an initiative that facilitates implementation of evidence-based practice? How can leadership skills be used to initiate this practice on one unit, additional units, and ultimately the entire organization? Successful implementation of the team and later positive outcomes demonstrate how the CNL can create opportunities to lead activities by engaging others through coalition building and establish positive outcomes.

High-performing leaders are astute and proficient communicators who advance the mission and values of their organization and develop personal and professional goals. Clearly organizational trust is built on and driven by effective communication. The next section focuses on major principles of effective communication.

Communication

Communication is fundamental in daily life and occurs within vast encounters and situations. It is the transmission of feelings, attitudes, ideas, and behaviors between persons. It is complex and involves numerous components, including verbal and nonverbal communication, active listening, assertiveness, conflict management, and communication issues unique to individuals and situations.

Maxwell (1999) described four essential qualities of effective communicators:

1. Keep it simple/convey a clear and simple message—communication extends beyond what is said and includes how a message is delivered. Keeping it simple helps one connect with others.
2. See the whole person—convey respect and belief in others. Use active listening skills.
3. Demonstrate credibility/show the truth—display confidence and belief in what is said.
4. Seek a response/clarification that the correct message is communicated. The goal of communication is action—give the recipient something to feel, think, remember, and do, and motivate others.

In today's rapidly changing world, communication is likely to be transmitted via technology rather than face to face. More and more people are communicating through social media, such as Facebook, Twitter, blogs, smartphones, text messages, email, and telephonic or video conferencing. Also, more and more consumers are receiving care through telehealth and other electronic devices including the Internet, cell phones, and virtual support groups where consumers with chronic illnesses network through informational chat rooms and blogs (Kaufman & Woodley, 2011). Regardless of the venue, communication occurs at many levels and requires skills that facilitate healthy work relationships, impart information, convey respect, and address consumer and organizational needs. An inconsiderate message or response to an email may be more damaging to a relationship than simply picking up the phone to call after abating one's anger or frustration. Technology takes away the human component of feelings, warmth, and eye contact and leaves the sender and recipient to decipher words rather than verbal and nonverbal cues. In contrast, face-to-face interactions provide a forum for body language and verbal communication to convey a message and clarify misinterpreted nonverbal cues. Verbal and non-verbal communication based on mutual understanding and respect is necessary if the CNL expects to support individuals, families, colleagues, and organizations.

Intrinsically, nurses are confronted with the daily challenge of deciphering verbal and nonverbal messages regarding the responses of others. Effective com-munication enables the CNL to realize the complexity of human interactions and form meaningful relationships with others. Whether interacting with the patient or family at the bedside or within a group of colleagues or presenting data to senior leadership, the CNL must command effective communication skills and use verbal and nonverbal cues to convey clear messages and respond to others appropriately. Both qualitative and quantitative studies have presented evidence of the bene-fits of effective communication, particularly in critical care settings (Engström & Söderberg, 2010; Papastavrou, Efstathiou, & Charalambous, 2011).

Communication styles are influenced by individual differences, which include developmental stage, gender, socioeconomic status, sexual orientation, values, reli-gion, spiritual beliefs, health practices, psychosocial factors, culture, ethnicity, and language. Changing societal demographics play a critical role in how messages are communicated and deciphered. These changes require nurse leaders to recognize personal attributes, beliefs, and values, and differences in others when communi-cating. A common communication error is failure to listen and trying to read others' minds or expecting them to read ours. In order for others to respond to our needs and ideas we must clearly communicate what they are and convey them in a manner that others understand and can respond to appropriately (see **Table 6-1**).

Body language or nonverbal communication, such as tone of voice, sweat on the brow or palms, dress, hygiene, facial expression, posture, and gait can also be mis-interpreted. Nonverbal communication must be clarified when in doubt to ensure accurate interpretation of a sender's message. Verbal and nonverbal messages must be congruent. For instance, if a person's voice tone is loud and his or her speech is rapid, receivers may conclude the speaker is anxious or angry. If one is confronted about anger, it is imperative to assess how messages are being conveyed rather than being defensive. The more congruent nonverbal cues are with verbal, the clearer the message. This is particularly important when communicating highly charged, con-troversial, or important results, issues, or requests.

Table 6-1 Giving Feedback and Receiving Feedback

- Clearly state your intentions
- Emphasize the positive
- Be specific
- Focus on the behavior rather than the person
- Refer to behavior that can be changed
- Be descriptive rather than evaluative
- Use "I" statements instead of "you" statements to reduce defensiveness
- Avoid using generalizations such as "always" or "never"
- Avoid giving advice

Verbal communication involves an exchange of words, both spoken and written, between people. A sender of a message cannot assume what is spoken and/or written is understood by the recipient of the message. It is imperative to look for verbal and nonverbal cues that ensure the correct message is heard and understood.

Verbal communication requires:

- An unhurried and confident approach
- Knowledge and preparation of subject matter
- Good eye contact
- Affording personal space
- Assertive posture (ample distance between self and others)
- Simple, clear explanations based on education, developmental stage, gender, culture, ethnicity, and cognitive function
- Active listening skills (Antai-Otong, 2008)

Active listening is interactive and requires full attention, notably suspending multitasking or other activities; appropriate verbal and nonverbal cues such as nods, moving forward, and appropriate responses. Body language or nonverbal communication defines whether the recipient is actively listening. Listeners must allow the person speaking to complete sentences and train of thought without interruptions. This is critical to fully hearing others' points of view, processing information, and being respectful. An effective listener concentrates and mentally summarizes content (sender's main points); listens for themes or a central point; and analyzes the evidence, integrates it into the communication process, and responds accordingly. Evidence that the message is clearly understood can be conveyed by paraphrasing, restating the central idea, or by asking a question that conveys understanding of the main idea. These techniques are excellent methods to check or validate assumptions about nonverbal and verbal communication. An easy way to remember relevant or salient points of exchange of a message is to recollect an encounter or situation in which you felt at ease, comfortable, and heard, and conveyed feelings, thoughts, and things that concerned you. What put you at ease—the person and/or environment?

Projecting these qualities results in effective communication:

- Use of self
- Genuineness
- Warmth and acceptance
- Shared values
- Assurance of your ability to solve your problem

Consider these factors during your next encounter. Self-awareness is critical to how individuals listen and communicate with others. Active listening is the heart of effective communication. The active listener is reflective, empathetic, and nonjudgmental and avoids blurring issues with guilt or put-down statements.

A poor listener is inattentive, lacks warmth or "connectedness" with the sender, and uses encounters and situations to advance personal agendas or values. Poor listening skills cause miscommunication. Miscommunication results from incongruent verbal and nonverbal cues, failure to use active listening skills, and a lack of interest in the encounter or situation. It is costly, nonproductive, and reduces productivity and consumer satisfaction. Miscommunication is also associated with passive and aggressive communication skills. In contract, effective leaders use assertive communication skills.

Assertive communication is based on the premise that everyone has a right to meet needs, believe in oneself, and express feelings, thoughts, and ideas with mutual respect for others. Assertiveness is learned, and it is difficult for some people. High self-esteem and self-worth, self-awareness, and confidence are the matrix of assertiveness. It is not the message that equates assertiveness, even though words must be carefully crafted; it is also nonverbal communication and congruence with verbal communication that constitutes this communication skill.

Stress impacts how messages are received and heard. Normally, high emotional states or stressful situations interfere with what listeners hear and interpret from the sender. Reduced attention is linked to stress, high anxiety, and tension. It is critical that individuals control their anxiety or stress by using deep breathing exercises to reduce heart rate and respirations, thus reducing stress reactions. Thoughts are clearer and more focused when anxiety levels decrease. A failure to manage stress reactions results in ineffective verbal and nonverbal communication manifested by yelling, sharp or curt responses, and an inability to convey messages in a clear and respectful manner. Yelling, shouting, and angry responses often produce the same negative response in others. Major benefits of assertive communication are:

- Enhances self-esteem and confidence
- Facilitates respect
- Reduces stress and anxiety
- Promotes overall health
- Allows one to say "no" without guilt
- Helps parties state ideas, thoughts, and feelings more clearly
- Allows expression of feelings, thoughts, and ideas without the intent of provoking others
- Engenders open and honest communication and mutual respect
- Promotes win-win outcomes, as detailed in **Table 6-2**

All in all, communication is an integral part of our lives. Its effectiveness is multifaceted and guided by mutual respect between parties, assertiveness skills, verbal and nonverbal communication, cultural factors, self-awareness, confidence, and

Table 6-2 Assertive Communication Techniques

- Control anger and strong emotions through deep breathing exercises or other stress reduction measures
- Use a firm yet friendly confident tone of voice
- Use nonthreatening body language, including eye contact (consider cultural factors and appropriate distance—usually leg's length)
- Use "I" statements
- Be specific
- State what you mean, for example:
  - ▲ "I am concerned that every time we are in a staff meeting you ignore me when I ask a question."
  - ▲ "When you ignore me I feel angry and insulted."
  - ▲ "In the future, when I ask a question I would appreciate it if you respond or answer my questions."
- Own your feelings, thoughts, and ideas (use "I" statements)
- Use active listening skills
- Allow the other person to complete sentences or thoughts
- Display respect

self-esteem. It promotes quality and healthy interpersonal relationships that are rich, genuine, honest, and open. Effective communication skills require constant fine tuning to ensure ideas and thoughts are conveyed in a respectful and clear manner, advancing health care using problem-solving and decision-making skills that produce positive outcomes (see **Table 6-3**).

Problem Solving and Decision Making

Much of what clinical nurse leaders do involves problem solving and decision making, as defined by professional and personal values, the organization, and consumers. It is imperative to involve the right people in the planning and implementation of problem solving. A natural reaction to problems is to respond quickly.

Table 6-3   Comparison of Assertive, Passive, and Aggressive Communication Styles

Assertive	Passive	Aggressive
Confident, displays self-respect, goal oriented	Puts others' needs above own	Puts personal needs over others with intent to intimidate, manipulate, demean, and threaten
Active listening	Low self-esteem	
A choice	Uses demeaning body language	Manipulative
Open and honest	Low voice tone	Angry
Direct	Lacks confidence	Vengeful
Trust	Helplessness	Distrustful
Focus on unacceptable behavior and not the person	Distrust	Focus on other (blame)
	Angry at self and others	Defensive and resentful
Based on mutual respect and meeting personal needs without compromising others' needs	Afraid to hurt others' feelings	Loud and threatening body language, intrusive
	Anxious demeanor	Righteous, derogatory
Requires congruent body language, such as normal voice tone, eye contact, appropriate distance	Poor eye contact	Win-lose position (win at all costs and at the expense of others)
	Lack of self-respect	
	Guilt-driven decision making	
Win-win positions	Lose-win positions	

However, some problems are not easily solved and require additional time and resources. Several guidelines can facilitate a thoughtful problem-solving process:

1. Define the problem with input from internal and external consumers, major stakeholders, and leadership. Evaluate complex problems and avoid being overwhelmed or intimidated by closely scrutinizing the real problem.
2. Evaluate underlying causes of the problem and seek opinions or input from others. This may occur within various venues using diverse approaches, including brainstorming and prioritizing the problems.
3. Explore options based on priorities, required resources, input from others, and timelines.
4. Determine an approach.
5. Develop a plan of action:
   a. Measurable, realistic, and attainable goals
   b. Strategies or activities
   c. Objectives
   d. Responsible person(s)
   e. Resources/budget
6. Implement the plan.
7. Monitor progress based on identified problems, resources, responsible persons, and timelines for completion.

Problem solving and decision making occur at all levels within an organization. The CNL plays an instrumental role in obtaining input from key team members, internal and external consumers, and other stakeholders to ensure relevant information and resources are used to implement action plans, trend and track data and outcomes, and resolve problems.

Cultural Sensitivity

Cultural sensitivity is a leadership quality that is an integral part of all encounters and situations. It influences organizational trust, communication, and problem solving. The complexity of cultural sensitivity requires a lengthier discussion than this chapter allows; a general overview is given here.

Multiple considerations are used to guide implementation, such as race, ethnicity, gender, age, religion, health practices, culture, language, sexual orientation, socioeconomic status, educational preparation, and country and region of origin. No approach fits all encounters or situations. Cultural sensitivity infers individualized approaches that ensure respect, acceptance, tolerance, and avoidance of humiliation and exploitation. Cultural sensitivity is consistent with individual wishes, strengths, abilities, preferences, beliefs, and values. Person-centered approaches are inherent to healthy interpersonal relationships and must be considered within social contexts and treatment planning for both patients and providers.

Coalition Building: An Essential Competency for the CNL

Consensus is emerging that integrated delivery systems provide strong support to care coordination teams and offer opportunities for improving quality of care and reducing costs (Scheetz, Bolon, Postelnick, Noskin, & Lee, 2009). Effective teams are based on effective communication and team-building skills, membership, and group dynamics.

Team collaboration involves developmental stages and processes that improve mutual performance. Similar to interpersonal relations, collaboration evolves over time and requires certain people and resources to facilitate organizational changes and outcomes. The effectiveness and efficiency of team collaboration is determined by the purpose of the team, team member composition, and participation. The role of the CNL in team formation ranges from informal to formal and is based on individual and organizational needs. Research indicates that collaborative teams provide an invaluable contribution to an organization (Palmer, Bycroft, Healey, Field, & Ghafel, 2012; Schoen et al., 2012). The efficiency and effectiveness of teams can be bolstered by the implementation of lean thinking or systems redesign methodologies (Zokaei et al., 2010).

Lean six sigma is often referred to as "lean thinking." Lean principles are largely recognized and have vast applicability, and increasingly organizations are implementing these models to develop efficient processes to reduce silos and fragmentation of services, improve access and consumer satisfaction, expand flow and speed, and effectively respond to dwindling healthcare resources. Successful implementation of lean six sigma requires executive leadership endorsement and investment that begins with training, planning, and selection of the right team members at all levels of the organization.

The following discussion focuses on the major principles of lean six sigma and research studies that demonstrate the effectiveness of team collaboration in the implementation of these principles. George, Rowlands, and Kastle (2004) described the four keys to lean six sigma as follows:

1. Increase consumer satisfaction by improving quality and speed.
2. Improve processes that eliminate waste, fragmentation, and variation and improve flow.
3. Promote team collaboration that engenders communication and sharing of ideas.
4. Ensure all decisions are data driven.

Growing evidence indicates the positive impact of lean six sigma methodologies on the efficiency of patient flow processes and increased access within clinical areas, such as primary care and the emergency department. Furthermore, studies have demonstrated that collaborative teams coalesce and identify waste, opportunities to improve efficiency, and clinical outcomes through lean thinking methodologies (Palmer et al., 2012; Schoen et al., 2012; Scott et al., 2011). One study examined several areas of concern including quality issues identified using a patient journey across the healthcare continuum (Scott et al., 2011). Throughout the patient's journey, team collaboration was used at various points on the healthcare continuum to identify problems, solutions, and evaluate processes using quality improvement cycles (e.g., plan-do-study-act). Information from these data, both successes and areas of improvement, were regularly communicated with all teams.

As an active member of collaborative teams, the CNL is poised to collaborate with various members of healthcare teams to eliminate waste, increase customer satisfaction, remove silos, and add value to collaborative teams. The end-point goal is to redesign healthcare systems and sustain them over time. Strategies to establish and maintain team collaboration fall into four domains:

1. Personal competencies—develop individual competencies; establish and understand shared processes
2. Interpersonal skills—improve group dynamics; engender common purpose and commitment
3. Organizational structure—resolve barriers between various services within the organization (e.g., turf issues)
4. Organizational environment—build a team with distinguishing characteristics within the larger organization

Successful team collaboration requires four essential qualities: trust, open and effective communication, member involvement, and clearly defined measurable goals/outcomes (Antai-Otong, 1997). Effective teams require appropriate member selection based on a willingness to participate, confidence, proven history of following through on previous committees or teams, and command of effective communication skills. The CNL must be competent to lead and participate as a team member and model these behaviors in various situations and encounters.

An important feature of successful team building is membership involvement. Member involvement is a sense of commitment to the team, respect for team members, and enthusiasm for understanding team dynamics. Involved members value diversity, genuineness and open-mindedness; they display empathy and are emotionally invested in the team and goal attainment. Team members feel linked to the larger system and are willing to collaborate and negotiate with others. Although they value their own role and contributions to the team, they perceive themselves as part of the whole, with the intent to reach common goals (Antai-Otong, 1997).

A team is a group that works towards a single, common goal even when the members have diverse individual goals. Teams can be informal or formal and include members from various parts of the healthcare system. Interdisciplinary teams and care planning are commonly found in specialty areas and are required to meet The Joint Commission and other national standards involving healthcare issues. These teams often include various disciplines, patients, families and/or significant others, and other stakeholders (Meltzer et al., 2009).

On the whole, team members possess vast technical skills and clinical expertise and are encouraged to develop new skills that foster versatility and adaptability and add value to the overall team. Team members are responsible for monitoring, trending, and tracking the overall process of goal attainment, along with delegating problem-solving tasks to members. Successful teams foster trust, creativity, and risk taking, creating an environment in which members listen to and share their thoughts and feelings without being reprimanded (Pype et al., 2012). Despite individual goals, those goals advance the higher collective one. For example, one Joint Commission team may track and trend tracers while another might conduct tracers, and another might participate on the Quality Executive Council. Yet all are accountable for preparation for a successful Joint Commission survey. Growing empirical data indicate that positive clinical outcomes are associated with self-directed teams. In a time of reduced resources, complex healthcare issues, and emphasis on positive clinical outcomes, teams provide a cost-effective approach to advancing implementation rates of proven safety outcomes (Palmer et al., 2012; Schoen et al., 2012; Scott et al., 2011).

Team Selection

The success of team and coalition building rests on the selection process. Coalition and team building involve using existing supporting relationships and establishing new relationships with key players, aligning with persons in positions of power, and mobilizing resources. The novice CNL must assess where power lies in the organization and align with persons in positions of power. The novice CNL must then observe how these individuals conduct meetings, respond to differences, and manage and control resources. Equally important is identification of mentors or individuals who are supportive, resourceful, and know how to navigate power and influence within the organization. Influential people in the organization are critical resources for the CNL and provide the following:

- Expertise—knowledge, experience, competencies
- Access to information—information technology; computers, software
- Status—level of power and influence in the organization
- Control—budgets, resources, and finances
- Loyalty—trustworthy, reliable, and supportive (Watkins, 2003)

Watkins (2003) described the following principles of coalition building:

- *Map the influence landscape.* A common mistake among new leaders is spending excessive time during transition within the vertical dimension (e.g., supervisor, senior leadership) of influence rather than the horizontal dimension (e.g., colleagues, peers). The most basic relationships must occur within horizontal dimensions among colleagues, interdisciplinary groups, and consumers. These relationships are more likely to yield early successes and build the infrastructure for vertical areas in the organization.
- *Identify key players.* Team composition is critical to effective problem identification, decision making, planning, and outcomes. Involving internal and external team members, consumers, and stakeholders must occur during early coalition building. Considerations for member selection should be guided by individual strengths, education, and expertise in a given area and should support professional and organizational values. Ground rules about behaviors, accountability, responsibility, and interpersonal and communication skills reduce normal time required to create and sustain group cohesiveness. Group cohesiveness is widely researched and a basic component of groups. It generates a sense of "we-ness," common values, and greater

solidarity, and it protects against internal and external threats and provides mutual support (Yalom & Leszcz, 2005).

Supporters share a vision for the future and common values and have mutual respect for professional and organizational goals. They are change agents with demonstrated effective interpersonal skills and team-oriented results. Normally opponents object no matter what; they resist changes and reject the proposed vision for the future. They perceive team goals as a threat to their influence or power, values, and goals. Oftentimes they are the informal leaders who exert power at the grassroots or unit level. Engaging opponents in the coalition-building process is critical to garnering buy-in through healthy interpersonal interactions, which minimizes energy used to address push back and resistance.

- *Use tools of persuasion.* The tools are generally effective communication skills, especially assertiveness and influential alliances within the organization (Watkins, 2003). It is imperative to use these tools to open doors, such as getting an agenda on various committees, garnering influence, and increasing visibility and credibility across the healthcare continuum. As the CNL navigates within various aspects of the healthcare continuum, it is imperative to understand the principles and value of group dynamics.

Group Dynamics

A common mistake made by the beginning CNL as team member or leader is delay in reaching expected outcomes within designated time lines due to poor planning, unrealistic goals, inappropriate membership, inadequate resources and organizational support, and lack of knowledge about group dynamics. To mitigate these mistakes, it is important to assess the organizational alignment with the team and use this to guide decision making, planning, and implementation. Strategies to achieve these goals can be created using the following questions:

1. What is the team's alignment with organizational values, goals, and outcomes?
2. What decisions are required to ensure that team goals, implementation, time lines, and outcomes are consistent with the organization's goals, mission, and values?
3. What is the game plan to meet mutual goals?
4. How do we implement or deploy the plan across the health continuum?

Answering these questions can assist in determining if the team is headed in the right direction or if it should revamp its course and focus. The novice CNL is most likely to lead or be a member of a unit-based or service group. Knowledge of how the organization uses teams to advance its mission, values, and goals is necessary.

Coalition or team building requires effective communication, interpersonal skills, and knowledge of group dynamics. Successful groups will be judged by outcomes and their impact on organizational efficiency, effectiveness, customer satisfaction, and cost savings.

Group dynamics is the interactive behaviors of individuals within the context of a group. Like other important interpersonal relations, group dynamics involve individuals and the group as a whole. Group cohesiveness evolves over time and is based on various issues previously discussed. Group dynamics extend beyond people meeting, during which time they agree or disagree and come to consensus about the purpose of the team, goal and outcome identification, time lines, and membership.

Empirical data on group development reveal an array of theories about group processes. Growing evidence also indicates that survival of groups is based on a natural process in which they go through various phases or stages. For example, most people want to know something about team members, form some degree of interdependence to achieve team and personal goals, and effectively manage conflict.

The most frequently cited model of the developmental process is that of Bruce W. Tuckman (1965). Tuckman's model and group stages are:

- Forming—orientation stage in which members define interpersonal boundaries and task behaviors.
- Storming—resistance to group influence and task requirements occurs and is characterized by interpersonal conflicts.
- Norming—resistance abates and group cohesiveness occurs, new expectations emerge, and new roles are accepted. Members feel free and comfortable sharing personal opinions, thoughts, and ideas.
- Performing—members become productive and work for the common good of the group. Interpersonal relations drive activities and results (Tuckman, 1965).
- Adjourning—dissolution stage; refers to termination of roles and the completion of tasks. The group has successfully attained its goals (Tuckman & Jensen, 1977)

This synopsis of Tuckman's (1965) model is helpful in understanding the normalcy of group dynamics and moving the team from the honeymoon period (forming) through storming, norming, and performing stages in which the group cohesiveness and outcomes emerge, respectively, and the adjourning stage in which the group terminates after it completes its purpose.

Developmental stages within organizations and interdisciplinary care coordination teams are useful in advancing the mission of the organization and health care. Group or team decision making involving tasks and strategies can be addressed by health promotion planning, education, policy development, and organizational support.

Conflict Management

Conflict occurs when two or more values, beliefs, and opinions are incongruous and reconciliation of differences has not occurred. Conflict frequently arises from stressful and emotional encounters or situations associated with diverse causes, such as culture, gender, religion, age, health practices, health, socioeconomic status, and education. Regardless of the cause of conflicts, they are a natural part of all relationships. Furthermore, they are necessary for health, personal development, and organizational growth. Resistance to change in healthcare systems is often led by individuals who are satisfied with the status quo and threatened by change, new ideas, and people. Societal and demographic changes increase the propensity for conflicts and opportunities to learn about others.

Predictably, unresolved conflict reduces productivity; it is costly, lowers morale and self-esteem, increases apathy, and often results in violence or other inappropriate responses. Avoidance of conflict management is shown in passive behaviors, ineffective communication skills, apathy, and an attitude of pretending it does not exist or is not worth resolving (see Tables 6-2 and 6-3).

Management of Healthcare Environments

The final discussion centers on the management of healthcare environments through delegation, supervision, and interdisciplinary coordination of care. Management of care has been discussed extensively in previous sections of this chapter, including the topics of leadership skills, effective communication, professional values, group dynamics, and conflict management. Specific issues that impact the new CNL within the organization vary and depend upon educational preparation, clinical expertise, and leadership skills.

Organizational management requires looking at the "big picture" and intricacies that evolve from within and outside the healthcare system. It also offers the CNL a chance to work within healthcare systems to explore strategies to better understand and discover new approaches to improve communication processes and advance strength-based practices. One such approach is appreciative inquiry (AI).

Cooperrider and Whitney (2005) describe AI as a constructive and person-affirming process that incorporates a "4-D" cycle—discovery, dream, design, and destiny. AI centers principally on human relatedness and relationships to distinguish the best in each other and the overall organization. Based on these principles, positive organizational change is most likely to occur when it engenders a strength-based culture that allows for identifying problems; analyzing successes; describing what currently works well; exploring possibilities; determining types of systems, processes, and strategies needed to make changes; and implementing and sustaining the dream (Cooperrider & Whitney, 2005). Advancing these principles must occur at all tiers within the organization, including unit and service levels.

The successful deployment of the CNL role is often contingent on bringing a "fresh set of eyes," competencies, and operating from a strength-based approach to staff at the unit and leadership level. These positive interactions enable the astute CNL to develop alliances at these levels to glean knowledge about basic standard operations and expectations within the role. For example, the CNL who chooses to work primarily as an administrator must have expert clinical skills to understand the daily issues of taking care of patients and working with interdisciplinary teams. In the case of a CNL with an advanced practice background in mental health, the clinical and administrative components of the role are likely to help him or her form effective relationships and lead interdisciplinary groups at the unit level, in specialty units, and organizationally.

In the case of an advanced practice nurse with a critical care background, the CNL can also integrate these competencies and work with staff at all levels within the organization. For instance, a new critical care nurse who has difficulty managing her time and completing assignments in a timely manner has been placed on a performance improvement plan. The CNL can use her expertise in critical care nursing and administration to work with this nurse to discern areas to improve while giving her assignments as a team member to explore ways to enhance her time management and clinical skills to meet the terms of the performance improvement plan. Administratively, the CNL can also work with the nurse manager to help identify her strengths and ways to strengthen her leadership skills to ensure a proactive response to staff who are not performing as expected.

Frequently, the integration of clinical and administrative responsibilities requires the CNL to supervise others, as mentioned with the nurse manager in critical care; the CNL delegates responsibilities and duties and facilitates interdisciplinary care coordination. Delegation is widely used in nursing. Delegation refers to the assignment of authority and responsibility to another person, usually a peer or subordinate, to perform specific activities. The individual who delegates is still accountable and responsible for the outcome of the delegated assignment. The decision to delegate infers that the person assigned to a specific task is competent to perform it. If it is a technical assignment, such as performing a procedure, the CNL must observe and deem the individual competent to perform the assignment in their absence. Competence to perform delegated assignments is also the responsibility of the individual who agrees to the delegation. For instance, if the CNL is responsible for reporting critical lab values or performing waived tests, it is critical for the designated individual to demonstrate through verbal communication, written records, and observation. The same principles apply to delegated administrative assignments.

The concept of interdisciplinary team coordination has been threaded throughout this chapter in various discussions about team building, leadership skills, and communication. As the CNL moves from novice to expert, communication and essential qualities remain the building blocks for team building, positive outcomes, and meeting the needs of internal and external consumers across the healthcare continuum.

Summary

- Regardless of role or practice setting, the CNL has an opportunity to establish alliances with individuals and consumers across the healthcare continuum.
- Effective communication will unlock many doors and facilitate organizational trust.
- Communication is a complex and interactive process.
- Social media and the digital age of communication present challenges and opportunities for the CNL to create innovative communication forums.

- CNLs lead to motivate others and generate change.
- Essential qualities are the foundation of nursing.
- Active listening is a critical communication tool.
- Assertiveness is an art that requires practice and fine tuning.
- Assertive communication is mutually respectful and helps the CNL meet personal needs without disrespecting the rights of others.
- Professional values direct the manner in which we treat others, respect ourselves, and guide our practice and decision making.
- Leadership skills provide vast opportunities to deploy the CNL role across the healthcare continuum.
- Team collaboration has demonstrated success and cost effectiveness in advancing the needs of internal and external consumers and organizations.

Reflection Questions

© Arenacreative/Dreamstime.com

1. What does the organization expect about health care, internal and external consumers, quality, and safety?
2. Are providers expected to develop and implement evidence-based interventions and clinical outcomes?
3. What healthcare models are in place to address and manage complex patient problems and ensure appropriate monitoring, tracking, and trending of quality improvement activities?
4. Does the organization embrace evidence-base practice? If not, why? By answering these questions the CNL can generate ideas and develop a niche within the organization that is consistent with its mission, values, and expectations.
5. How can this knowledge guide the CNL to lead an initiative that facilitates implementation of evidence-based practice?
6. How can leadership skills be used to initiate this practice on one unit, additional units, and ultimately the entire organization?

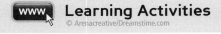 Learning Activities

© Arenacreative/Dreamstime.com

1. Select a mentor with strong leadership skills and shadow him or her during administrative or interdisciplinary group meetings.

2. Observe group dynamics in an interdisciplinary care coordination team and determine which of the developmental stages in Tuckman's model applies.
3. Attend a new employee orientation session with senior leadership; listen to their discussion about organization mission, values, and expectations from staff.
4. Shadow an advanced practice nurse in a leadership role, such as consultative liaison; observe for active communication skills among patient, family, and staff.
5. Visit a community-based clinic; shadow the administrative officer and learn how he or she monitors and tracks quality indicators. Inquire about patient satisfaction scores (review trends and action plan to address low satisfaction scores).

References

Antai-Otong, D. (1997). Team building in a healthcare setting. *American Journal of Nursing, 97*, 48–51.

Antai-Otong, D. (2008). Therapeutic communication. In D. Antai-Otong (Ed.), *Psychiatric nursing: Biological and behavioral concepts* (pp. 149–175). Albany, NY: Delmar Thomson Learning.

Barker, A. M. (1992). *Transformational nursing leadership*. New York, NY: National League for Nursing Press.

Barnett, L., & Kendall, E. (2011). Culturally appropriate methods for enhancing the participation of Aboriginal Australians in health-promoting programs. *Health Promotion Journal of Australia, 22*(1), 27–32.

Biddle, B. J. (1986). Recent development in role theory. *Annual Review of Sociology, 12*, 67–92.

Chummun, H., & Tiran, D. (2008). Increasing research evidence in practice: A possible role for the consultant nurse. *Journal of Nursing Management, 16*, 327–333.

Cooperrider, D. L., & Whitney, D. (2005). *Appreciative inquiry: A positive revolution in change*. San Francisco, CA: Berrett-Koehler Publishers, Inc.

Cummings, G. C., Hutchinson, A. M., Scott, S. D., Norton, P. G., & Estabrooks, C. A. (2012). The relationship between characteristics of context and research utilization in a pediatric setting. *Bio Med Central (BMC) Health Services Research, 10*, 168. doi: 10.1186/1472-6963-10-168

Engström, A., & Söderberg, S. (2010). Critical care nurses' experiences of follow-up visits to an ICU. *Journal of Clinical Nursing, 19*, 2925–2932.

George, M., Rowlands, D., & Kastle, B. (2004). *What is lean six sigma?* New York, NY: McGraw-Hill.

Ginory, A., Sabatier, L. M., & Eth, S. (2012). Addressing therapeutic boundaries in social networking. *Psychiatry, 27*, 40–48.

Hauck, S., Winsett, R. P., & Kuric, J. (2012). Leadership facilitation strategies to establish evidence-based practice in an acute care hospital. *Journal of Advanced Nursing, 69*(3), 664–674. doi: 10.1111/j.1365-2648.2012.06053.x. [Epub ahead of print]

Kajermo, K. N., Undén, M., Gardulf, A., Eriksson, L. E., Orton, M. L., Arnetz, B. B., & Nordström, G. (2008). Predictors of nurses' perceptions of barriers to research utilization. *Journal of Nursing Management, 16*, 305–314.

Kaufman, N. D., & Woodley, P. D. (2011). Self-management support interventions that are clinically linked and technology enabled: Can they successfully prevent and treat diabetes? *Journal of Diabetes Science and Technology, 5*, 798–803.

Lloyd, J., Wise, M., Weeramanthri, T., & Nugus, P. (2009). The influence of professional values on the implementation of Aboriginal health policy. *Journal of Health Services Research & Policy, 14*, 6–12.

Maxwell, J. C. (1999). *The 21 indispensable qualities of a leader.* Nashville, TN: Thomas Nelson, Inc.

McIntosh, J., & Tolson, D. (2009). Leadership as part of the nurse consultant role: Banging the drum for patient care. *Journal of Clinical Nursing, 18,* 219–227.

Melnyk, B. M., Fineout-Overholt, E., Gallagher-Ford, L., & Kaplan, L. (2012). The state of evidence-based practice in US nurses: Critical implications for nurse leaders and educators. *Journal of Nursing Administration, 42*, 410–417.

Meltzer, L. J., Steinmiller, E., Simms, S., Grossman, M., Complex care consultation team, & Li, Y. (2009). *Patient Education Consultants, 74,* 77–83.

Moubarak, G., Guiot, A., Benhamou, Y., Benhamou, A., & Hariri, S. (2011). Facebook activity of residents and fellows and its impact on the doctor-patient relationship. *Journal of Medical Ethics, 37,* 101–104.

Palmer, C., Bycroft, J., Healey, K., Field, A., & Ghafel, M. (2012). Can formal collaborative methodologies improve quality in primary healthcare in New Zealand? Insights from the EQUIPPED Auckland Collaborative. *Journal of Primary Healthcare, 4*, 328–336.

Papastavrou, E., Efstathiou, G., & Charalambous, A. (2011). Nurses' and patients' perceptions of caring behaviours: Quantitative systematic review of comparative studies. *Journal of Advanced Nursing, 67,* 1191–1205.

Patterson, K., Grenny, J., McMillan, R., & Switzler, A. (2011). *Crucial conversations tools for talking when stakes are high* (2nd ed.). New York, NY: McMillian.

Pype, P., Symons, L., Wens, J., Van den Eynden, B., Stess, A., Cherry, G., & Deveugele, D. (2012). Healthcare professionals' perceptions toward interprofessional collaboration in palliative home care: A view from Belgium. *Journal of Interprofessional Care.* 2012 Nov 27. [Epub ahead of print]

Scheetz, M. H., Bolon, M. K., Postelnick, M., Noskin, G. A., & Lee, T. A. (2009). Cost- effectiveness analysis of an antimicrobial stewardship team on bloodstream infections: A probabilistic analysis. *Journal of Antimicrobial Chemotherapy 63*, 816–825.

Schoen, C., Osborn, R., Squires, D., Doty, M., Rasmussen, P., Pierson, R., & Applebaum, S. (2012, November 15). A survey of primary care doctors in ten countries shows progress in use of health information technology, less in other areas. *Health Affairs (Project Hope).* [Epub ahead of print]

Scott, I. A., Wills, R. A., Coory, M., Watson, M. J., Butler, F., Waters, M., & Bowler, S. (2011). Impact of hospital-wide process redesign on clinical outcomes: A comparative study of internally versus externally led intervention. *British Medical Journal of Quality and Safety, 20,* 539–548.

Tuckman, B. W. (1965). Developmental sequence in small groups. *Psychological Bulletin, 63,* 384–399.

Tuckman, B. W., & Jensen, M. A. C. (1977). Stages of small group development revisited. *Group and Organizational Studies, 2,* 419–427.

Watkins, M. (2003). *Critical success strategies for new leaders at all levels: The first 90 days.* Boston, MA: Harvard Business School Publishing.

Watson, J. (1988). *Human science and human care, a theory of nursing.* New York, NY: National League of Nursing (originally published by Appleton & Lange).

Yalom, I. D., & Leszcz, M. (2005). *The theory and practice of group psychotherapy* (5th ed.). New York, NY: Basic Books.

Zokaei, Z., Elias, S., O'Donovan, B., Samuel, D., Evans, B., & Goodfellow, J. (2010). Lean and systems thinking in the public sector: Report for the Wales Audit Office. Wales, U.K.: Lean Enterprise Research Centre, Cardiff University. http://www.wao.gov.uk/assets/englishdocuments/Systems_Thinking_Report_eng.pdf

The Clinical Nurse Leader: Utilizing Effective Communication and Lateral Integration to Meet the Care Needs of a Dying Patient

■ Beth VanDam

Key Terms: lateral integration, coordination of care, communication, nurse/patient advocate

It was a typical morning as I stepped onto the unit as a CNL. I reviewed the unit census in an attempt to prioritize my day. Kim would be my first patient to meet as her story and plan of care were complicated and her physical condition was tenuous. Ensuring the newly assigned nurse had a clear understanding of Kim's plan of care would be essential to providing the best care. I had met Kim and her family the day before when she was admitted. I had listened carefully as she shared her journey with cancer. Kim, a 35-year-old mother of two young children, struggled with end-stage cancer, now requiring a hospital admission due to dehydration. Her request, as well as the wish of her family, was to remain a full code. She was alert and pleasant but obviously suffering with emotional distress. Physically she was extremely cachectic; unlike I had ever seen before.

As the events of the day transpired there were many opportunities as a CNL to not only impact the patient/family care experience but also provide support for the nursing staff as Kim transitioned from being extremely ill to dying. First, I facilitated continuity of care by communicating Kim's cancer story and plan of care to changing caregivers. Kim's husband and both sets of parents were present; however, due to recent traumatic experiences, there were different levels of acceptance around the reality of Kim's rapidly changing condition. At times the nursing staff was also troubled by the physician orders and focus of care as Kim remained a full code in spite of the fact that she became unresponsive and had mottling. Knowing the patient story, I was able to help connect the dots for the staff and share the plan of care along with the reasons why we were still providing some non–life-sustaining treatments. Laterally integrating the team was essential to ensure a smooth transition of care took place for the patient/family as well as point-of-care support for the nursing staff.

Coordination of care became an increasing need throughout the day. As CNL, I evaluated and involved key members of the interdisciplinary team. Palliative care was called for assistance in managing changing symptoms; a cancer resource specialist was called for psychosocial support for the family, including the two young children; and ongoing clinical support for nurses regarding when and how to verbalize changing patient needs/conditions to the physician was provided. Kim remained a full code until a few minutes before dying. She remained comfortable in her room with family close by, as well as key members of the oncology interdisciplinary team who cared for her throughout her cancer journey.

My role continued after Kim expired. It was a very emotional time, not only for the family but also for the staff. Being a resource to ensure time and emotional support for the staff was instrumental to allowing the team to grieve appropriately. Supporting and encouraging the staff to take the time to grieve enabled them to once again carry on with providing excellent care to our other patients.

Communication and Handoff in the Emergency Department

Madalyn Frank-Cooper
Winthrop University Hospital, Mineola, NY

The emergency department in our facility has a holding area for admitted patients. Because the two areas are within one department, the handoff between staff tended to be informal and inconsistent, which frequently has resulted in delays or omitted doses of medication. We asked the staff to identify flaws with the handoff process, with the goal of providing standardization and decreasing chances of error. We created a template for a report, which gave the nurses a regular reporting format. It also provided accountability for the report, as signatures were required. The challenge was not to teach staff how to give an accurate report, but to change the culture to become consistent in providing specific information during a handoff. Implementing a new tool and the expectation of staff compliance was a challenge, but the new procedure was incorporated into daily practice in conjunction with direct observation and positive reinforcement.

In the preimplementation period, 13 reports regarding medication/fluid error were reviewed. Of those reported, 7 were due to communication issues. In the postimplementation period, 10 reports were reviewed. Of those reported, 4 were due to communication issues. Not only was there a slight decrease in errors secondary to communication, there was also a slight decrease in total reported occurrences.

Collaboration of a Clinical Nurse Leader and Clinical Nurse Specialist

Mary Harnish

A hospital system seeking to improve the care of patients with diabetes facilitated the collaborative work of its CNL for diabetes and its clinical nurse specialist (CNS) for medicine, diabetes, and renal service line. The CNL and CNS roles complemented and enhanced one another through the joint efforts to implement evidence-based practice to improve efficiency and patient safety. Both the CNL and CNS were integral members of a hospital-wide diabetes operations team.

The CNL and CNS joined forces to attain The Joint Commission accreditation for advanced in-patient diabetes care for the hospital. The CNS performed a gap analysis to determine the current state prior to beginning the process of accreditation. The CNL, also a certified diabetes educator, utilized her knowledge and expertise of diabetes while simultaneously applying her knowledge of systems to work toward meeting the needs identified in the analysis. The CNL developed a standardized tool to assess the comprehension and competencies of patients with regard to their diabetes to facilitate educating patients to meet these identified needs. The CNL and CNS collaborated on developing education material for patients and staff. They educated multiple disciplines on best practices. The hospital was the first in the state to receive the Joint Commission accreditation for advanced in-patient diabetes care.

The CNL and CNS collaborated on implementing the use of computer software to assist in the dosing of intravenous insulin. The preexisting process involved a paper protocol, allowing for nursing discretion in titrating insulin doses. The CNL and the CNS became system administrators for the software, educating the staff in the software use and problem solving. The increased safety outcome of this software implementation was evidenced by the decrease in hypoglycemia rates from 2.1% on the paper protocol to less than 0.5% with the new software.

SEVEN

The Nurse Manager and the Clinical Nurse Leader
Delineating Roles, Competencies, and Responsibilities

 Greg Eagerton

www Learning Objectives

- Discuss the current drivers affecting the healthcare environment, the role of managers, and the nurse manager/clinical nurse leader dyad
- Identify why managers can benefit from collaboration, persuasion, coordination, and engagement with clinical nurse leaders

> Skate to where the puck is going . . . not to where it has been.
>
> **Wayne Gretzky**

- Identify and discuss the clinical nurse leader competencies that complement manager role and functions
- Differentiate between manager administrative leadership and clinical nurse leadership
- Identify and discuss barriers and opportunities associated with nurse manager/clinical nurse leader dyads

Key Terms

Nurse manager/CNL dyad   Collaboration   Coordination   Persuasion
Engagement   Integration   Core competencies
Administrative leadership   Clinical leadership

CNL Roles

Leadership   Evidence-based practice   Design and implementation
Lateral integral   Outcomes manager   Educator
Life-long learner

CNL Professional Values

Social justice   Accountability   Altruism   Ethics   Advocacy

CNL Core Competencies

Communication   Collaboration   Leadership   Critical thinking
Risk anticipation   Team management

Introduction

Planning for the future in any business or within any organization is difficult even under the best of circumstances. When environments are dynamic, the challenges multiply exponentially, and unfortunately, few environments have been more unpredictable in the 21st century than health care (Huston, 2008). Unpredictable environments lend themselves to unpredictable outcomes, which, in healthcare environments, are not acceptable. Traditional management solutions no longer apply, and a lack of strong leadership in healthcare organizations has limited the innovation needed to create solutions to the new and complex problems that the future will bring (Marquis & Huston, 2009).

However, these challenges also present an opportunity for the nursing profession to take the lead in initiating change. This lead can be most effectively taken by teams of nurses at the points of patient care, whether in primary care settings, outpatient procedure settings, inpatient acute care settings, long-term care settings, or other points of care where patients and families are receiving nursing care. In today's complex, dynamic healthcare management environment, it is imperative that nurse managers take a more focused look at nursing leadership within the arena of direct patient care in organizations (Downey, Parslow, & Smart, 2011). However, with the volume and complexity of administrative duties, nurse managers must partner with clinicians, such as the clinical nurse leader (CNL) to ensure that patient care is afforded the same level of attention, if not greater, than issues of an administrative nature.

It is imperative that administrative and clinical leaders within healthcare organizations clearly delineate the competencies, roles, and responsibilities of the nurse manager and the CNL. Failure to recognize the vast differences between the roles will lead to significant confusion and subsequent failure to fully utilize the roles. It is also important to note how the two roles complement each other and serve as a source of collaborative support for the staff and patients being served and led.

This chapter identifies the core competencies and essential roles and responsibilities of both the nurse manager and CNL. Individual healthcare organizations can use these as they further define the specific roles within their healthcare delivery system(s). The competencies identified in this chapter were developed and implemented by professional organizations and are used as the basis for professional practice and education curricula. The roles and responsibilities, as outlined here, can help healthcare organizations begin to explore how to delineate them within their organizations and to explore how these shared responsibilities can help build an engaging and integrated administrative and clinical team for the patient care areas where the CNL role is implemented.

Competencies

As with all roles in the nursing profession, the roles of the nurse manager and CNL have their unique sets of competencies. These competencies have been established by professional organizations based on education and practice standards and through practice and experience in the roles. The American Organization of Nurse Executives (AONE) established the competencies required for nurse executives in 2004

(AONE, 2011). Nurse managers are expected to acquire the same competencies at the unit, or micro, level within assigned administrative responsibility. CNL competencies were identified by the American Association of Colleges of Nursing (AACN) in the landmark *White Paper on the Role of the Clinical Nurse Leader* (AACN, 2007). Nurse educators and nurse leaders have used these established competencies as the basis for the development of formal and informal education curricula and clinical experiences for the nurse manager and CNL.

Table 7-1 identifies the competencies of the nurse manager and CNL. At first review, it appears that many of the competencies are the same; however, a more thorough review of each competency helps differentiate the two roles.

Nurse Manager Competencies

American Organization of Nurse Executives (AONE) established the competencies required for nurse executives in 2004. The competencies identified by AONE describe the skills common to nurses in executive practice, regardless of their educational level or title in different organizations, and they can be used by aspiring nurse leaders in planning personal preparation for their careers (AONE, 2011). There are five major categories of competency for the nurse managers: communication and relationship building, knowledge of the healthcare environment, leadership, professionalism, and business skills. Each of these competencies is further defined here in an effort to differentiate, or acknowledge the similarities between, the competencies of the CNL.

Nurse Manager Competency #1: Communication and Relationship Building

AONE (2011) and the AACN (2007) identify communication and relationship building as a required competency for nurse managers and CNLs. AONE further defines this competency by identifying specific skills and knowledge the nurse leader must demonstrate, including:

Effective Communication: competence demonstrated by successfully preparing and presenting professional oral presentations, producing effective written materials, and by managing and resolving conflict

Relationship Management: competence demonstrated by successfully building trusting, collaborative relationships with peers, supervisors, subordinates, and internal and external stakeholders

Table 7-1   Nurse Manager and Clinical Nurse Leader Competencies

Nurse Manager Competency	Clinical Nurse Leader Competency
Communication and relationship building	Critical thinking
Knowledge of the healthcare environment	Communication
Leadership skills	Assessment
Professionalism	Nursing technology and resource management
Business skills	Health promotion, risk reduction, and disease prevention
	Illness and disease management
	Information and healthcare technologies
	Ethics
	Human diversity
	Global health care
	Healthcare systems and policies
	Provider and manager of care
	Designer/manager/coordinator of care
	Member of a profession

Sources: American Organization of Nurse Executives. (2011). The AONE nurse executive competencies. Retrieved from http://www.aone.org/resources/leadership%20tools/nursecomp. shtml; American Association of Colleges of Nursing. (2007). White paper on the role of the clinical nurse leader. Retrieved from http://www.aacn.nche.edu/publications/white-papers/cnl

Influencing Behaviors: competence demonstrated by creating, sharing, and gaining buy-in for a shared vision; by developing, communicating, and monitoring behavior expectations with appropriate reward and recognition for adherence to expectations when confronting and managing inappropriate behaviors

Diversity: competence demonstrated by creating an environment that fosters and values differences in the people nurses work with and the patients they serve; by defining diversity for their organization in terms of gender, race, religion, ethnicity, sexual orientation, age, and other factors; by defining cultural competence and ensuring its permeation throughout the organization; by incorporating cultural beliefs into care; and by effectively managing inappropriate behaviors and attitudes toward diverse groups

Shared Decision Making: competence demonstrated by creating a work environment where staff and others are involved in decision making, where staff are comfortable with opinion sharing, and where decisions about the organization are patient centered

Community Involvement: competence demonstrated by being an active member in the community, representing the profession and employer to nonhealthcare constituents; by serving as consultant to the community as needed; and by serving on community and/or professional boards and organizations

Medical/Staff Relationships: competence demonstrated by building and maintaining relationships with medical staff; by representing nursing at board meetings and on committees; by collaborating with medical staff to identify patient care needs, programs, and equipment; and by facilitating disputes between physicians, nurses, and other disciplines

Academic Relationships: competence demonstrated by ongoing assessment of current and future supply and demand for nursing care; by identifying educational needs of current and future nursing staff and working with academic partners to develop strategies to meet these needs; and by serving on academic councils, collaborating with academic partners in nursing research, and incorporating this research into nursing practice

Nurse Manager Competency #2: Knowledge of the Healthcare Environment

As with nurse manager competency #1, there are several subcategories, some of which may also be components of the CNL competencies. However, it should be noted that this competency requires the nurse manager to approach the healthcare environment from an administrative perspective rather than a clinical perspective.

Clinical Practice Knowledge: competence demonstrated by maintaining knowledge of current nursing practice and the roles of patient care team members; by understanding and enforcing patient care standards and standards of nursing practice established by boards of nursing, the American Nurses Association, and others; and by establishing and enforcing appropriate policy and procedure

Delivery Models/Work Design: competence demonstrated by maintaining and enhancing knowledge about patient care delivery models and appropriately redesigning an organization's delivery system when needed

Healthcare Economics: competence demonstrated by knowledge and ability to articulate federal, state, and private-payer system regulations and issues, as well as the impacts on organizations

Healthcare Policy: competence demonstrated by knowledge and ability to articulate local, state, and federal policy that affects provision of patient care; the ability to educate other healthcare team members about these policies

Governance: competence demonstrated by knowledge and ability to articulate the role of the governing body and have the ability to represent nursing and the needs of patient care at board meetings

Evidence-Based Practice/Outcome Measurement: competence demonstrated by the ability to interpret information from research and use findings to establish standards, practices, and patient care models for the organization; participate in studies that provide outcome measurements

Patient Safety: competence demonstrated by actively supporting the development and implementation of an organization-wide patient safety program that supports a nonpunitive reporting environment and that encourages continuous learning with new and improved patient safety modalities

Utilization/Case Management: competence demonstrated by the ability to articulate the model employed by the organization, by involving physicians in ongoing utilization of management practices, and by designing continuum of care options for managing patient throughput

Quality Improvement/Metrics: competence demonstrated by determining patient care quality improvement goals and objectives, monitoring outcomes metrics, changing practice as needed based on outcomes, and using benchmarking as appropriate

Risk Management: competence demonstrated by ability to identify areas of risk/liability, taking actions to decrease the potential for these areas of risks/liabilities, and educating staff on risk management and compliance issues

Nurse Manager Competency #3: Leadership

It is essential to note that leadership is a competency that is linked to the nurse manager role, but that is not specifically identified in the competencies for CNLs. This does not indicate that the CNL does not have leadership responsibilities; however, the nurse manager has an essential competency to provide administrative leadership, whereas the CNL has implied competency to provide clinical leadership. The essential elements of the nurse manager leadership competency are:

Foundational Thinking Skills: competence demonstrated by addressing ideas, beliefs, and viewpoints that should be given serious consideration while recognizing one's personal method of decision making

Personal Journey Disciplines: competence demonstrated by placing value and acting on feedback that is provided about personal strengths and weaknesses and demonstrating the values of life-long learning

Systems Thinking: competence demonstrated by promoting systems thinking as a value in the nursing organization and considering the impact of nursing decisions on the overall healthcare organization

Succession Planning: competence demonstrated by serving as a professional role model and mentor to future nurse leaders, by promoting nursing management as a desirable specialty, and establishing mechanisms for identifying staff with leadership potential

Change Management: competence demonstrated by using change theory to plan for the implementation of organizational change, serving as a change agent, and assisting others through change; adapting leadership style to situational needs

Nurse Manager Competency #4: Professionalism

The professionalism competency crosses both the nurse manager and CNL pathway. The primary difference is that the CNL has the responsibility of managing individual professional practice and responsibilities, whereas the nurse manager has individual responsibilities to manage and guide the professionalism of other nurses and interprofessional team members.

Personal and Professional Accountability: competence demonstrated by creating an environment that facilitates the team to initiate actions that produce results, holding self and others accountable for actions, and answering for one's behaviors and actions

Career Planning: competence demonstrated by developing a personal career plan and measuring progress according to that plan; coaches and mentors others in developing career plans and creates an environment in which professional and personal growth is an expectation

Ethics: competence demonstrated by integrating high ethical standards and core values into everyday work activities and creating an environment that has a reputation for high ethical standards

Evidence-Based Clinical and Management Practice: competence demonstrated by advocating the use of documented best practices and teaching and mentoring others to routinely use evidence-based data and research

Advocacy: competence demonstrated by ensuring that the clinical perspective is included in organizational decisions and that nurses are actively involved in decisions that affect practice

Active Membership in Professional Organizations: competence demonstrated by personal involvement in a professional organization and encouraging others to participate in professional organizations

Nurse Manager Competency #5: Business Skills

This competency is specific to the nurse manager role and is not identified as a competency for the CNL. This does not indicate that the outcomes of the CNL role will not impact the business aspects of the organization, but it is not an essential competency of practice. The specific components of this competency are:

Financial Management: competence demonstrated by the ability to articulate and use business models for healthcare organizations; analyzing financial statements, developing business plans, and educating patient care teams on financial implications of patient care decisions

Human Resource Management: competence demonstrated by the ability to participate in workforce planning and employment decisions; using corrective discipline to mitigate workplace behavior problems, reward and recognize exemplary performance, and implement ergonomically sound work environments to prevent worker injury and fatigue

Strategic Management: competence demonstrated by the ability to analyze the situation and identify the strategic direction; conduct gap analysis; and formulate objectives, goals, and specific strategies related to the mission and vision

Marketing: competence demonstrated by the ability to analyze and develop marketing opportunities and strategies and to use public relations and media outlets to promote the organization

Information Management and Technology: competence demonstrated by basic use of email and common word processing, spreadsheet, and Internet programs; recognizing the relevance of nursing data for improving practice; participating in system change processes and utility analyses; and reading and interpreting benchmarking, financial, and occupancy data

This section identified the competencies of the nurse manager according to AONE (2011). As noted, there are competencies that apply to both the nurse manager and CNL; however, the competencies identified for the nurse manager can be quite broad and encompass the individual, the staff the nurse manager leads, and the assigned work area. The competencies for the CNL will be explored next to assist in delineating that role from the role of the nurse manager.

Clinical Nurse Leader Competencies

The *White Paper on the Role of the Clinical Nurse Leader* (AACN, 2007) is a landmark document identifying the educational requirements for CNLs. This document identifies several components of education that are necessary to adequately prepare the nurse for the CNL role. These components are liberal education, professional values, core competencies, core knowledge, and role development (AACN, 2007).

Clinical Nurse Leader Competency #1: Critical Thinking

Critical thinking involves independent and interdependent decision making using evidence gathered through personal experiences and through the research of others in evaluating and designing modes and plans of care.

Clinical Nurse Leader Competency #2: Communication

Communication is the use of complex and interactive processes that form the basis for building interpersonal relationships with other interdisciplinary team members, peers, supervisors, and the patient. This requires the effective use of face-to-face communication skills, the use of technological modalities to communicate, the ability to present formally and informally, and to communicate effectively in divergent group situations.

Clinical Nurse Leader Competency #3: Assessment

This competency requires the use of evidence-based practice to build assessment skills to create realistic patient plans of care. These assessments must include the patient's family, community, or population and data from organizations and systems in planning and delivering care. Outcomes databases must be established to adequately measure the effectiveness of the plans of care.

Clinical Nurse Leader Competency #4: Nursing Technology and Resource Management

The CNL must have an understanding of the technology nurses use in the care they provide for patients, but more importantly, they must have the ability to teach, delegate, and supervise the performance of skilled tasks that others perform. Ongoing learning of new technologies and concepts is required for the CNL to be effective in the role, and the ability to transfer this knowledge to others is a basic requirement.

Clinical Nurse Leader Competency #5: Health Promotion, Risk Reduction, and Disease Prevention

Knowledge of theories of health promotion, disease prevention, and health maintenance of patients is an essential competency for the CNL role. Effective management of these concepts requires effective teaching and evaluation skills and knowledge, including knowledge and use of available resources, teaching and communication methods, and learning principles.

Clinical Nurse Leader Competency #6: Illness and Disease Management

This competency requires knowledge of pharmacology, the pathophysiology of disease, and assessment and management of symptoms across the life span with particular emphasis on the chronic nature and sequelae of illness. There must be an understanding and appreciation for the impact that social, physical, psychological, and spiritual aspects have on patients' illness and healing.

Clinical Nurse Leader Competency #7: Information and Healthcare Technologies

Information technology includes current and future technologies that assist CNLs in obtaining, processing, and using information to better care for patients. This not only includes technology related to retrieving information such as the most recent literature or evidence-based information but also includes technology such as patient care equipment (e.g., cardiac monitors, IV pumps, and vital sign machines). Again, the CNL role not only requires knowledge about the application of the technology, but also teaching others about the proper use of this technology.

Clinical Nurse Leader Competency #8: Ethics

The AACN's (2006) definition of ethics includes values, codes, and principles that govern decisions in nursing practice, conduct, and relationships. The CNL should be able to identify actual or potential ethical issues arising within the healthcare team and with patients and deal with them effectively. In addition, the CNL serves as the patient's advocate.

Clinical Nurse Leader Competency #9: Human Diversity

The CNL must recognize and synthesize ways that cultural, ethnic, socioeconomic, linguistic, religious, and lifestyle variations are expressed and how these factors may impact health and healing. Age-related competencies are also an integral piece of the CNL's portfolio.

Clinical Nurse Leader Competency #10: Global Health Care

Due to the extensiveness of travel, both domestic and international, the CNL must be cognizant of the implications associated with disease transmission, health policy, and healthcare economics. Again, cultural competence is important as communication across disciplines, cultures, and geographic boundaries is an everyday reality in today's mobile society.

Clinical Nurse Leader Competency #11: Healthcare Systems and Policy

Although the CNL's primary role is that of clinician, those in the role must also evidence an understanding of the organization and environment in which nursing and health care is provided and how policy shapes health systems. In addition, the CNL must have a basic understanding of the business principles of the organization in order to effectively manage patients' care and throughput in the system.

Clinical Nurse Leader Competency #12: Provider and Manager of Care

Evidence-based knowledge is the basis for the design, coordination, and evaluation of the delivery of patient care. The CNL must lead the interprofessional healthcare team to ensure that the plan of care is patient focused and includes not only the patients but also their families and caregivers.

Clinical Nurse Leader Competency #13: Designer/Manager/Coordinator of Care

The CNL serves as the responsible leader in the design, coordination, and management of health care across the life span, including all types of healthcare settings (e.g., primary care, acute care, and long-term care). Utilizing multiple skill sets—including expert communication, collaboration, negotiation, delegation, persuasion, coordination, and evaluation of interprofessional work—is pivotal to success.

Clinical Nurse Leader Competency #14: Member of a Profession

The CNL understands and demonstrates the traits of a professional and consistently role models the aspects of professionalism of life-long learning, the incorporation of professionalism into practice, and identification with the values of the profession. Mentoring and coaching for the next generation is essential to sustaining and continuing to develop the role of CNL.

Conclusions: Nurse Manager and Clinical Nurse Leader Competencies

As discussed in this chapter, professional organizations, based on education and practice, have identified the core competencies for the nurse manager and CNL. It is evident that the roles share several of the same competencies; however it is imperative that each role identify the method(s) by which it demonstrates compliance with the competencies, as the demand is very different for the roles in most cases. The nurse manager must demonstrate *administrative competence* with specific, well-defined aspects of clinical knowledge, whereas the CNL must demonstrate *clinical competence* with specific, well-defined aspects of administrative knowledge. Working collaboratively in a specific clinical setting can be the basis for a strong administrative and clinical leadership team that can enhance the care of the patients in that setting.

Roles and Responsibilities

As the CNL role is implemented in healthcare organizations, the roles and responsibilities of the CNL will need to be delineated from that of the nurse manager. This can be done before implementation of the role, but it can be expected that as the CNL role matures in the clinical area where it is being implemented, the associated role and responsibilities will evolve, and the roles of the CNL and the nurse manager will become clearer.

Table 7-2 is an example of how the roles and responsibilities of the nurse manager and CNL can be delineated in an effort to decrease confusion about the differences between the two. The AACN's 2006 *Working Statement Comparing the Clinical Nurse Leader and Nurse Manager Roles* may also assist in developing an organization's list of roles and responsibilities. The AACN document not only identifies broad roles and responsibilities of each role but also identifies shared role characteristics of the nurse manager and CNL. Each nursing care unit where the CNL is employed can develop its own list based on the specific needs of the patients served and services provided. Clearly defining the roles and responsibilities of the nurse manager and the CNL can lead to a more successful partnership between the two and can lead to stronger administrative and clinical dynamics, with the goals of improving patient outcomes, creating higher staff satisfaction, and improving effectiveness and efficiencies in patient care delivery.

Table 7-2   Roles and Responsibilities of the Nurse Manager and CNL

Nurse Manager Roles and Responsibilities	Clinical Nurse Leader Roles and Responsibilities
Provides administrative leadership and oversight for a defined clinical unit(s)	Provides clinical leadership and guidance for patient care for a defined clinical unit(s)
Provides resources for staff education and clinical training	Conducts staff education; provides for individual and/or group of nurses and/or interdisciplinary team members
Identifies and secures staffing and resources for staffing the unit(s) for which they are administratively responsible	Leads teams of care providers in day-to-day patient care delivery; works with nurse manager to identify staffing needs and delivery model(s)
Works with committees and interdisciplinary teams at the organization level; typically long-term committee assignments	Works with interdisciplinary team on unit where assigned; may at times work with small work groups at organizational level for short-term assignments such as process action teams, time-limited special focus teams, etc.
Identifies and maintains daily staffing requirements and needs	Works with staff on duty to provide care for patients on their unit
Creates and manages budget	Provides input about budget requests based on the patient care needs identified through practice
Evaluates employee performance	Provides educational support and guidance to staff during orientation and/or for performance deficits that require reeducation; provides feedback to nurse manager regarding employee clinical practice and/or conduct issues
Responsible for the overall nursing care provided on the unit(s) under his or her supervision	Provides leadership in the development of patient-specific plans of care and works with interdisciplinary team to deliver patient care

Summary

- Nurse managers and CNLs are essential elements of a successful administrative and clinical leadership team.
- To maximize the skill sets of both the nurse manager and the CNL, it is imperative to delineate the competencies and roles and responsibilities of each position, thus eliminating barriers and role confusion.
- Clearly defining each role can lead to a successful collaboration between the administrative and clinical leadership dyad in which patients, families, and the member of the healthcare delivery team benefit.

 Reflection Questions
© Arenacreative/Dreamstime.com

1. What roles of the nurse manager and CNL are complementary?
2. What benefits occur when CNLs are introduced to the microsystem and subsequently to the meso- and macrosystem?

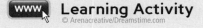 **Learning Activity**
© Arenacreative/Dreamstime.com

- Compare and contrast the roles of the nurse manager and the CNL, identifying which, if any, are duplicative.

References

American Association of Colleges of Nursing. (2006). *Working statement comparing the clinical nursing leader and nurse manager roles: Similarities, differences and complementarities.* Retrieved from apps.aacn.nche.edu/CNL/pdf/tk/roles3-06.pdf

American Association of Colleges of Nursing. (2007). *White paper on the education and role of the clinical nurse leader.* Retrieved from http://www.aacn.nche.edu/publications/white-papers/cnl

American Organization of Nurse Executives. (2011). The AONE nurse executive competencies. Retrieved from http://www.aone.org/resources/leadership%20tools/nursecomp.shtml

Downey, M., Parslow, S., & Smart, M. (2011). The hidden treasure in nursing leadership: Informal leaders. *Journal of Nursing Management, 19,* 517–521.

Huston, C. (2008). Preparing nurse leaders for 2020. *Journal of Nursing Management, 16,* 905–911.

Marquis, B., & Huston, C. (2009). *Leadership roles and management functions in nursing: Theory and application* (6th ed.). Philadelphia, PA: Lippincott, Williams, and Wilkins.

Clinical Nurse Leader and Manager Collaboration

Beth VanDam

Key Concepts: team collaboration, patient satisfaction, evidence based

Our unit leadership team, nursing service line director, unit manager, CNL, clinical nurse specialist, and case managers review patient satisfaction scores each month. As a team we are always looking for ways to improve the patient care experience.

Last April the unit manager and I, as CNL, reviewed evidence-based literature on posthospitalization discharge phone calls. We collaborated regarding information we had gathered from the literature. Our first step was to formulate questions to ask patients in the phone calls. Most of the questions came from Quint Studer, and we added a couple others that the manager and I felt were specific to our unit.

As the CNL, I was responsible for leading a team with the purpose of designing a process change for discharge phone calls and developing a plan to measure the effects of the change on the patient care experience. While I was working on the process, the manager was determining staffing needs to incorporate dedicated time to making the follow-up calls to patients. Once the details of the process were determined, the manager and I again collaborated closely as we initiated the new process. Each day the manager and I would support the staff. I would assist the staff member to help gain a clear understanding of the process. I ensured the staff member knew where to gather the list of patients to call, which questions to ask, where to document patient feedback, and where to document a call in the electronic medical record, as well as where to put the completed forms. The manager was instrumental in working with the charge nurse in identifying staff who would be available to making discharge phone calls each day.

The unit manager and I have found this collaboration with each other to be enjoyable and successful because the staff sees us working together to support a common goal. As a result, patient satisfaction scores on our unit have improved as well.

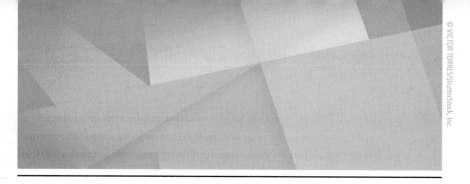

EIGHT

Preparing Preceptors for CNL Immersions

■ Susan Wilkinson

 Learning Objectives

- Define preceptor and preceptee and identify core competencies of each
- Define clinical nurse leader immersion in the clinical setting and the requisites for a successful immersion
- Define and discuss the significance of a dedicated learning environment for the clinical nurse leader's clinical experiences and life-long learning trajectory
- Identify steps in developing meaningful and sustainable clinical immersion projects
- Provide examples of clinical immersion projects and discuss the impact on the healthcare system

> The dictionary is the only place that success comes before work. Work is the key to success, and hard work can help you accomplish anything.
>
> Vince Lombardi, Jr.

159

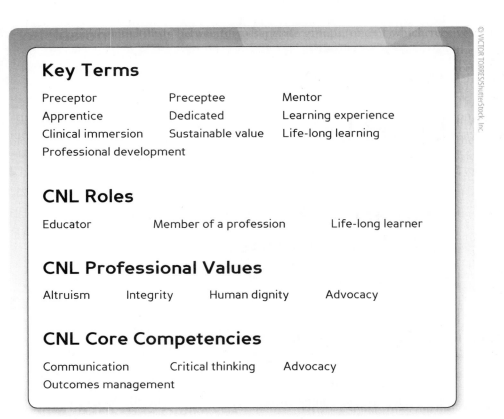

Key Terms

Preceptor

Preceptee

Mentor

Apprentice

Dedicated

Learning experience

Clinical immersion

Sustainable value

Life-long learning

Professional development

CNL Roles

Educator

Member of a profession

Life-long learner

CNL Professional Values

Altruism

Integrity

Human dignity

Advocacy

CNL Core Competencies

Communication

Critical thinking

Advocacy

Outcomes management

Preceptors, Preceptees, and Core Competencies of Each

The clinical immersion experience consists of two central participants: the *preceptor,* who leads, manages, directs, teaches, and oversees the clinical immersion experience, and the *preceptee,* who observes, listens, learns, engages, and transforms into the clinical nurse leader (CNL). The relationship between these two individuals is critical to a successful clinical immersion experience. Creating an environment in which both parties feel they can communicate openly, express ideas freely, and plan objectives equally helps to ensure a positive experience for both. Conversely, an environment where one individual makes all the decisions; is not forthcoming, honest, or reliable; or does not consider the goals and objectives of the other creates a stressful and agonizing environment in which barriers that adversely impact both preceptor and preceptee are created, and neither individual benefits from the experience. Dynamic and operative relationships between preceptor and preceptee create bonds that remain in place long after the clinical immersion experience has ended.

The Preceptor

A preceptor can be defined as a teacher, tutor, instructor, professor, or any other of the myriad terms that mean "to instruct." The role of the CNL preceptor can be more accurately defined as that of mentor. Merriam-Webster defines a mentor as "a trusted counselor or guide, tutor or coach" (2012). With more than half of all CNL students emerging from a Model C program, a master's degree program designed for individuals with a baccalaureate degree in another discipline (American Association of Colleges of Nursing [AACN], 2012), many preceptees have never even worked as a nurse, and if they have, it has been for only a very short time. The preceptor often functions as the ambassador of the healthcare profession to the preceptee and serves as the foundational cornerstone for the clinical immersion experience.

Ideally, the preceptor for the CNL student should be a CNL (AACN, 2007). The *White Paper on the Role of the Clinical Nurse Leader* (AACN, 2007) states, "an extended clinical experience, prior to graduation, mentored by an experienced Clinical Nurse Leader, is critical to the effective implementation of the role." However, the reality of finding an "experienced" CNL and pairing one with every student enrolled in a CNL program can be difficult. As of September 13, 2012, 2,325 registered nurses had sat for the CNL exam is, of which 340 were serving as CNL faculty (AACN, 2012). However, this number does not reflect those individuals actually certified as a CNL and practicing in the role. Furthermore, due to the skill set that CNLs acquire, develop, and master over time, many CNLs are often recruited quickly into other positions and roles within the organization, leaving vacancies in the CNL positions.

Out of necessity, many schools of nursing have resorted to coupling CNL students with preceptors who serve in other roles, such as nurse managers or case managers. There is danger in this practice if the preceptor does not fully understand the extent and latitude of practice of the CNL. Caution should be used when assigning a CNL student to a non-CNL preceptor, because no other role exists in health care that focuses and practices from a generalist's view across the healthcare spectrum as does the CNL. Nurse managers must recognize the differences that exist between managers and leaders. Case managers should understand that the objectives for the CNL include more than actual or anticipated needs of the patients; they also encompass the actual or anticipated needs of the associates, managers, physicians, and professionals of the microsystem, as well as the directors and administrators at the macro level.

Identifying qualified individuals to serve as mentors for CNL preceptees can be challenging for schools of nursing. Lack of time, competing demands of serving as mentor and providing patient care, and lack of protected time for mentoring are all barriers to successful preceptorships (Veeramah, 2012). Nurses everywhere are busy, very busy. The bedside nurse is overwhelmed with the increasing responsibilities and tasks of providing safe and quality care, acquiring and mastering the ever changing complexities of technology, improving patient satisfaction scores, policing physicians, serving on various teams and committees, increasing efficiency while reducing costs—all during an 8- or 12-hour shift so that they clock out on time to maintain budget limits and eliminate shift overage. Nurses who do not work at the bedside have been stretched so thin by reductions in the workforce that they are now serving on or have been appointed to serve on so many diverse and multidisciplinary teams and task forces that by the time they actually get down to doing the work assigned, there are no more hours left in the day. However, there are certain qualities and traits that make for excellent preceptors, regardless of job position or title, that should be sought after when establishing CNL preceptors.

The core competencies of a CNL preceptor include that of advocate, member of a profession, team manager, information manager, life-long learner, systems analyst/risk anticipator, clinician, outcomes manager, and educator—the roles and functions of the CNL. A competent preceptor also possesses the ability to value and recognize the significance of self-evaluation, has a willingness to serve as a role model, assists students in developing critical thinking skills, adapts and accepts the different ways in which students learn and function, and provides positive reinforcement (Lichtman et al., 2003). Preceptors who are actively involved in interdisciplinary teams and practice are desirable if the preceptee is to understand, engage in, and maximize the full learning experience (AACN, 2007). Other competencies include the ability to give feedback, experience, availability of time, and a positive attitude (Huybrecht, Loeckx, Quaeyhaegens, De Tobel, & Mistiaen, 2011). Schools of nursing must recognize and acknowledge the crucial role that dedicated preceptors play in ensuring the success of the CNL student and they must pursue individuals possessing such competencies and professional values as altruism, integrity, and respect for and acknowledgment of human dignity. The support and backing that the preceptor offers to the preceptee, along with modeling successful interdisciplinary team relationships, is imperative for the student to reach his or her full potential and thrive (Goode, 2012).

The Preceptee

The preceptee, simply defined, is the student. The preceptee learns and develops under the direction and guidance of the preceptor, in much the same way an apprentice integrates knowledge learned from classroom instruction with on-the-job training. In the clinical immersion experience, the preceptee has the responsibility of assuming accountability for the learning process. Most schools of nursing, colleges, and universities have defined universal core competencies for students such as oral and written skills, information technology, and professional values. Core competencies that the CNL preceptee should possess, like that of the CNL preceptor, are serving as an advocate and a member of a profession, being dedicated to lifelong learning, and showing commitment to professional development. Acquiring and cultivating these key proficiencies determines the level of success of the clinical immersion experience.

There are also certain behaviors the CNL preceptee can exhibit that will foster positive clinical immersion experiences, such as coming prepared for clinical days with a clear list of short-term and long-term objectives. The preceptee should involve the preceptor in the didactic course of study and homework assignments so that he/ she can follow along with the preceptee. He or she should actively engage in and participate in the microsystem structure by becoming an effective and functional team member. He or she must remember to exercise patience and recognize that the preceptor will have job responsibilities that must be prioritized and juggled throughout the CNL immersion. The preceptee should communicate openly with the preceptor about what is working well and what areas may need further attention or tweaking.

The CNL Clinical Immersion and Requisites for a Successful Immersion

The culminating educational experience for the preceptee is the CNL clinical immersion, which is a 300–400 hour concentrated practicum in which the preceptee enters the healthcare environment and begins incorporating the knowledge and skill sets gained throughout the educational process, including previous didactic and clinical proficiencies. During this time, weekly opportunities to discuss experiences, ask questions, and reflect on events with other CNL students, faculty, or mentors should be made available (AACN, 2007). Practice environments in which staff understand and have embraced the CNL role should be given first priority for placement of CNL students embarking on the clinical immersion experience. Requisites for ensuring successful immersions between schools of nursing and healthcare settings include collaborative partnerships and agreements, education about the role, thoughtful planning and pairing of preceptor and preceptee, and support and backing of the CNL role by nurse administrators and nurse managers.

Successful immersion begins long before the CNL preceptee actually enters the doors of the chosen healthcare environment. Academia should have already laid the groundwork for enriching clinical immersions by educating, having dialogue, interviewing, recruiting, and developing and nurturing relationships with potential preceptors, especially those who are not CNLs, to explain the history, framework, and competencies of the CNL role. Candidates for preceptor should be made aware of and understand the level of commitment and guidance required before agreeing to serve in this role. Academia should assess and thoughtfully consider if potential preceptors are a good fit for their institutional goals. Once preceptors have accepted the responsibility and school of nursing faculty have deemed these preceptors a good fit, careful pairing of student to preceptor should occur.

In many ways, the pairing of a preceptor and preceptee is like forming a business partnership. Successful partnerships usually have common threads, such as clearly defined goals and purposes, awareness and understanding of either other's roles and responsibilities, and planned deliberate reviews of performance through ongoing observation, communication, and evaluation (Hunter & Perkins, 2012). Considering personality traits, strengths and weaknesses, and teaching and learning styles of both individuals also contributes to effective relationships.

Prior to the clinical immersion commencing and throughout the duration of the clinical immersion, regular and periodic meetings should be held between the schools of nursing, preceptors, and preceptees to ensure that a clear understanding of the CNL role is maintained and the core competencies are being achieved. When possible, on-site visits should occur, or if on-site visits are not practical for CNL programs that provide online distance learning, conference calls should be scheduled. This time should be used to evaluate progress toward and attainment of both long- and short-term goals, to discuss and remove barriers, to celebrate successes, and to chart direction. The projected course curriculum, in-class assignments, and clinical opportunities should also be reviewed.

Successful immersions require the assistance and backing of senior nursing leadership. In a qualitative study of CNLs, failure of nurse administrators to provide support to the role was identified as the chief barrier to achieving success. Moreover, nurse administrators who reinforce and uphold the role and objectives of the CNL increase the sustainability of the role (Weaver Moore & Leahy, 2012). Nurse managers also play a role in determining whether or not clinical immersion experiences are effective. Because the focus of the CNL is the microsystem, the unit manager of that microsystem must have a clear understanding of the CNL competency objectives and project goals. Unit managers who are confident and secure in their own role are much more apt to welcome and support improvement projects and embrace change processes than unit managers who are insecure or afraid of upsetting the status quo. Faculty should evaluate hindrances created by nursing leadership that might impede successful project plan implementation of the CNL and be prepared to intervene and facilitate when events such as this occur.

Dedicated Learning Environment and Life-Long Learning Trajectory

Ideally, schools of nursing should partner with healthcare organizations committed to dedicated learning environments for the CNL's clinical immersion. In a dedicated learning environment, educators and clinicians work together to create an atmosphere in which all members have a concentrated focus on teaching and learning (Fourie & McClelland, 2011). Also known as dedicated education units, these environments are created for the express purpose of facilitating experiential learning and positive student experiences (Mullenbach & Burggraf, 2012). Key factors contributing to satisfying and successful student learning experiences include the quality of planning, welcome and orientation of the student to the unit, peer encouragement and teamwork, cooperation of the unit manager and charge nurses, and support of clinical and faculty preceptors (Fourie & McClelland, 2011).

When preceptees begin the clinical immersion journey, it is usually with fear and trepidation. How will I be received? Will the nurses on the unit welcome me? How can I earn the respect of staff and management? These questions are frequently asked by both novice and experienced CNL students. In dedicated learning environments where staff and management routinely work with CNL students, there exist clear and identifiable learning objectives, anticipated trajectories, formation, development and acquisition of CNL core competencies, and a concluding CNL project plan. Staff is acclimated to the role of the CNL student, and the student perceives that careful and thoughtful planning of this immersion was completed beforehand.

Time should be allocated early in the immersion experience for the CNL student to orient with charge nurses and staff nurses, unit secretaries, patient care associates, and the unit manager in order to learn each member's role and how this role contributes to the overall function and purpose of the unit. Furthermore, time spent orienting with individual associates helps to create and establish relationships that enable the CNL student to work freely in the environment, become part of the "team," and assume accountability and responsibility for unit performance, outcomes, and opportunities. This engagement and evolution of becoming a team member is beneficial to the student experience and critical for the overall success of the immersion experience, as well as the project plan implementation and sustainability.

Data about unit performance should be accessible and shared freely with the CNL student. Transparency is the hallmark of a high-reliability organization, and any attempt to cover up or hide weaknesses within the system can hinder effective and meaningful project plans. There is a responsibility on the part of the student and faculty to ensure that any sensitive information that could in any way be disparaging to the institution remain confidential. Agreements between schools of nursing and healthcare organizations where CNL preceptees complete clinical immersions should be obtained prior to the clinical experience to ensure confidentiality. Organizations that are not willing to share necessary information and data prevent the CNL preceptee from achieving maximum results and create a culture of distrust and futility. Careful selection and partnering with institutions, providing ongoing education, and maintaining close relations promotes an environment of trust, clarity, and openness.

Developing Meaningful and Sustainable Clinical Immersion Projects

The culminating assignment for the CNL student is the clinical immersion project. The clinical immersion project is often viewed as a nemesis or the bane of the

Project (*)

preceptee's existence. However, the intent of requiring the CNL student to complete a process or quality improvement project is to provide the student with a means to demonstrate all objectives, course work, competencies, and experiential learning acquired throughout the CNL program of study. Thus, the project is scheduled at the end of the learning experience, after the CNL has acquired the knowledge and developed the necessary skill set to execute such a challenge. Completing a diverse and multidisciplinary orientation lays the groundwork for maneuvering throughout the system. Diligently checking off the CNL competencies day by day empowers the CNL student with the skill set and knowledge necessary for implementing a successful project. Conducting the microsystem assessment and performing a gap analysis hones in on disparities and inconsistencies within the microsystem that can be potential project plan ideas.

Tip

Common mistakes made among CNL students are attempting to identify a project plan too early in the clinical immersion experience or selecting a project that is so broad or far reaching that there is not sufficient time or resources to allow for adequate education, implementation, and measurement. There are ordered steps, which if applied correctly and adhered to, can ensure successful project plan implementation. Identifying and selecting the appropriate project plan, setting measurable and attainable goals, developing a realistic step-by-step time-line for implementation and evaluation, and summarizing events are key factors for accomplishing desired targets.

Identifying and Selecting a Project Plan

Identification and selection of an appropriate project plan is the most important decision in implementing a successful process or quality improvement change. It is also the most difficult step of the endeavor. Many students enter into the healthcare setting with their own ideas and agendas for what the project plan will be and how it will be implemented before they even become familiar with the culture or goals of the organization and microsystem. This is a misstep and usually results in failure. Egos should be checked at the door, and students should approach project plan ideas first as observers.

Six steps that safeguard effective project plan selection include (1) completing an overview of the organization, (2) recognizing the importance and value of the introductions and orientations to the facility, (3) listening, (4) conducting thorough literature researches, (5) seeking feedback, and (6) determining buy-in.

6 steps for project

Fall

Step 1

Complete an overview of the designated healthcare organization prior to entering the clinical immersion setting. Formulate an impression by driving by the facility, talking to people, asking questions, and conducting online searches to determine the history, development and progress, and purpose of the institution. Learn the mission, vision, and values of the organization and discern if those values line up with your own. If not, know that going in and be prepared for situations that may prove challenging during the immersion experience. Commit the mission, vision, and values to memory or save them to a location where they can be reviewed throughout the year and assess periodically if the organization "walks the walk" of the vision. Conduct a self-evaluation and see how your time spent there will impact the organization and also how time spent at the organization will impact you. Students who complete some degree of background homework first usually are able to begin contemplating project plan ideas that align with organizational goals; they also experience a much less stressful transition into the clinical setting.

Fall

Step 2

Acknowledge the value and importance of introductions and orientation to the clinical immersion setting and microsystem. Introductions to personnel during the orientation period is the time when the CNL student learns the who, what, and where of obtaining information and support, and serves as the formative time for establishing underpinnings necessary for building and developing interdepartmental relations. Spending time with and learning the roles of key personnel in other departments enables the CNL student to identify the "go-to" people and resources readily available, which will be beneficial as project plan ideas and implementation evolve. Orientation with associates in the microsystem helps form alliances and bonds that will be instrumental as the time for project plan identification and implementation approach. Attending organizational, multidisciplinary, and interdisciplinary team meetings, as well as unit meetings within the microsystem, provides a plethora of information pertaining to goals and objectives for future reference for project ideas.

Fall

Step 3

The most important undertaking for developing meaningful and sustainable clinical immersion projects is to just simply listen. What is everyone talking about? What is the organization talking about? What are the leaders talking about? What are you hearing as you spend time with infection control, outcomes managers, nursing leadership, and quality? What are the associates talking about? Are there resounding themes and topics being heard over and over again? Are any of these themes being discussed locally? Nationally? Do these recurring themes apply to the microsystem where you are completing your clinical immersion? Do you personally have a passion for these themes? Listen until you can identify the aims of the organization, pinpoint objectives of the chief nurse officer and director of nursing, and ascertain the goals and aspirations of the unit manager, CNL, and associates of the microsystem. Then begin a list of possible project plan ideas and continually add to this list as the clinical immersion progresses. Do not be afraid to ask questions and seek clarification. Above all, do not try to establish the project plan too early. Be patient. Allow the course work, guided curriculum, and clinical time to develop, and project plan ideas will emerge.

Step 4

Conduct literature reviews and research the recurring themes that have been identified. Determine if studies have already been done in this area and if there are any evidenced-based best practice standards for the project plan ideas. Review as much literature as necessary until the point of saturation occurs. Afterwards, conclude if the project plans offer sustainable value and can be successfully implemented within the microsystem. Consider the costs involved and determine if the project plan requires capital, manpower, supplies, or resources that simply may not be available. Ensure that the scope of the project is not so large that it cannot be implemented, evaluated, or sustained within the time constraints of the immersion. Determine if the project plan creates or reduces work for associates. Ascertain if the manager, CNL, or associates have an interest in this idea or a burden for this process improvement. Once the research has been completed and thoughtful contemplation given to all contributing factors, eliminate those ideas that are not feasible, and hold onto those ideas that remain possibilities.

Step 5

Seek feedback. Discuss project plan ideas, how they were identified and arrived at, and the results of your literature review with your designated preceptor at the clinical facility. Identify the goals and expected outcomes of each project plan idea, as well as limitations, anticipated obstacles, potential barriers, and roadblocks. Be flexible and open minded. Trust your preceptor and foster open communication so that both preceptor and preceptee can talk through whether or not the microsystem is ready for and open to this change process. Allot time for interactive discussion, questions, dialogue, and careful and deliberate consideration. Allow time after the initial conversation for both parties to mull over thoughts and views expressed, and make an appointment to revisit these project plan ideas at a later date. Time spent away from the discussions for processing thoughts and exploring new ideas produces fruitful and insightful results.

Step 6

Determine buy-in. The most excellent project plan ideas can crumble and deteriorate if buy-in isn't obtained prior to implementation, and while it would be unrealistic to expect support and backing from the entire team within the microsystem, it is essential that buy-in exist among key stakeholders. The unit manager, preceptor, appointed and derived leaders within the unit, and the CNL student should all believe in the project plan selected and share in the development and implementation of the identified goals. Furthermore, when project plan goals are aligned with the microsystem, organizational, and system objectives, it is very difficult to reject or discount actions that will directly impact and improve desired aims.

Set Measurable and Attainable Goals

Setting measurable and attainable goals is essential for implementing a successful project or quality improvement change process. It is important to be realistic in what one can hope to accomplish or achieve in the time frame allotted. Change is slow, and sustained change requires a conscience effort of others to practice a rote task or behavior differently than might have been practiced the same way for years. Establishing a baseline time frame for education and implementation and a due date for measuring results allows the CNL preceptee to see the degree of improvement and success.

Selection of the baseline data is critical and requires careful thought and realistic planning. For example, a project aim statement *to reduce central line–associated bloodstream infections (CLABSIs) by 50% over a 2-month period as compared with the previous year* may not be practical if the microsystem only had four CLABSIs last year and three CLABSIs this year. With the baseline data selected in this example, you have already failed at your project goal. Furthermore, a 2-month period of measurement should not be compared to a year's worth of data. Instead, when selecting a baseline, consider the amount of time you have for project implementation and measurement. If you are lucky enough to have an entire quarter of a year (three months) for project implementation, then select a quarter of data from a previous time frame as the baseline. If you only have 1 month to implement a project and measure results, consider getting an average of the last 6 or 12 months and set a goal to reduce or improve performance by a certain percentage of that number.

Selection of attainable goals must also be considered. There is a tendency for CNL students to set their sights high and aspire to lofty goals that usually cannot be reached within the designated time allotted. Avoid the tendency to "conquer the world" and instead, set your sights on improving one small piece of it. Change is more easily accomplished when it is simple, entailing one or two steps that do not require additional work, or even better yet, reducing extraneous efforts or tasks. Do not belittle any project idea that creates additional time for a nurse, decreases steps in work flow, or helps to improve an overall goal, even if the project is but one small step in the change process. K·I·S·S·

Develop a Step-by-Step Time-Line

Developing a realistic step-by-step time line is imperative. Be smart and think through everything going on in your life throughout the clinical immersion experience. Create a calendar and include every day of the week, including weekend days, that runs until the clinical immersion is complete. Plug in test dates and assignment due dates for classwork, any events required outside of clinical time, clinical days and work days. Divide readings so that there is approximately the same amount of material to read on a daily basis. Then add important personal events such as birthdays or holidays, children's events if you are a parent, and extracurricular activities you may participate in such as hobbies or church events, until a clear picture emerges delineating the expected time and obligations required to meet and fulfill deadlines. Remember to include some downtime and strive to maintain some type of balance between work, home, and school. Remind yourself that while free time will be minimal, it is only temporary. You will, eventually, get your life back.

Once the calendar is completed, plan an outline with an accompanying time frame for project plan goals. Do not be afraid to ask your preceptor to help you with your planning. This individual has sat right where you sit now and can offer suggestions to help alleviate stressors you might be going through. Work backwards for project plan due dates. Determine the time frame you will want to collect and analyze all concluding data and plug this into your calendar. Then determine how long the project plan or process change needs to be in effect after education is provided and mark that time. Consider the time required to educate associates about the project plan, and remember that some healthcare settings offer "7 on/7 off" shifts, which will require 2 weeks of education before implementation. Once all data is added to the master calendar, you will be able to identify a due date for project plan selection.

Implementation and evaluation of the project plan is usually the time when the hard work ceases and the oversight and reinforcement begins. Observing daily for compliance, reinforcing objectives, and collecting and logging data as often as possible becomes the focus of the remaining clinical days. Meetings with the preceptor should occur regularly, and findings, deviations, barriers, and successes should be discussed. Do not be afraid to tweak the project plan along the way if unforeseen obstacles occur that hinder project goal attainment.

Summarize Findings and Results

Finally, summarize findings and results of the project plan. Go back to the baseline and demonstrate progress made toward goal attainment and trends noted; do not forget to include unforeseen barriers that presented roadblocks along the project's course. Consider using graphs, pie charts, run charts, or line charts. Brief summaries with picture boards and educational material developed to promote project plan goals are interesting to the reviewers and should be included in the summary.

Examples of Clinical Immersion Projects and Impact on the Healthcare System

Exemplars of CNL clinical immersion projects can be located in various books and textbooks written for the CNL, poster presentations from previous CNL summits and CNL conferences via the Web, and from the Clinical Nurse Leader Association (CNLA) website. Additionally, ongoing monthly continuing education units (CEUs) provided by the CNLA offer a variety of CNL topics, including projects CNLs or former CNL students have completed or are presently working on within their organization. The book, *Project Planning and Management: A Guide for CNLs, DNPs, and Nurse Executives* (Harris, Roussel, Walters, & Dearman, 2011) is an excellent resource for guiding the CNL student through project plan selection and implementation. Networking with other CNL students and CNLs also can provide ideas for meaningful and sustainable clinical immersion projects.

An example of a successful clinical immersion project conducted in one acute care hospital setting was to improve patient outcomes by reducing the number of catheter-associated urinary tract infections (CAUTIs) within a microsystem. According to the APIC *Guide to the Elimination of Catheter-Associated Urinary Tract Infections* (2008), a CAUTI event can cost $44,043 per hospital stay. CAUTIs can also create discomfort for the patient, and they are associated with increased length of stay, mortality, and morbidity (Centers for Disease Control and Prevention, 2012).

Because the CNL is responsible for a cohort of patients within a microsystem, drilling down on each CAUTI event to determine if the cause of the CAUTI was related to insertion, maintenance, or both was a meaningful way to improve patient outcomes and significantly impact the healthcare system by reducing hospital-acquired infections and increasing reimbursement rates for high-achieving performance. Knowledge gained from drilling down to the root causes of how and why the infections occurred allowed the CNL preceptor and preceptee to identify and focus on areas for improvement.

For example, if results show that CAUTIs are a result of improper insertion technique, then the skill level of healthcare associates inserting catheters can be assessed and evaluated, demonstrations for proper catheter insertion can be provided one on one or in group settings, or competency check-offs can be required and conducted for associates who routinely insert catheters. Likewise, if the causes of the CAUTIs are related to maintenance, regular rounding on patients with indwelling urinary catheters can be performed to ensure a securement device is in place, that the catheter is properly cleaned and maintained in the correct position and removed when no longer necessary. In-service training can also be provided to educate associates about proper maintenance of the indwelling urinary catheter.

Another example of a CNL project that directly impacted a healthcare system was to improve patient satisfaction scores related to communication about medications. The Hospital Consumer Assessment of Healthcare Providers and Systems (HCAHPS) Survey is a standardized tool used by many hospitals to evaluate patients' viewpoints on hospital care received; it is also used as a scorecard, rewarding hospitals with financial incentives for high ratings (HCAHPS, 2012). There are eight key topics addressed in the HCAHPS survey; the component related to communication about medication and side effects was particularly low for this one microsystem. To improve the patients' level of understanding, several plans of action were developed, including having the nurse write down new medications and side effects on

> To each there comes in their lifetime a special moment when they
> are figuratively tapped on the shoulder and offered the chance to
> do a very special thing, unique to them and fitted to their talents.
> What a tragedy if that moment finds them unprepared or unquali-
> fied for that which could have been their finest hour.
>
> Winston Churchill

the whiteboard in each patient's room, creating and providing small preprinted drug
classification information cards to be handed out to patients with each new medication, and accessing and printing medication fact sheets from medication databases
to be distributed during routine rounds. These measures improved patient satisfaction scores for this microsystem and in turn, improved the overall ratings for the
hospital.

Summary

- The preceptor and preceptee are the two key players in the CNL clinical
  immersion experience. Both have core competencies that facilitate the
  mutual success of each other.
- Clinical immersion sites that partner with academia and understand the
  role of the CNL foster an enriching learning environment and help pave the
  way for future CNL immersions.
- Dedicated learning environments where CNL preceptees are welcomed and
  routinely complete clinical rotations instill life-long learning trajectories
  and shape professional development. Meaningful and sustainable CNL
  immersion projects can be identified and implemented by following established guidelines.
- Identifying and selecting the appropriate project plan, setting measurable and attainable goals, developing a realistic step-by-step time line for
  implementation and evaluation, and summarizing events are key factors for
  achieving project plan success.
- Examples of former successful CNL projects can be located through CNL
  books, textbooks, websites, organizations, and networking. Hard work is
  rewarded with success.

www. Reflection Questions
© Arenacreative/Dreamstime.com

1. How are core competencies of the CNL preceptor and the CNL preceptee alike? How are they different?
2. What requisites are important to you for achieving success in the clinical immersion experience?
3. What barriers could prevent you from achieving success in the clinical immersion experience?
4. Why is it important for a CNL or member of a profession to commit to life-long learning?
5. What do you feel constitutes meaningful and sustainable clinical immersion projects?

www. Learning Activities
© Arenacreative/Dreamstime.com

1. Complete a self-evaluation to determine your preferred methods of communication and feedback and be prepared to discuss these methods with your preceptor. Ask your preceptor about his/her preferred method of communication and ascertain what type of feedback he/she needs to maintain open lines of communication and exchange of ideas. Work together to establish means and frequency of communication acceptable to both parties.
2. Identify your strengths and weaknesses in your roles as student, preceptee, nurse, and a member of a profession. In one column list strengths, and in the other column list weaknesses. Identify ahead of time strategies for handling weaknesses that are part of your individual make-up prior to the clinical immersion experience, acknowledging that these weakness will be magnified during peak times of stress, fatigue, and weariness.
3. Assess your ability to organize and prioritize events in your life. Pinpoint events and triggers that cause you to go astray and lose focus. Research ways to minimize these triggers. Think of events in your past that made you want to give up and quit, and analyze those events to identify the mitigating factors that caused these feelings and/or actions. Develop an action plan to recognize when these situations are threatening and how to prevent and halt their progression.

References

American Association of Colleges of Nursing. (2007). White paper on the role of the clinical nurse leader. Retrieved from http://www.aacn.nche.edu/publications/white-papers/cnl

American Association of Colleges of Nursing. (2012). *CNL certification exam data*. Retrieved from http://www.aacn.nche.edu/leading-initiatives/cnl/cnl-certification/pdf/CNLStats.pdf

APIC. (2008). *Guide to the elimination of catheter-associated urinary tract infections (CAUTIs): Developing and applying facility-based prevention interventions in acute and long-term care settings*. Retrieved from http://www.apic.org/Resource_/EliminationGuideForm/c0790db8 -2aca-4179-a7ae-676c27592de2/File/APIC-CAUTI-Guide.pdf

Centers for Disease Control and Prevention. (2012). *Catheter-associated urinary tract infection (CAUTI) event*. Retrieved from http://www.cdc.gov/nhsn/pdfs/pscmanual/7psccauticurrent .pdf

Fourie, W., & McClelland, B. (2011). *Enhancing nursing education through dedicated education units*. Wellington, New Zealand: The National Centre for Tertiary Teaching Excellence. Retrieved from http://akoaotearoa.ac.nz/download/ng/file/group-1658/enhancing-nursing -education-through-dedicated-education-units.pdf

Goode, M. L. (2012). The role of the mentor: A critical analysis. *Journal of Community Nursing 26*(3), 33–35.

Harris, J. L., Roussel, L., Walters, S. E., & Dearman, C. (2011). *Project planning and management: A guide for CNLs, DNPs, and nurse executives*. Burlington, MA: Jones & Bartlett Learning.

Hospital Consumer Assessment of Healthcare Providers and Systems. (2012). Home page. Retrieved from http://www.hcahpsonline.org

Hunter, D., & Perkins, N. (2012). Partnership working in public health: The implications for governance of a systems approach. *Journal of Health Services Research & Policy, 17*(Supple.), 45–52.

Huybrecht, S., Loeckx, W., Quaeyhaegens, Y., De Tobel, D., & Mistiaen, W. (2011). Mentoring in nursing education: Perceived characteristics of mentors and the consequences of mentorship. *Nurse Education Today, 31*(3), 274–278.

Lichtman, R., Burst, H. V., Campau, N., Carrington, B., Diegmann, E. K., Hsia, L., & Thompson, J. E. (2003). Pearls of wisdom for clinical teaching: Expert educators reflect. *Journal of Midwifery & Women's Health, 48*(6), 482–484.

Merriam-Webster's Dictionary. (2012). Mentor definition. Retrieved from http://www.merriam -webster.com/dictionary/mentor

Mullenbach, K. F., & Burggraf, V. (2012). A dedicated learning unit in long-term care: A clinical immersion for student nurses. *Geriatric Nursing, 33*(1), 63–67.

Veeramah, V. (2012). What are the barriers to good mentoring? *Nursing Times, 108*(39), 12–15.

Weaver Moore, L., & Leahy, C. (2012). Implementing the new clinical nurse leader role while gleaning insights from the past. *Journal of Professional Nursing, 28*(3), 139–146.

The CNL as a Mentor

Bridget Graham

In February 2011, our hospital opened a 32-bed acuity-adaptable senior adult unit (3 Lacks). Staff members who had a passion for working with senior adults were hired for the unit. The majority of staff that was hired was competent in medical–surgical nursing but did not have any intermediate experience. In fact, fewer than 12% of the staff members were intermediate competent. CNLs and the unit's clinical nurse specialist (CNS), teamed together to develop and execute registered nurse (RN) intermediate education in order to provide the professional development, education, and coaching required to ensure safe and excellent patient care.

Our first objective was to determine the minimum competencies for an RN to be considered intermediate trained. The criteria were as follows:

- RNs must understand, verbalize, and demonstrate the use, effects, and monitoring requirements for the vasoactive drips used on our unit.
- RNs will understand, verbalize, and demonstrate the use of hemodynamic monitoring.
- RNs will recognize the signs/symptoms of and care for patients with respiratory and cardiac failure.
- RNs will understand, verbalize, and demonstrate continuing assessment and reassessment of the intermediate patient.
- RNs will verbalize and demonstrate the knowledge and ability to access additional resources during their shift (e.g., rapid responder, e-library, unit literature, CNLs, and CNS).
- RNs will complete 3 Lack's specific intermediate competency checklist.
- All nonintermediate RNs will have telemetry/EKG classes and 4 hours of didactic intermediate training.

A unit-specific intermediate competency tool was developed, which was to be completed by the end of training. This served as a record of completion. Charge nurses were the priority group to receive intermediate training. All RNs were paired with a CNL or the CNS for three 8-hour shifts. We worked one on one at the bedside to ensure education and monitor progress. The CNLs and the CNS worked the schedule of the nurse, whether it was days or nights. After three shifts, the RN and/

or the CNL and CNS could determine the need for continued education. Training would continue if the RN required additional education. Intermediate education binders were also placed on the unit as a resource for staff.

When we began our training and mentoring, only 11.76% of our RN staff members were intermediate trained. Currently, 76% of our RN staff members are intermediate trained. The CNLs and the CNS continue to mentor staff. We have increased the level of trust between staff and the CNLs/CNS. RNs who have completed intermediate training verbalize that they feel empowered to teach new RNs on the unit intermediate skills.

By training our staff to care for the intermediate patient, we have prevented transfers to a higher level of care. Handoffs to RNs on a higher level of care were decreased by 32%.

The financial impact of training the nurses was minimal. One-on-one training and mentoring with CNLs or the CNS came at no additional cost to the unit. We paired with staff on their already budgeted shifts and therefore incurred no cost.

The CNLs on 3 Lacks played an instrumental role in the mentoring and training of intermediate RNs for the new unit. Through collaboration, education, evidence-based practice for seniors, and application of clinical skills, the CNLs impacted patient safety on the unit and helped to ensure a higher standard for the level of care expected. Working closely with the RNs fostered the growth of knowledge and skills for the bedside nurse.

CNL Preceptor Role Satisfaction on a Dedicated Education Unit

Sherry Webb and Tommie Norris

Key terms: preceptor, satisfaction, clinical nurse leader, dedicated education units, clinical teachers

Aim: To describe CNL preceptor role satisfaction

The role of the preceptor is critical to the achievement of the end-of-program competencies for Model C master's entry-level CNL students. Preceptor role satisfaction ensures preceptor continuity for students in adult health, pediatrics, acute care, leadership, target population diagnosis, and clinical leadership practicum courses.

Expert staff nurses on the dedicated education unit (DEU) were selected by the nurse manager, trained by the faculty at the university, and evaluated as DEU preceptors by students and faculty. Surveys of the DEU preceptors indicated overwhelming satisfaction with their role in working with CNL students, and preceptors expressed interest in serving in future courses. They believed that they provided realistic clinical opportunities, which helped students achieve their course outcomes, and they were proud of their students' successes. The DEU preceptors valued the relationships that they formed with their students and faculty and believed that the DEU partnership bridged the gap between academia and practice. They reported that they learned about quality, safety, risk reduction, and evidence-based practice from the students, which made them interested in returning to college to advance their education. Faculty served as ambassadors of the college and provided letters of recommendation for the CNL program. In addition, the DEU preceptors became more interested in pursuing achievement in the hospital's clinical ladder program for advancement. DEU preceptors received recognition from their colleagues, nursing leadership, hospital staff, patients, and families through verbal feedback, hospital newsletters, performance appraisals, and site visits by other organizations. Six clinical teachers received the preceptor of the year award presented during the College of Nursing Alumni Day awards celebration. DEU preceptor satisfaction is critical to the success of CNL student education.

NINE

The Clinical Nurse Leader Advisory Council: An Opportunity for Partnership and Synergy

■ Karen M. Ott

www Learning Objectives

- Define a clinical nurse leader advisory council
- Describe the importance and relevance of partnership and collaboration to the sustainment of the clinical nurse leader role
- Describe the role of the clinical nurse leader advisory council
- Develop a clinical nurse leader stakeholder advisory council charter that includes outcomes and deliverables

> An Advisory Board is composed of people with a genuine interest in your work and desire to see it done well.
>
> Susan Ward

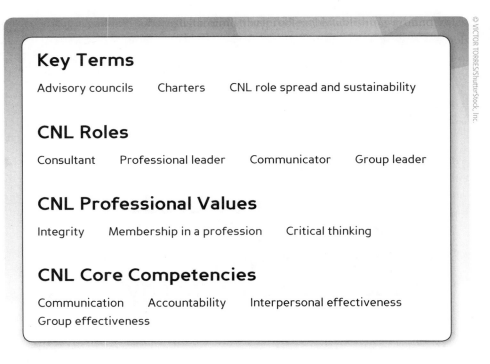

Key Terms

Advisory councils   Charters   CNL role spread and sustainability

CNL Roles

Consultant   Professional leader   Communicator   Group leader

CNL Professional Values

Integrity   Membership in a profession   Critical thinking

CNL Core Competencies

Communication   Accountability   Interpersonal effectiveness
Group effectiveness

Introduction

A healthcare organization's decision to create an advisory council may be the single most important one made to ensure the spread and sustainability of the CNL program and create venues for mutual sharing among faculty, students, and other stakeholders. Many challenges are faced by organizations daily, especially when a major change is introduced. Introducing a change to the nursing profession presents no less of a challenge given that staff roles are often duplicative, overlapping, and steeped in tradition. An advisory council can be a valuable asset, providing both the authority and influence for organizational change.

Using the CNL Advisory Council to Enhance Partnership and Collaboration

A CNL advisory council that provides a forum for academics, students, and healthcare members to engage in synergistic partnership and collaboration is an invaluable resource that increases the visibility of the CNL role. The council's combined knowledge, experience, and vision positions an organization to achieve the best course of action for the spread and sustainment of its CNL program.

> **Your Advisory Board members serve as a sounding board, offering ideas and expertise and giving you honest advice.**
>
> Susan Ward

CNL advisory councils may be established for distinctly different purposes. For example, the council may provide the vision, objectives, and goals; actively lead the development and formation of policies and processes; or advise, guide, and direct the CNL implementation program. The council provides a forum for CNL stakeholders to share expertise and serves as a resource network.

This chapter provides information and guidance for the establishment and maintenance of CNL advisory councils that serve one or more of these described purposes. Examples presented throughout the chapter describe aspects of a CNL advisory council established by a corporate office of a multisystem healthcare organization.

The concept of the CNL advisory council provides a vision and actionable goals and leads to the formation and implementation of policies and processes intended to assist and support individual medical facilities in spreading, adapting, adopting, and sustaining the CNL program. In addition, the CNL advisory council provides the following:

- An external assessment of the state of the CNL role implementation, including practice patterns and barriers
- Prioritization of CNL goals and help setting boundaries
- Identification of viable internal and external partnerships to provide post-graduate curriculum support and synergy
- Oversight of transition-to-practice programs to support synergy
- Oversight of a systems redesign (spread-adapt-adopt) implementation approach to create synergy
- Development of effective communication venues

Advisory Council Responsibilities

An advisory council's leader, facilitator/consultant, and members all have distinct roles. The following sections identify key responsibilities.

The Leader

The leader drives the council's organization and development and serves as its primary point of contact with the organization's formal leadership. Additionally, the leader's responsibilities include:

> The art of nursing requires us to alter the environment safely.
>
> Florence Nightingale

- Overseeing the development and implementation of the council charter, including the goals (this responsibility may be shared with a facilitator)
- Recruiting and interviewing members
- Identifying the meeting schedule
- Overseeing council operations
- Ensuring effective council structure, roles, and processes
- Evaluating the effectiveness of the council

The Facilitator/Consultant

According to Geoff Ball & Associates, an advisory council is best served when there is an environment of collaborative tension. A facilitator with expertise in process and organizational work may also provide consultation and balance the effectiveness of interactions (process) and initiatives/action items (content) to achieve a synergistic partnership (Geoff Ball & Associates, n.d.). See **Table 9-1** for factors the leader should consider when making the decision about whether to use a facilitator.

The Members

Advisory councils typically do not function independently or have legal authority; therefore, the initiatives and action items of the members may require leadership approval before goal implementation (McNamara, n.d.). Members' responsibilities include the following:

- *Program Planning and Review.* A small group of members may be valuable advisors in the early stages of CNL program planning and design. Council membership can be expanded at a later time.
- *Policy and Protocol Creation.* Members agree to take responsibility for the development of policies and protocols that will provide direction and support for the CNL program goals.

Table 9-1   Considerations for the Use of a Facilitator

Facilitator Is Needed When:	Facilitator Is Not Needed When:
Council members are not a previously formed group, accountable to each other, nor will likely work interdependently on a regular basis	Council members are a formed and cohesive team
The purpose and the goals are not clearly understood	Members share a solid and recognized commitment to the purpose and goals
Neither group process nor content is clearly understood	Members understand group methods, tools, and the topics under discussion
The leader does not possess facilitation skills	The leader is skilled in negotiating, evoking response, and recognizing group dynamics
The leader wants to maximize his or her participation in all aspects of the meeting	The leader is able to fully participate, observe, and orchestrate process and content to meet desired outcomes
There are complex issues with multiple possible solutions and potential for conflict	The leader can remain objective and has no vested interest in one course of action over another

Source: Adapted from Geoff Ball & Associates. (n.d.). *Making facilitation work for you: A guide to using facilitation and selecting facilitators.* Retrieved from http://www.geoffballfacilitator.com/ClientAwareness Guide.pdf

- *Subcommittees.* Members agree to establish and lead subcommittees to accomplish assigned tasks in specific areas, in specified time frames.
- *Marketing and Communication.* Members can be effective and influential champions for the CNL role both within and outside of the organization.

Subcommittees

It is advisable to establish subcommittees to assist with the development of council goals, especially goals that are complex or long term. Subcommittees should be led by a council member, with additional council members participating as needed. Each subcommittee must have a specific charge or set of tasks to address. All subcommittee recommendations for policy and process changes should be approved by the entire council. Whether established as continuing (for the duration of the goal) or ad-hoc (one time), subcommittees can provide valuable expertise and diversity for the council (McNamara, n.d.). As the aforementioned example of the CNL advisory council at a corporate office of a multisystem healthcare organization matured, a CNL implementation and evaluation service was formed to provide consultation services to facilities, patient care units, and to individuals, as well as to academic partners.

Getting Started

Draft the Charter

A charter serves two main objectives: to formally establish a council and clarify its purpose, and to indentify its goals. A typical charter contains seven headings: (1) Purpose, (2) Charge (outcomes and deliverables), (3) Chair, (4) Membership, (5) Strategies Used (methods/approach), (6) Meeting Requirements (types/frequency), and (7) Reporting Requirements (interaction with the organizational leadership). See **Figure 9-1** for an example.

Recruit Members

As previously stated, the strength and effectiveness of an advisory council lies in the commitment, contribution, and influence of its members. Leaders must recruit and select members with diverse opinions and experiences who can think strategically about the CNL role to "engage with the topic, build understanding, create new ideas, support each other, bring the outside world into the group, and the work of the group to the outside world" (Geoff Ball & Associates, n.d.).

The following recruiting guidelines from Carter McNamara can make the recruitment process more effective (McNamara, n.d.). The leader should consider the following actions:

> **Develop and distribute a questionnaire or application form that will serve to recruit prospective council members.** In addition to asking for basic biographical information, include questions that will elicit their purpose in applying for membership, their relevant skills, interests, personal and professional goals, and their value to the council and to its goals. Identify the terms and conditions of membership—for example, term length, role, and responsibilities.

Figure 9-1   Sample CNL Advisory Council Charter

Purpose: Develop and implement processes to engage, guide, and support individual medical facilities to spread, adapt, adopt, and sustain the CNL program at all medical facilities by 2016; provide consultative assistance to individuals for CNL implementation; and develop a CNL transition-to-practice program pilot to augment the postgraduate orientation and mentoring of newly graduated CNLs

Charge: Outcomes and deliverables
- Create conditions and build on staff skills that lead, promote, and support high-performing microsystems within facilities
- Empower facility macro- and microsystems leaders through a systems redesign spread-adapt-adopt approach centered on the CNL role
- Create a CNL implementation and evaluation service to provide consultation, guidance, and other assistance to facilities
- Develop a formal CNL residency/transition-to-practice program pilot to begin in 2012

Chair: Chief nursing officer and medical director

Membership: Practice representatives from the corporate office, program manager for the CNL implementation and evaluation service, facility nurse executives and microsystems staff from two to three facilities, staff from a regional engineering resource center (RERC) to lead the systems redesign work, and academic representatives

Strategies Used: Methods/approach
- Use cohorts of four to eight medical facilities that represent early CNL adopters, midway CNL adopters, and those that have not started to implement the role to lead and support systems redesign through projects that improve the work at the microsystems level
- Use staff and fiscal resources to deliver a wide range of consultative services to individuals, nurse managers, and nurse executives, as well as to local academic partners for the implementation and sustainment of the CNL role

Meeting Requirements: Types/frequency
- Initial "kick-off" meeting with cohort facility leadership followed by three collaborative virtual module sessions using virtual Blackboard technology to assist the staff to complete the work
- Weekly meetings to provide updates from the subcommittee to the leaders and to receive feedback and necessary support

Reporting Requirements: Reporting schedule details
Updates provided to the chief nursing officer quarterly until the advisory council's 2016 strategic goal of implementing the CNL role systemwide is attained

Keep an updated list of prospective council members. Interview the nominees who are being considered for selection to acquaint them with the role and responsibilities of the members and to identify any conflicts of interest or potential negative issues.

Invite prospective members to council meetings. Help the prospective member become acquainted with other council members and with council business.

Contact prospective members afterward. Determine whether the member is still interested in becoming an advisory council member and provide appropriate follow-up actions with organizational leadership if higher concurrence is required.

Provide new member orientation. Describe short- and long-term council purpose, authority, goals, and objectives, current activities, and past successes and challenges. Notify council members of actions taken.

Advisory Council Meetings

Plan and Organize the Meeting

The leader (or coleaders), along with the facilitator if applicable, agrees on meeting goals and deliverables, intended audience, meeting time frames, and all required logistical support.

When planning the meeting, (Burke et al., 2002) recommend that the leader consider the following:

Goals
- What are the overarching goals for the meeting?
- What specifically needs to be accomplished at the meeting?
- How much time is needed for each goal or task to be accomplished?

Participants
- Are the right people invited?
- Can everyone participate as needed?

Logistical Support
- What meeting space and A/V equipment needs to be obtained?
- Are members required to travel? If so, does lodging need to be reserved?
- Do conference call lines need to be established?

Meeting Agenda
The agenda should:

- Identify the goals, date, time, location, and list of tasks to be accomplished

- Be distributed 1 to 2 weeks before the meeting to allow members to understand the expectations and prepare for what is ahead
- Allocate a block of time for each group of participants and group of tasks to create an environment of energy and interest and to stimulate ideas
- Ensure adequate time to achieve meeting goals

See **Figure 9-2** for a sample advisory council meeting agenda.

Conduct the Meeting

The leader (or coleaders), along with the facilitator/consultant, must be present throughout the entire meeting to set the purpose and welcome the group. Specific actions include the following at every meeting (Burke et al., 2002):

- Reviewing the charter, goals, and time lines to assist the members in understanding the purpose of the collaborative
- Using a collective exercise to identify members' expectations and desires
- Identifying members' challenges and successes at subsequent meetings. Ask, "What do you need to get to the next step/complete this task?"
- Refocusing the group when situations impede the program, such as the following:
  - Persistent sidebar conversations
  - Never-ending discussion
  - Continual delay in returning from breaks
  - Negative conflict
  - Group is not staying on task
- Not intervening to refocus the group if all the participants are engaged in productive discussion to redefine goals, initiatives, or time lines, particularly when sufficient and valid information is present
- Assisting the group to develop a clear scope of practice for the CNL role from a leadership, practice, and strategic perspective to identify the benefits and value, using kickoff slides to create contexts that include the following:
  - Identify ways to perceive the benefit and value of the role
  - Define opportunities and ways to improve CNL practice and role implementation
  - Identify strategies to get leadership buy-in and support as opposed to lip service

Figure 9-2   Sample CNL Advisory Council Meeting Agenda

CNL Advisory Council Meeting Agenda
Initial Meeting
[Date]

Meeting Purpose:
1. Undertake a collective exercise (office of nursing services leader)
   a. Discuss the CNL role from a leadership, practice, and strategic perspective to iden-tify the benefits and value, with kickoff slides to create context
   b. Identify ways sites can perceive the benefit and value of the role
   c. Define opportunities and ways to improve CNL practice and role implementation
   d. Identify strategies to get leadership buy-in and support as opposed to lip service
2. Discuss the spread collaborative design (regional engineering resource center [RERC] leader)
   a. Understand the purpose of the collaborative: Work with early adopter/champion sites, sites that are making progress, and sites that are unable to adopt the role
   b. Understand the "pilot" and the subsequent team goals/purpose: Enable pilot sites to initiate the role with success; enable subsequent team sites to take advantage of the spread initiative
3. Develop the collaborative team agenda framework (RERC and chief nursing officer as facilitators)
4. Develop key metrics for each collaborative to measure the success of their CNL program (RERC)
5. Clarify management responsibilities (RERC leader/facilitator)
   a. Periodic monitoring and oversight
   b. Commitment

Meeting Deliverables:
1. Develop the collaborative team agenda framework:
   a. Premeeting agenda for medical facility nurse executives/chief medical officer before the beginning of each new collaborative cohort ("voice of the customer" exercise)
   b. Establish collaborative team meeting frequency
   c. Identify collaborative team goals, objectives, purpose, and responsibilities
   d. Identify facility leadership responsibilities

~~~~~~

AGENDA:

10:00–10:15—Welcome/Group Introductions:
• Members introduce themselves and identify their experience

10:15–11:30—Collective Exercise (nurse leaders):
• Discuss the CNL role from a leadership, practice, and strategic perspective to identify the benefits and value, with kick-off slides to create context
• Identify ways sites can perceive the benefit and value of the role
• Define opportunities and ways to improve CNL practice and role implementation
• Identify strategies to get leadership buy-in and support as opposed to lip-service

Figure 9-2   Sample CNL Advisory Council Meeting Agenda (continued)

11:30–1:00—Working Lunch:
Discuss the spread collaborative design (RERC leader):
- Understand the purpose of the collaborative: Work with early adopter/champion sites, sites that are making progress, and sites that are unable to adopt the role
- Understand the "pilot" and the subsequent team goals/purpose: Enable pilot sites to initiate the role with success; enable subsequent team sites to take advantage of the spread initiative

1:00–2:00—Develop Collaborative Team Agenda Framework (corporate office and RERC leaders/facilitator)

Develop an agenda for the facility nurse executive/chief medical officer premeeting to be scheduled before the beginning of each new learning session cohort
- Establish collaborative team meeting frequency
- Identify collaborative team goals, objectives, purpose, and responsibilities
- Identify facility leadership responsibilities

2:00–3:00—Develop Key Metrics for Each Collaborative Team to Measure CNL Program Success (RERC leader)

3:00–3:30—Clarify Member Responsibilities (RERC leader)
- Periodic monitoring and oversight
- Commitment

3:30–4:00—Wrap-up/Identify Next Steps (All)

Evaluate the Meeting

The leader (and facilitator/consultant) should objectively evaluate the meeting as close to the conclusion as possible.

Follow Through

The leader should communicate periodically with council members to clarify tasks, identify obstacles, reset priorities, and provide support for the completion of all action items. Leaders may ask the question of the members, "Where do we go from here?" (from a policy, clinical, and healthcare perspective) or, "What will the CNL role look like and where does it fit?"

Evaluate the Effectiveness of the Council

It is suggested that the leader (with the facilitator) perform an annual self-assessment of the council to determine whether or not the goals and objectives of the council are being met (Campaign Consultation, Inc., n.d.). See **Figure 9-3** for a sample meeting evaluation.

Figure 9-3   An Advisory Council Self-Assessment Sample

Sample Meeting Evaluation

Name (optional):

Date: __/__/__

Please evaluate the clarity and relevance of the following elements:

Meeting objectives:

_____Excellent

_____Above average

_____Average

_____Poor

Comments:

Meeting tasks:

_____Excellent

_____Above average

_____Average

_____Poor

Comments:

Time dedicated to each task:

_____Excellent

_____Above average

_____Average

_____Poor

Comments:

Please evaluate the knowledge and skill of the facilitator:

_____Excellent

_____Above average

_____Average

_____Poor

_____Not applicable

Comments:

Maintaining and Sustaining the Council

It is advisable to undertake periodic maintenance measures to ensure the group sustains its value to the organization. The leader should intermittently:

- Ensure that the council goals remain relevant and aligned with the organization's overall mission and vision
- Engage new members to inject fresh energy into the group
- Review the structure and schedule to ensure appropriate alignment with members' sense of purpose, goals, contributions, and outside workload
- Provide the members with individual recognition and thanks and feedback on the progress of meeting the group goals (U.S. Department of Education, 2008)

Summary

- The decision to use an advisory council to enhance and sustain the CNL role is paramount to the success of an organization's CNL program.
- The first critical step is the development of a charter with a clearly defined purpose and identification of major goals.
- Recruiting and sustaining a diverse group of qualified, visionary, committed members to create and lead an effective course of action does not have to be complicated.
- Involving interprofessional stakeholders to facilitate meetings can be beneficial in promoting the CNL role beyond nursing domains and engaging other disciplines.

www Reflection Questions
© Arenacreative/Dreamstime.com

1. What are key goals or action steps that can be achieved by a CNL advisory council?
2. What types of academic and clinical members are best suited for a CNL advisory council?
3. What other types of members can add value to the council's work?
4. What synergy can exist between practice and academia, CNLs and nurse managers, and CNLs and physicians?

Learning Activities

© Arenacreative/Dreamstime.com

1. Request to observe a CNL advisory council meeting
2. Describe potential advisory group goals for:
   a. Clinical team expectations for safety and quality
   b. Patient and the healthcare expectations for care
   c. Provider expectations for clinical outcomes and teamwork
   d. The CNL role in a team-centered healthcare system

References

Burke, D. W., Donahoe, M., Hirzel, R., Mather, L., Morgenstern, G., Ruete, N., Smith, E., Starzynski, D., & Stoddard, J. (2002, May). *Basic facilitation skills.* The human leadership and development division of the American Society for Quality. The association for quality and participation. *The international association of facilitators.*

Campaign Consultation, Inc. (n.d.). *Advisory council member self-assessment.* Retrieved from http://vistacampus.org/file.php/1/viewfinder/external_documents/Board-Advisory_Council _Self-Assessment.pdf

Geoff Ball & Associates. (n.d.). *Making facilitation work for you: A guide to using facilitation and selecting facilitators.* Retrieved from http://www.geoffballfacilitator.com/ClientAwareness Guide.pdf

McNamara, C. (n.d.). All about facilitation, group skills and group performance management. Retrieved from http://managementhelp.org/grp_skll/facltate/facltate.htm

U. S. Department of Education. (2008, April). Building an effective advisory council. Mentoring Resource Center, No. 21. Retrieved from http://educationnorthwest.org/webfm_send/232

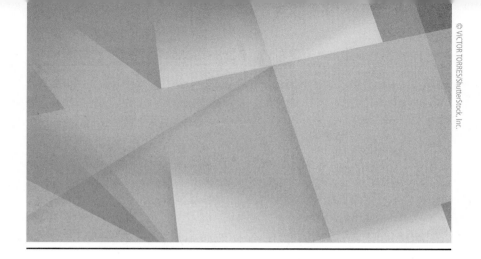

UNIT 3
Achieving a High-Reliability Organization

TEN

Creating a Value-Driven Approach to Care in a High-Reliability Organization

■ Laura Archbold and Patricia L. Thomas

---

www **Learning Objectives**
© Arenacreative/Dreamstime.com

- Define high-reliability organization
- Discuss key strategies for creating a high-reliability organization
- Discuss the characteristics of a high-reliability organization and evidence-based practice culture
- Define value and discuss the relevance of safety and economics for the clinical nurse leader role in a high-reliability organization
- Define enterprise risk management, identify key benefits, and discuss the relationship to value-driven care
- Discuss the role of the clinical nurse leader in value-driven, high-performing microsystems

> In healthcare, we get results from people's exceptional efforts in the face of imperfect circumstances.
>
> **Mark Graban**

Key Terms

High-reliability organization   Evidence-based practice   Value

Value-driven care   Safety   Economic value   Risk management

Enterprise risk management   Root cause analysis (RCA)

CNL Roles

Advocate   Catalyst   Integrator

Broker   Risk averter   Member of a profession

CNL Professional Values

Accountability   Outcome management   Quality improvement

Integrity   Financial stewardship

Social justice   Interprofessional teamwork

CNL Core Competencies

Data analysis   Critical thinking   Assessment

Ethical decision making   Communication   Resource management

Information and healthcare technologies

Design/manage/coordinate care

Creating a Value-Driven Approach to Care in a High-Reliability Organization

The "triple aim," as defined by the Institute of Healthcare Improvement, calls for "improving the individual experience of care; improving the health of populations; and reducing the per capita costs of care for populations" (Berwick, Nolan, & Whittington, 2008, p. 759). The only means by which this can be accomplished is through improving existing care delivery systems across the continuum of care. Although multiple care providers should be involved in these efforts, in multidisciplinary teams CNLs are uniquely positioned by their organizational skills and clinical education to be key players in such improvement efforts.

A triad of organizational constructs contributes to the environment in which the CNL functions; those concepts involving high reliability, evidence-based medicine, and process excellence provide a sound performance framework from which to function. High-reliability organizations (HROs) need to focus on mindfulness and perfection, according to the June 2012 report from The Joint Commission. Evidence-based medicine (EBM) "means integrating individual clinical expertise with the best available external clinical evidence from systematic research" (Sackett, Straus, Richardson, Rosenberg, & Haynes, 2000). Process excellence entails continuous improvement through the elimination of waste and the reduction of variation. As the CNL embraces and employs the constructs of HRO, EBM, and process excellence, the capacity for enhancing the value of the organization improves.

In process excellence terms, items are identified as adding value when the customers' needs are met. Often this entails meeting the following three challenges:

1. *Identifying the customer.* Customers in health care are the patient, families, healthcare providers, the community, and payers. The challenge, in light of reform, is to redefine the true value of the service to be delivered to each customer.
2. *Defining value in terms of the whole product or service.* The delivery of a product or service occurs across a continuum. The Affordable Care Act challenge is to improve care across the care continuum, providing it to an increased percentage of the population.
3. *Achieving target cost.* When the target cost is identified, the key stakeholders across the continuum works collaboratively to maintain or lower the target (Womack & Jones, 2003, pp. 31–36).

The concept of value is important in today's healthcare landscape, as the economic model transforms from a focus on volume (quantity) to a focus on activities that contribute to high-value outcomes (quality). The CNL has the capability and capacity to greatly impact value-based purchasing, which is defined as the unification of "information on the quality of health care, including patient outcomes and health status, with data on the dollar outlays going towards health. It focuses on managing the use of the health care system to reduce inappropriate care and to identify and reward the best-performing providers" (Meyer, Rybowski, & Eichler, 1997).

The CNL's role in creating a value-driven approach to care in an HRO is dependent on the optimized environment of high reliability, the incorporation of EBP (evidence-based practice) concepts, and the CNL's ability to help create those two constructs. The CNL's role in creating value is further enhanced when the principles of process excellence are applied. This chapter explores how each of the constructs of the environment contributes to value and the role that the CNL plays in the formation of both. The highly customized CNL process excellence program is defined from a curricula and application perspective.

A High-Reliability Environment

The constructs of high reliability, EBM, and process excellence, when present in an organization and utilized by the CNL, contribute to making it value driven. Each of the constructs contributes distinctive elements to the environment; the constructs are interdependent and synergistic. For the CNL to be successful in the pursuit of delivering value, the organization must support these constructs and the CNL must be knowledgeable about their application.

HROs, as discussed earlier, need to focus on mindfulness and perfection. These foci are outcomes of several core principles that move organizations toward the ultimate goal of high reliability; consistent quality results, in every location, every time. Multiple industries possess characteristics that challenge their ability to deliver such consistency. From the aviation industry to correctional services, the constructs of high reliability exist. In health care, HROs deliver an outcome of "exceptionally safe, consistently high quality care" (Agency for Healthcare Research and Quality [AHRQ], 2008, p. 6). An exploration of the characteristics and principles will assist in the understanding of the CNL's approach to creating value-driven HROs.

Organizations face myriad challenges that contribute to their ability to perform consistently. Healthcare organizations are not unique in that they demonstrate many, if not all, of these challenges, including the following identified by AHRQ:

- Hypercomplexity: multiteam systems that must coordinate processes and performance to provide consistent results.
- Tight coupling: closely aligned teams whose members are dependent upon one another for the completion of tasks contributing to overall performance.
- Extreme hierarchical differentiation: well-defined roles requiring extensive coordination; those team members considered "expert," regardless of rank, assume the position of "decision-maker" during times of crisis.

- Multiple decision makers in a complex communication network: many positions that make decisions that are interdependent and interconnected.
- High degree of accountability: high level of responsibility and liability when errors occur.
- Need for frequent, immediate feedback: continuous need for communication and feedback, presenting ongoing opportunities to make adjustments.
- Compressed time constraints: processes, systems, people, and culture to identify when time is needed to consistently perform as desired (AHRQ, 2008).

Health care is replete with these challenges. The CNL, as the leader of the microsystem, is immersed within them and must be well armed both with awareness of the challenges and with strategies to mitigate them.

Respecting the following five core principles can help in addressing the challenges that most complex organizations face on their journey to becoming highly reliable:

1. *Sensitivity to operations*: HROs continuously monitor processes and systems to identify and eliminate errors. Developing associates with "situational awareness" and a sensitivity to operations facilitates an environment that promotes consistent performance. CNLs in their microsystems are well positioned for early identification of defects to address upstream impacts. By engaging his or her team members in process and quality improvements, the CNL uses their knowledge of systems, quality improvement, and measurement to lead interdisciplinary teams to address concerns that could lead to errors.

2. *Reluctance to simplify*: HROs understand that their work is complex and realize that one-dimensional systems will not suffice to resolve the challenges. Associates in HROs recognize that processes and systems evolve and can fail in new and unimaginable ways. With the recognition of complexity and the acceptance that many of the systems cannot be simplified, healthcare associates in HROs remain vigilant and simplify those processes that they can, using multidisciplinary teams trained in systems design. CNLs consider this when they examine and streamline processes.

3. *Preoccupation with failure*: HROs continually consider the prospect that their systems may fail and that errors may occur. Healthcare organizations anticipate that these errors will put patients at risk and therefore when the errors or "near misses" occur, they are investigated and systems are redesigned to

mitigate future errors. CNLs use this knowledge when they engage in process redesign.

4. *Deference to expertise*: HROs respect knowledge and reinforce a culture where the associates with the greatest knowledge take the lead in resolving issues. In such a culture, the leadership defers to those with the best understanding; in this culture, it is also the responsibility of those with the knowledge to share it. In creating teams to address practice and process concerns, CNLs use this strategy to engage all the parties that touch a process, recognizing that clinicians, support staff, and ancillary department team members influence outcomes and need to be involved in process design and improvements.

5. *Resilience*: HROs strive to develop a capacity to respond quickly to errors. HROs are dependent on the result of honoring expertise and a relentless attention to process. CNLs, possessing nursing expertise and a foundational knowledge of process excellence, are integral stakeholders in the creation and sustainability of high reliability in their organizations.

Evidence-Based Practice

A second factor that shapes the CNL's environment is EBP, earlier defined as an integration of "individual clinical expertise with the best available external clinical evidence from systematic research"; initially this concept was termed evidence-based medicine (EBM; Sackett et al., 2000). Additional components of EBP are patients, who have their own expectations for care and the value to be derived from the encounter. Clearly a contributing factor in the creation of an HRO, EBP places emphasis on knowledge and expertise. And just as clearly, the CNL is in a position to play an active role in each of the HRO and EBP environments.

Sackett and colleagues identified five essential steps in the EBM/EBP process that facilitate the integration of internal practice, external practice, and the expectations of the patient:

1. Assess the patient: Start with the patient—the clinical problem or question arises from the patient.

2. Ask the question: Construct a well-built clinical question derived from the case.

3. Acquire the evidence: Select the appropriate resource(s) and conduct a search.

4. Appraise the evidence: Appraise the evidence for its validity (closeness to the truth) and applicability (usefulness in clinical practice).
5. Apply: Talk with the patient. Return to the patient—integrate that evidence with clinical expertise and patient preference and apply it to practice. (Sackett et al., 2000).

The outlined process embeds a discipline and standardization that impels high reliability. The CNL, through education and practice, develops the expertise to accurately assess the patient and ask appropriate questions. Through the acquisition of evidence and appraisal, the CNL, proficient in the microsystem, determines the degree of usefulness. To close, the CNL, through the relationship established with the patient, integrates the determined evidence with the patient's preference to deliver EBP.

Process Excellence

Just as healthcare HROs are synergistic with EBP, so are they with process excellence. Process excellence can be appreciated as the vehicle for enhancing HROs and EBP, through a continuous improvement cycle using proven methodologies that span all industries. Process excellence represents the embodiment of all types of process, quality, or performance improvement: Lean, Six Sigma, and total quality management (TQM). Process improvement practitioners have long understood that the persons who are most effective in leading quality initiatives are those who understand the principles of improvement and are closest to the work that requires improvement. The CNL, enhanced with process excellence skills, becomes that effective person who leads quality initiatives as they work within their microsystems.

A microsystem is defined as the smallest unit on the front line of healthcare delivery systems. The clinical microsystem provides direct care to patients and families, establishing the essential building blocks of the organization. It is within this microsystem that the quality of care is defined and the reputation of the organization is created (Nelson, Batalden, & Godfrey, 2007). To prepare CNLs to become process excellence practitioners for microsystems, an understanding of improvement methodology within the construct of microsystems and integration of improvement methodology into the CNL curriculum is essential. The creation of HROs in health care depends on EBP and a culture that embraces continuous improvement through process excellence. The CNL, as a practitioner of EBM and process excellence, is seen as a leader of the movement toward high reliability. A further discussion of the CNL process excellence curricula will be explored later in this chapter.

Healthcare Economics

More than in any other time in history, the cost of health care has become current household conversation. As health reform and the implementation of the Affordable Care Act have gotten under way, the cost of care in the United States has come into question. Compared to other civilized countries, the United States lags in clinical care outcomes but nevertheless has the distinction of being the most costly system in the world. The Institute of Medicine (IOM) conducted a workshop series, *Healthcare Imperative: Lowering Costs and Improving Outcomes*, which found that, "The United States spends far more on health care than any other nation. In 2009, health care costs reached $2.5 trillion—nearly 17 percent of the GDP. Yet despite this spending, health outcomes in the United States are considerably below those in other countries." (IOM, 2011). In light of this data, the relationship between process, structure, and outcomes takes on greater importance, especially as we strive to reduce errors, bring greater consistency to care delivery, and develop process improvements to decrease waste. Likewise, as we look at principles of high reliability and value, the need for evidence-based interventions and desired outcomes will be key. Elements of pay for performance rest on the assumption that consistent EBP is the most cost-effective care, building the line of sight between high reliability, cost, error prevention, risk reduction, and the role of the CNL.

Risk Management

The definition of high reliability implies a parallel path of assessment of risk and risk management in managing microsystems. Once it is recognized that clinical operations need interdependent microsystems to deliver safe, appropriate, and consistent care, risks can be managed through a lens of preoccupation with error. Traditionally, risk assessment and risk management have been retrospectively viewed in clinical situations that did not produce a desired outcome. The landscape of healthcare delivery today is focused on quality and safety and is dedicated to understanding systems and processes that result in outcomes. Commitment to value, rather than volume, and strategic initiatives aligned for reliability, consistency, and safety are gaining attention as organizations strive for seamless, efficient, error-free care. With the development of the CNL role, organizations have embraced that those closest to the patient (in a microsystem) have unique and desirable insights about where gaps exist in our current processes, which are ripe for contributing to errors.

In designing the CNL role, the AACN (2007) established risk anticipation, or the ability to critically evaluate and anticipate risks to client safety, as a critical component of the role. At the systems level (risk to any client) and the individual level (by review of patient history and comorbidities), CNLs anticipate risk when new technology, equipment, treatment regimens, or medication therapies are introduced (AACN, 2007). Tools for risk analysis, for example failure mode evaluation analysis, root cause analysis, and quality improvement methodologies, are important for the CNL. Because CNLs are embedded in a microsystem, their knowledge of systems, leadership, quality improvement, and measurement uniquely qualifies them to scan the clinical environment to identify potential risk.

The CNL Role

The role of the CNL is that of a leader in the delivery of care to patients, in sickness and in wellness, across the continuum of care. In this assigned leadership position, the CNL is responsible for myriad accountabilities that are inclusive of care design and delivery, quality monitoring and improvement, collaboration and team management, education, and advocacy (AACN, 2007). Through the application of the EBP model, the CNL provides appropriate care to individuals, groups, and the community. Plans of care are evaluated for efficacy. The CNL is intentional with regard to the identification of performance metrics and outcome monitoring. As a team leader, the CNL provides management and is a model for interdisciplinary collaboration. The CNL influences the team and provides stewardship of resources— human, material, and financial. Information management and technology are tools used by the CNL to perform their work. In total, the CNL is responsible for integrating the care of a specified group of patients at the point of care.

In order to optimally fulfill the role, the CNL must be prepared to meet the assigned responsibilities. The AACN lists the following 10 assumptions for preparing the CNL:

1. Practice is at the microsystems level.
2. Client care outcomes are the measure of quality practice.
3. Practice guidelines are based on evidence.

4. Client-centered practice is intra- and interdisciplinary.
5. Information will maximize self-care and client decisionmaking.
6. Nursing assessment is the basis for theory and knowledge development.
7. Good fiscal stewardship is a condition of quality care.
8. Social justice is an essential nursing value.
9. Communication technology will facilitate the continuity and comprehensiveness of care.
10. The CNL must assume guardianship for the nursing profession. (AACN, 2007, pp. 6–10)

These assumptions for preparing the CNL are important to note, as they reflect the relationship to EBP and the desire to embed process excellence training into the CNL curriculum in order to best facilitate success.

Process Excellence Training

The AACN, in collaboration with nurse executives, health systems, and educators, proposed the CNL as a nursing solution to address gaps in healthcare quality by addressing patient needs, safety, and quality improvement through a systematic and deliberate approach to implementing EBP, quality management, and clinical leadership at the point of care. CNLs are prepared as advanced generalists accountable for identifying outcomes of practice on their units. This can be accomplished by participating in a range of quality improvement projects aimed at collecting and creating evidence, leading multidisciplinary teams, and incorporating interventions with the greatest likelihood of producing high-quality care outcomes (AACN, 2007; Bowcutt, Wall, & Goolsby, 2006).

For the CNL to function in this manner—to lead through quality and process improvement—foundational knowledge is needed. Microsystems, as the smallest unit of the frontline healthcare delivery system, can also be considered the smallest unit of a value stream. In process excellence terms, a value stream is defined as all of the activities that are required to bring a specific product, whether it be goods or a service, to the customer; in health care, the product is often a combination of goods and services. Critical tasks for managing the value stream are problem solving, information management, and transformation. Problem solving entails following an idea from detailed design through to product launch. Information management includes order taking, scheduling, and creating detailed documentation. Transformation entails the movement from raw materials to delivery of the completed product to the customer (Womack & Jones, 2003, p. 19).

Individual value streams may be composed of multiple microsystems, all of which contribute to the products or services of the whole system. It is important to note that products and services may also be produced at the microsystem level.

The Value Stream Leadership Course

With the understanding that the CNL is a key leader of microsystems and that microsystems are an elemental structure within a value stream, the decision was made to create customized curricula for the CNL. The Value Stream Leadership course, cocreated by Trinity Health and the University of Detroit Mercy, was structured to deliver on the process excellence constructs of efficiency and value, thus promoting quality, customer service, and cost effectiveness. The following topics were core to the curricula:

- Value: Concepts of value contribution, Kano model; waste
- Flow: Continuous flow versus batching, push, pull
- Problem solving: Five "whys," decision trees, Ishikawa diagrams
- Value streams: Components, mapping
- Metrics: Appropriate identification of process and outcomes measures

These concepts were taught over a period of 2 days through a combination of lecture, table exercises, and simulation as part of the health systems leadership course. A second component of project management was added to the course to support the leadership and quality components of the CNL curriculum. Each student was required to complete a process improvement project over a 15-week semester in the microsystem leadership course and the quality management course. An 8-hour day focused on project management assisted the CNL in understanding the phases of a project and the components of managing teams, financial aspects and metrics, and time lines. Projects for these courses were identified by the chief nursing officer and the clinical department directors as a means to support organizational learning. Each CNL selected projects he or she was most interested in and then developed a project plan, starting with problem identification, and then proceeding through implementation and sustainability using the organization's quality improvement philosophy.

Conclusion

The era of high-reliable care that is effective, efficient, seamless, and cost effective is the CNL's playground! Positioned as a clinical leader in microsystems that span the continuum of care, the CNL has the opportunity to emerge as a leader in creating HROs. CNL education has focused on quality improvement, risk anticipation, measurement, monitoring, and assessing care practices. Additionally, CNLs serve as mentors and team leaders in pursuit of improvements in the patient care experience. CNLs have the opportunity to optimize the care environment of HROs and EBP to create value when the principles of process excellence are applied.

Summary

- The principles of high reliability, EBP, and process excellence are integrated into the CNL role and serve as the foundational elements to improve quality and patient safety.
- Continuous systematic assessment of the clinical environment is essential for situational awareness in HROs.
- Hypercomplexity is a characteristic of health care, and respect of this complexity is essential for meaningful quality improvement.

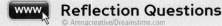

WWW   Reflection Questions

© Arenacreative/Dreamstime.com

1. If you were having lunch with a nurse on your unit and were asked to define high reliability, how would you answer?
2. Think about a recent experience on your unit where an error occurred. Can you identify elements of high reliability that were enacted? Are there elements of high reliability that might have prevented the error?
3. Consider a "near miss" that you or a coworker has experienced. What process was undertaken to review the incident? Were any tools used to document it? What recommendations would you make based on the principles of high reliability and risk anticipation?

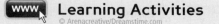

Learning Activities

1. Consider your most recent work shift. Identify a process that would benefit from a process excellence value stream review.

2. Obtain a copy of a policy or procedure that is commonly used on your work unit. Is there an evidence base that supports the steps in the policy or procedure? Were the references from literature published less than 5 years ago? Who was involved in the development of the policy or procedure?

References

American Association of Colleges of Nursing (AACN). (2007). White paper on the role of the clinical nurse leader. Retrieved from http://www.aacn.nche.edu/publications/white-papers/cnl

Agency for Healthcare Research and Quality. (2008). Becoming a high reliability organization: Operational advice for hospital leaders. Retrieved from http://www.ahrq.gov/qual/hroadvice/

Berwick, D., Nolan, T., & Whittington J. (2008). The triple aim: Care, health, and cost. *Health Affairs, 27*(3), 759–769.

Bowcutt, M., Wall, J., & Goolsby, M. J. (2006). The clinical nurse leader: promoting patient-centered outcomes. *Nursing Administration Quarterly, 30*(2), 156–61.

Institute of Medicine (IOM). (2011). The healthcare imperative: Lowering costs and improving outcomes. Workshop series summary. Retrieved from http://www.iom.edu/Reports/2011/The-Healthcare-Imperative-Lowering-Costs-and-Improving-Outcomes.aspx

Meyer J., Rybowski L., & Eichler R. (1997). *Theory and reality of value-based purchasing: Lessons from the pioneers.* Rockville, MD: Agency for Health Care Policy and Research. AHCPR Publication No. 98-0004.

Nelson, E., Batalden, P., & Godfrey, M. (2007). *Quality by design: A clinical microsystems approach.* San Francisco, CA: Jossey-Bass.

Sackett, D., Straus, S., Richardson, S., Rosenberg, W., & Haynes, R. (2000). *Evidence-based medicine: How to practice and teach EBM* (2nd ed.). London, England: Churchill Livingston.

Womack, J. P., & Jones, D. T. (2003). *Lean thinking.* New York, NY: Free Press/Simon & Schuster.

Interdisciplinary Collaboration: The Role of the Clinical Nurse Leader

Miriam Bender

Aim: To explore the feasibility and acceptability of a CNL role to improve interdisciplinary collaboration within a fragmented acute care microsystem.

Background: Fragmented patient care is associated with preventable adverse healthcare outcomes. Interdisciplinary collaboration decreases fragmentation and improves patient care quality. The CNL role is theorized to provide the necessary leadership and competency skill base to impact interdisciplinary collaboration at the optimal organizational level, the point of care where most healthcare decisions are made.

Methods: This study used a descriptive nonexperimental design. CNL daily work-flow was developed to target empirical determinants of interdisciplinary collaboration. Descriptive data were collected from multiple stakeholders using an investigator-developed survey.

Results: Findings indicated that the integration of the role is feasible and acceptable to the microsystem healthcare team.

Conclusions: Preliminary evidence suggests that the CNL role may be an effective intervention to facilitate interdisciplinary collaboration. More research is needed to support the CNL role's association with microsystem interdisciplinary collaboration.

Implications for nursing management: The CNL role presents an innovative opportunity for clinical and administrative leadership to partner together to redesign a healthcare delivery system and improve patient care quality.

Bender, M., Connelly, C. D., & Brown, C. (2013). Interdisciplinary collaboration: The role of the clinical nurse leader. *Journal of Nursing Management, 21*(1), 165–174.

Reducing Fall Rates Using an Interdisciplinary Team Approach

▨ Bridget Graham

Falls are classified as a never event by Centers for Medicare and Medicaid Services (CMS). Falls can result in devastating and debilitating injury for the hospitalized senior adult, leading to increased lengths of stay and increases in healthcare costs. The total number of falls for fiscal year 2011 was 49. The fall rate for the 3 Lacks unit in FY2011 was 5.52 per 1,000 patient days, compared to the national benchmark of 3.88 per 1,000 patient days. The goal on 3 Lacks was to eliminate patient falls with injury by the end of FY2012 and to reduce the overall fall rate by 25%.

The CNL formed an interdisciplinary team that included registered nurses (RNs), patient care assistants (PCAs), leadership, a CNL, and a pharmacist. Using the Lean process and a DMAIC (define, measure, analyze, improve, control) process improvement method, the group started by defining the problem and measuring the current state. The next steps included a root cause analysis using the "6 Ms." The 6 Ms are materials, man, mother nature (environment), method, measurement, and machine. The root cause analysis assisted the group in getting to the causes that were contributing to our increased fall rate. After the root cause analysis was complete, the group proceeded to the improve phase and implemented several intereventions:

1. Staff must do 1:1 education with family and patient and document.
2. Implement the following standards of care on 3 Lacks:
   a. Use bed alarms and chair alarms for anyone with Morse scale > 45.
   b. Educate staff on the use of gait belts (provided in each room).
   c. Use bedside commode if patient gait unstable.
   d. Staff stay with the patient while in the bathroom.
   e. RN/physical therapist to complete white boards with specific plan such as up with 1 or 2, must use walker, etc.
   f. Create an individualized plan for each patient.
3. Pharmacist is reviewing medication lists daily of any patients with Morse Scale > 45 to identify meds that may be contributing to fall risk. Pharmacist will discuss changes with physician.

4. Discuss all falls in leadership group, getting to cause of the falls. Super huddles completed immediately after a fall with all staff on the unit.

5. CNLs to monitor and ensure that daily Morse scale is completed and safety actions are in place.

6. Hold staff accountable for lack of following standards/actions that put patients at risk.

7. Institute intentional hourly rounding.

8. Have targeted "lunch and learn" with PCAs specific to patient readiness for transfer, use of gait belts, etc.

9. Provide targeted education to student nurses.

Each intervention was assigned to someone and given a start and completion date. The group followed up on each interevention and its effectiveness.

In FY2011, our fall rate on 3 Lacks was 5.52. At the end FY2012, our fall rate was 4.03. This is a 27% reduction in our fall rate. We had no falls with injury in FY2012. The total number of falls in FY2011 was 49, compared to 38 in FY2012.

Our interdisciplinary falls team was able to positively impact our unit fall rate. A Lean process was utilized to help frame and direct the work group. As the group is now in the control phase of the project, we will continue to examine our compliance with the listed interventions; we are striving for the ultimate goal of zero patient falls.

ELEVEN

Quality Care and Risk Management

■ Patricia L. Thomas

- Demonstrate an understanding of the clinical nurse leader's role in microsystem quality improvement
- Gain confidence in assessing microsystems, gathering tools, and collecting information necessary to implement systematic quality improvement efforts
- Establish the linkage between organizational goals, strategies, measurement, and communication of the clinical nurse leader's quality improvement efforts
- Articulate the clinical nurse leader's role in achieving a culture of safety and efficiency through process and quality improvement
- Evaluate quality improvement strategies in the clinical nurse leader's clinical immersion experience

> Quality without science and research is absurd. You can't make inferences that something works when you have 60 percent missing data.
>
> **Peter Pronovost**

Key Terms

Organizational learning   Culture of safety   Quality improvement
Planning   Quality patient care and safety   Cyclical review
Needs assessment   Metrics and measurement
Evidence-based practice   Microsystems

CNL Roles

Member of a profession   Outcomes manager   Team manager
Information manager   Systems analyst/risk anticipator
Coordinator of care

CNL Professional Values

Accountability   Outcome measurement   Quality improvement
Interprofessional teams   Integrity   Financial stewardship
Microsystems management   Evidence-based practice
Social justice   Quality patient care and safety

CNL Core Competencies

Critical thinking   Ethical decision making
Member of a profession   Team leader   Communication
Assessment   Information and healthcare technologies
Healthcare systems and policy designer/manager/coordinator of care
Assessment environment of care manager
Nursing technology and resource management

Introduction

The American Association of Colleges of Nursing's (AACN's) role expectations
for the clinical nurse leader (CNL) place an emphasis on the need to redesign care

delivery for improved patient safety, effectiveness, and efficiency (AACN, 2007). Integral to the care delivery redesign process are multidisciplinary team members committed to excellence and quality improvement quantified through metrics and measurement. By acknowledging the need to decrease fragmentation of care in the delivery system, processes underlying care delays, redundancy or gaps in service, and dissatisfaction within provider, patient, and stakeholders groups, quality improvement offers a framework and methods to support changes in interrelated systems aimed toward better clinical and financial outcomes.

> **There is a bell curve for quality— a wide gap between the best care and the worst. There is another bell curve for costs— again, a wide gap. Surprisingly, the two curves do not match. And that means there is hope. Because if the two curves did match—if the best care were the most expensive—then we would be talking about rationing.**
>
> Gawande

Several landmark studies have influenced the trends in quality improvement to address real and pressing concerns in the U.S. health system. In 1999 the Institute of Medicine (IOM) published *To Err Is Human: Building a Safer Health System*, which stated that between 44,000 and 98,000 Americans die each year as a result of medical errors; this exceeds the loss of lives from car accidents, breast cancer, and AIDS. Additionally, the cost of preventable errors resulting in injury was reported at between $17 and $29 billion dollars. The fragmentation of the healthcare delivery system was identified as a major contributor to these errors. In response to these findings, building a safer, outcomes-driven care delivery system relying on quality improvement tools to increase efficiency, cost effectiveness, and high performance became a focus (AACN, 2007; The Joint Commission, 2008).

A second IOM report, *Crossing the Quality Chasm: A New Health Care System for the 21st Century* (2001), made an urgent call for change that emphasized safety, effectiveness, patient-centeredness, and care that is timely, efficient, and equitable. This landmark study stressed the environment of care and systems issues as pivot points that negatively impact safety and effectiveness, noting that the care patients receive in today's healthcare delivery system has become increasingly complex, with nurses simultaneously interacting with multiple systems, processes, and technologies (Nelson, Batalden, & Godfrey, 2007; Wiggins, 2008). In a follow-up report,

Health Professions Education: A Bridge to Quality, the IOM (2003) recommended that health professionals be educated to deliver patient-centered care as members of an interdisciplinary team, emphasizing implementation of evidence-based practices, quality improvement practices, and informatics (AACN, 2007).

In 2008, The Joint Commission published a report, *Health Care at the Crossroads: Guiding Principles for the Development of the Hospital of the Future*, which emphasized the increasing complexity of care delivery and the pace of change and innovations that make it difficult for clinicians to keep up. Recognizing that hospitalized patients have higher acuity, more comorbid conditions in need of management, and shortened hospital stays, The Joint Commission report stated that the average length of stay has decreased 25% since the 1980s. At the same time, the Food and Drug Administration has approved more than 500,000 new medical devices. Advances in pharmaceuticals and genomic developments have exploded into the health delivery landscape during this time period as well. Although advances in technology help improve patient outcomes, the volume of technology and the requisite knowledge to manage new technology have made care delivery more complex, with sometimes unforeseen opportunities for error. This multifaceted complexity weighs heavily on conscientious clinicians. To respond to these demands, The Joint Commission identified the CNL as the clinician best suited to manage the "real time" care of patients within the microsystem to ensure the use of evidence-based practices and quality improvement principles, measurement, and evaluation to improve patient care outcomes.

The CNL role creates an opportunity for new care models and team configurations in every delivery setting. Regulatory and accreditation pressures to increase safety and reduce costs are mounting as we examine health outcomes. Unprecedented attention to cost, dwindling human and financial resources, and acknowledgment of increasing complexity underpin the desire to systematically address historical practices that present threats to patient safety (The Joint Commission, 2008; Newhouse, 2006; Rusch & Bakewell-Sachs, 2007). The assumptions underpinning the CNL role competencies are translated into daily operational performance in a microsystem where the CNL interacts at the point of care across the care continuum. Cost evaluation, return on investment, and cost–benefit analyses will be essential to validate the CNL's impact on cost reductions in an environment where pay for performance and the expectation of reducing errors and improving safety and efficiency are paramount to future organizational success (Haase-Herrick, 2005; Hwang & Herndon, 2007). Anticipating risks that influence safety and care outcomes, the CNL is positioned to scan the practice environment to identify system issues that could result in error, harm, or added costs based on the underlying processes embedded in care delivery. CNLs are uniquely qualified by their education in advanced clinical knowledge, understanding of systems, attention to measurement and outcomes, and firm grounding in quality improvement principles to lead teams of clinical professionals through risk identification, assessment, and planning to improve patient safety.

Background

The AACN—in collaboration with nurse executives, health systems, and educators—proposed the CNL as a nursing solution to address gaps in healthcare quality by addressing patient needs, safety, and quality improvement through a systematic and deliberate approach to implementing evidence-based practice, quality management, and clinical leadership at the point of care. CNLs are prepared as advanced generalists who are accountable for identifying outcomes of practice on their units. CNLs can accomplish their goals by participating in a range of quality improvement projects aimed to collect and create evidence, by leading multidisciplinary teams, and by incorporating interventions with the greatest likelihood to produce high-quality care outcomes (AACN, 2007; Bowcutt, Wall, & Goolsby, 2006).

In 2008, Berwick, Nolan, and Whittington articulate the "triple aim" for health care, "improving the experience of care, improving the health of populations, and reducing per capita costs of health care" (p. 579). The preconditions include enrollment of an identified population, a commitment to universality for members, and the existence of an organization (an "integrator") that accepts responsibility for all three aims for that population. The organization's responsibilities highlight partnerships with patients and families, redesign of primary care, population health management, fiscal responsibility, and macrosystem integration. The CNL is positioned to address the triple aim and support organizational integration through meticulous application of quality and risk management principles and processes in microsystems to support the macrosystem integration.

Supporting a Culture of Safety

Given the general agreement that patient safety needs improvement, it is important for healthcare providers to have a consistent, clear, and concise definition of what quality is. Lohr (1990) defined quality as "...the degree to which health services for individuals and populations increase the likelihood of desired health outcomes and are consistent with current professional knowledge" (p. 4). Systematic, deliberate, and defined methods will be needed to measure, understand, improve, and communicate internal progress at the unit and organization level. Regulatory agencies and groups external to the organization (including professional organizations, payers, and policy makers) will also need this information to make policy decisions based on clear measurements, shared goals, and systematic approaches toward improvement (Hwang & Herndon, 2007; Newhouse, 2006).

CNLs are situated to mentor, coach, and guide multidisciplinary teams to enact the paradigm shift necessary to sustain a culture of safety found in the application of evidence-based practices and quality improvement. In addition to advanced clinical knowledge, CNLs examine the care delivery system from the perspective of individual patients or a microsystem population framework, recognizing the interrelated functions of process, information management, and outcomes (AACN, 2007; Nelson, Batalden, & Godfrey, 2007).

Risk Anticipation, Risk Assessment, and Risk Management

For many clinicians, discussion of "risk" conjures up visions of litigation, malpractice, and blame. Whereas risk management historically focused on reducing liability, in recent years risk management has been closely aligned to quality improvement through the identification of processes to reduce errors, increase communication, and develop standardization in processes to establish consistency in care. The American Society of Healthcare Risk Management (ASHRM, affiliated with the American Hospital Association) defines risk management as, "The identification, analysis, and evaluation of risk and the selection of the most advantageous method of treating it" (CHUBB, 2004, p. 4). This process involves risk identification, risk analysis, risk treatment, and evaluation of risk treatment strategies. Risk management encompasses the monitoring, identification, and prevention of situations that could result in injury, financial loss, or regulatory noncompliance (CHUBB, 2004). Common elements of risk management programs include review of policies, procedures, and protocols; incident reporting; claims management; review of standards of care; and awareness of regulatory and accreditation requirement.

"Enterprise risk management," as defined in the *Risk Management Handbook for Health Care Organizations*, "is a structured analytical process that focuses on identifying and eliminating the financial impact and volatility of a portfolio of risks rather than on risk avoidance alone. Essential to this approach is an understanding that risk can be managed to gain competitive advantage" (ASHRM Taskforce, 2005, p. 1). Risk anticipation becomes part of a systematic process review found in process redesign or process flow diagramming in quality improvement projects.

Enterprise risk management (ERM) uses a process or framework to complete a comprehensive assessment and measurement of risk throughout an organization. It relies on stratification of risk into domains, looking for interrelatedness or interdependencies that allow the development of strategies to manage each risk. The domains include clinical operations, finance, human, strategic, legal/regulatory, and technological risks (ASHRM Taskforce, 2005).

Two principles guide ERM: the recognition that risk represents capital or potential for loss, and the belief that holistic or comprehensive approaches are critical to manage diverse risks. This framework requires awareness that risks are not isolated; although organizations are often structured in operational silos, the risks do not occur in isolation. Traditional healthcare risk management takes a clinically focused approach and examines risks individually. The ERM model defines risks in terms of the probability that adverse events will occur and result in financial losses. Risk management focuses on protecting the organization's assets. Instead of handling risk in functional silos where measurements of success are variable, an enterprise-wide risk management approach employs common metrics across risk domains to determine the effectiveness of risk management strategies that focus on both opportunity and risk (ASHRM Taskforce, 2005).

Risk assessment is often undertaken as a vehicle to improve safety. Recent initiatives to reduce hospital infections and falls, to improve and increase effective communication between healthcare team members, and to reduce errors have been showcased in regulatory requirements, reimbursement policies, and patient satisfaction results. Improvement activities highlight the ways organizations leverage opportunity in replicating successes achieved in different parts of an organization or microsystems, stressing that quality, safety, and cost can all be improved when we address a risk, not to avoid legal action but rather to improve care outcomes.

Many clinicians view the mitigation of risk in the context of quality improvement activities for good reason. Many of the tools used in quality improvement work, like root cause analyses, fishbone diagrams, failure mode and effects analyses

(FMEAs), and monitoring of outcome metrics, are common to risk management. Regulatory bodies also advocate risk anticipation and management through expectations of high reliability in healthcare organizations.

CNLs have an opportunity to identify high-risk processes in their assessment of the microsystem. Because CNLs have knowledge of process streams in the clinical environment and awareness of inputs and outputs from other units or departments and patterns or gaps in care delivery, they can lead efforts to manage risk and process improvements.

Quality Improvement, Evidence-Based Practice, and the CNL Role

Quality improvement is known by many names but holds in common the real life experiences and data within an organization to rapidly cycle through a defined process to evaluate outcomes (McLaughlin & Kaluzny, 2005; Newhouse, 2007). The terms continuous quality improvement, total quality management, performance improvement, and process improvement are often used interchangeably to describe efforts geared toward data-driven, process-oriented, outcome-focused activities. These efforts were originally established in the business world and have recently been applied in the healthcare industry. Oftentimes, quality improvement is offered as a framework to examine long-standing clinical and systems issues in a different way (McLaughlin & Kaluzny, 2005; Nelson, Batalden, & Godfrey, 2007).

The key feature of quality improvement is the cyclical nature of the process, which is designed to evaluate workflow, and processes built from value-added actions that are performed by work teams in a system (Hedges, 2006; McLaughlin & Kaluzny, 2005; Newhouse, 2007). Quality improvement processes do not meet the standards of rigor found in scientific research and have neither theoretical underpinnings nor an aim to generate new knowledge. Rather, quality improvement aims to bring individuals who work together into a venue where systematic review and evaluation of work processes can be examined in a cyclical fashion as a means to evaluate and improve established practices and outcomes (Hedges, 2006; Newhouse, 2007).

Philosophical Elements of Quality Improvement

Continuous quality improvement has several characteristics that are evident in organizations. According to McLaughlin and Kaluzny, they include the following:

1. Strategic focus drawing on the mission and values of the organization
2. A customer focus directed toward patients, providers, and stakeholders
3. A systems perspective, revealing emphasis on the interdependence of inter-acting processes that influence outcomes
4. Data driven analysis emphasizing the gathering of objective data to influence decision making
5. Team involvement inclusive of representatives that implement current work processes and those who will implement the resulting workflow change
6. Multiple causations requiring identification of root causes
7. Sets of solutions identified to enhance system functions and outcomes
8. Process optimization supported by alignment of tools and structures to evaluate interventions
9. Continuous improvement supported by ongoing analysis of outcomes directed toward ongoing modification of processes to enhance system performance
10. Organizational learning so the capacity to generate future improvements is enhanced (McLaughlin & Kaluzny, 2005)

Several quality improvement methodologies reside in health systems, identified as Lean, Six Sigma, or total quality management structures. Irrespective of the quality improvement methodology selected by an organization, there are eight common steps in quality improvement. They are as follows:

1. A clear and defined aim or purpose
2. A review of the literature
3. Examination of current resources to facilitate quality improvement
4. Mapping the current processes
5. Root cause analysis
6. Selecting appropriate tools for process analysis
7. Selecting measures and metrics (baseline and outcome)
8. Rapid cyclical review of the plan, data, interventions, and outcomes (McLaughlin & Kaluzny, 2005, Newhouse, 2006)

Defined Aim or Purpose

Having a clear purpose or aim in any project seems logical, but this is a part of quality improvement that can lead to frustration when project teams engage in work. Because the team is composed of individuals from varied disciplines, many assumptions are behind the way individuals define and view clinical issues. Additionally, because processes are complex and interrelated, it is easy for a team to lose focus or expand the project scope if the aim or purpose is not clearly and explicitly defined.

When creating an aim or purpose for a quality improvement team, answering the "who, what, when, where, and how" of a project is key. *Who* refers to the people affected by the concern; *what* refers to the problem identified; *when* refers to the timing of the issue; *where* refers to the specific unit or location of the concern; and *how* refers to the measures, metrics, or standards that alert the team to an issue. Once the team can establish these parameters, elevator discussions or concise yet informative language suitable to a conversation that lasts the duration of an elevator ride can be crafted. Additionally, when the team starts to drift into processes or topics that do not relate specifically and directly to the purpose or aim of the team, these issues for the "parking lot" can be documented for future discussion or communication to other project teams.

Review of the Literature

Newhouse (2007) defined evidence-based practice (EBP) as a problem-solving approach to clinical decision making that ingrates the best available scientific evidence with the best available experiential evidence from patients and practitioners; it incorporates the organization's culture, internal and external influences on practice, and critical thinking that supports judicious application of the evidence to the care of an individual, a population of patients, or the system. EBP and research inform quality improvement through review of the literature. By providing interventions with great likelihood of success, both research and EBPs inform quality improvement (Newhouse, 2007).

Central to the CNL role is the expectation that clinical practice and interventions will be evidence based. Driven from past experiences in not achieving consistent and sustainable improvements and increasing regulatory demands to demonstrate the inclusion of evidence in processes, protocols, and policies, EBPs are gaining attention. National patient safety goals based on the Joint Commission's requirements and supported by the National Quality Forum set the overarching goal for establishing EBP as the norm in clinical care (Department of Health and Human Services, 2009; The Joint Commission, 2008).

Resources to Facilitate Improvement

When undertaking a quality improvement initiative, it is important to explore, examine, and establish both internal and external resources for support. Internal resources can include individuals from quality management departments, finance, information services, the library, and the education department. Books, websites, and discussions with members of the interdisciplinary team who have experience with quality improvement activities can provide important resources to support a team's efforts. External resources include professional organizations, Internet resources, quality improvement organizations, and members of other industries with knowledge of quality management or root cause analysis.

Mapping Current Processes
Several methods for mapping current processes exist. When initiating the mapping process, CNLs will engage members of the interdisciplinary team in exercises to identify, define, and document process steps, decision points, and inputs from other departments or disciplines that lead to the current outcomes (McLaughlin & Kaluzny, 2005). This stage involves a detail-specific discussion between members of the team to capture the complexity of the process intended for improvement.

Root Cause Analysis
The Joint Commission established expectations for organizations to proactively identify high-risk processes that are likely to contribute to errors. Within this process is the realization that systems and processes contribute to adverse events and errors. Because quality improvement initiatives are focused on addressing processes, it is important to use systematic approaches to guide teams in identifying the root cause or process that breaks down and leads to an undesired result. Once a process flow is completed, further analysis of each process is required to identify the underlying cause or step in a process that sets into motion a cause and effect that drives an occurrence or problem. Drilling down on process steps to identify a root cause can be accomplished using different tools, but cause and effect or fishbone diagrams are most common. Fishbone diagrams delineate the causes of a situation centered on predefined categories of people, materials, methods, machinery, and policy (McLaughlin & Kaluzny, 2005; Shaw, Elliott, Isaacson, & Murphy, 2003).

Selecting Appropriate Tools
There are several tools used to represent data collected before, during, and after quality improvement efforts are undertaken. Each tool has a distinct purpose and provides a fact-based approach to identify concerns, propose solutions, and monitor outcomes of the process changes. The most common tools include brainstorming,

cause and effect diagrams, Pareto charts, control charts, process flow diagrams, fishbone diagrams, surveys, pie charts, histograms, and run charts (McLaughlin & Kaluzny, 2005; Newhouse, 2007; Shaw et al., 2003).

Selecting Measures and Metrics

Measurement and metrics are the foundation of quality improvement, as they are the basis for evaluating the impact of quality improvement activities. Defining the metrics at baseline is the starting point for quality activities, as these measures typically inform and define how a problem was recognized. Equally important are the primary and secondary metrics the quality improvement team selects as they modify processes to achieve the team's goals and purpose. Metrics can include clinical indicators of care and process or business metrics (McLaughlin & Kaluzny, 2005; Nelson et al., 2007; Newhouse, 2006).

Technology, and therefore electronic medical records and informatics, has been infused into the care arena at a rapid pace during the last decade. Clinicians are often bombarded with more data than could possibly be analyzed and reviewed. With this in mind, it is important to CNLs to consider how information is gathered, where it is stored, and what tools, methods, and resources are available to access data. When reviewing data stored in data warehouses, repositories, and databases, it is important to clarify terms and data definitions to ensure consistency and understanding of how data will be used in the quality improvement process (Bakken, Cimino, & Hripcsak, 2004).

Nurses are generally comfortable assessing clinical outcomes and indicators of care, but it is also important for CNLs to incorporate business metrics and measurements when planning quality improvement projects. These measures are important to the administrators and regulators of care accustomed to quantifying and articulating value at a systems level (Haase-Herrick, 2005; Hwang & Herdon, 2007). Quantifying the return on investment, impacts on costs of care, and articulating system improvements could establish the value of the CNL role in organizations. With rising pressures regarding pay for performance, trended outcomes of care in public reporting, and rising interest from accreditation and consumer groups, selection of business indicators aimed at cost effectiveness and efficiency are essential.

Rapid Cycle Review

A cornerstone and distinguishing characteristic of quality improvement is rapid cycle review, which encourages continuous and ongoing efforts to improve outcomes. The plan-do-check-act (PDCA) cycle is frequently referenced in quality improvement methodologies. Discussed by Deming (and attributed to Shewhart's work at Bell Laboratories), the PDCA cycle of improvement offers a cyclical process to structure tests of change identified by team members as being most likely to improve outcomes in a disciplined and rapid manner (McLaughlin & Kaluzny, 2005). *Plan* involves the definition of the problem, examination of the processes that contribute to it, and devising a plan to address the problem. *Do* involves identifying the steps in a plan and carrying them out. *Check* involves analyzing the data collected to summarize what was learned. *Act* involves examining outcomes with an eye toward further modifications so that the cycle can be initiated again to refine and bring further improvements ((McLaughlin & Kaluzny, 2005; Nelson et al., 2007).

Relevance of the Microsystem

Microsystems are defined as the smallest functional unit on the front line of healthcare delivery systems. The clinical microsystem provides direct care to patients and families, establishing the essential building blocks of the organization. It is within this microsystem that the quality of care is defined and the reputation of an organization is created (Nelson et al., 2007).

Microsystems include members of the interdisciplinary team in various roles who work together on a regular basis to provide care to discrete subpopulations of patients. A microsystem has business and clinical aims, linked processes, and a shared information environment that produces performance outcomes (Nelson et al., 2007). Microsystems are represented in all practice settings and specialties and evolve over time, but they always have a patient at the center. Microsystems vary widely in terms of quality, safety, and costs because they are embedded in a context where providers, support staff, information, and processes converge to support individuals who provide care to meet the unique and individual health needs of patients and families. Microsystems are loosely or tightly connected to one another and are the functional, interdependent systems that create an organization or macrosystem (Nelson et al., 2007).

Tornabeni, Stanhope, and Wiggins (2008) noted that, "the CNL role focuses on understanding the interdependency of all disciplines providing care and the need to tap into the expertise of the team, rather than individual providers" (p. 107). By understanding the roles of the interdisciplinary team, the CNL laterally integrates the team to provide patient-centered care. CNLs use their interpersonal communication skills, clinical leadership skills, and knowledge of group dynamics to facilitate care, leveraging their knowledge of internal and external resources to provide lateral integration.

Assessment of the Microsystem for Selection of Quality Improvement Projects

Many tools have been created to support CNLs in the assessment of their microsystems. Irrespective of the tool selected, a thorough and systematic assessment is needed before embarking on a quality improvement project. The microsystem assessment elements to be examined include: unit descriptors; skills, composition, and competence of team members; presence of formal and informal leaders; interdisciplinary team relationships and communication; accountability and control over practice; support for education; experience with quality improvement processes and resources; and readiness for change.

The "5 Ps" framework offers a deliberate framework for clinicians to assess microsystems in a systematic manner. The 5 Ps are purpose, patients, professionals, processes, and patterns. Each P has a definition associated with it, and these categories set a framework to inform the selection of improvement themes and aims. To be most effective, the exploration of the 5 Ps should include all the members of a clinical microsystem. Nelson and colleagues (2007) offer a series of questions and exercises to lead interdisciplinary teams through the microsystem assessment to establish the "health" of the microsystem, making obvious the areas that require attention (diagnosis) and solutions (treatment) to be evaluated by the team (follow-up) (p. 265).

Systematic and Purposeful Identification of Quality Improvement Initiatives

When considering initiatives to improve quality and safety, project selection in an organization is of paramount importance. By using a gap analysis or microsystem assessment, CNLs can align quality improvement efforts in the microsystem to strategic initiatives and organizational goals while simultaneously focusing attention on the front lines to impact change. The CNL is in a unique position to manage change, apply quality improvement methods, and incorporate team learning by leading interdisciplinary members through a disciplined, systematic approach of problem identification, process analysis, measurement, and evaluation that is meaningful in daily operations.

A potential pitfall for CNLs is the identification of quality improvement projects that extend beyond the microsystem. Scoping a project through a defined aim or purpose at the onset of quality improvement activities is essential to success. Because there are many priorities that overlap at the organizational level, concentrating on improvements at the microsystem level is key. Problem identification through brainstorming with members of the microsystem team is a mechanism to support unit-level activities that will be meaningful and appropriate for CNL intervention (Rusch & Bakewell-Sachs, 2007; Thompson & Lulham, 2007).

Structure for Monitoring Quality Improvement Projects

Many organizations have quality departments that distribute quality reports monthly, quarterly, and annually as a part of a quality dashboard, benchmarking, or quality report card process. In addition to these contributions, many quality departments distribute reports for quality improvement initiatives and regulatory obligations. There is a wealth of knowledge contained in these departments, and before engaging in a quality improvement project, the CNL team leader should explore what tools, report development, and distribution supports are available.

Team Leader Tools for Success

Once the philosophy of quality improvement has been embraced and the tenets of quality improvement have been articulated, the progress toward improvement needs to be monitored and evaluated. Irrespective of the methodology selected to guide the organizational quality improvements, team member roles, responsibilities, and ground rules need to be discussed and documented. This step is commonly avoided or driven by assumptions, but failing to explicitly address it is a critical mistake. If CNLs are going to embrace quality improvement, setting team expectations and responsibilities from the onset of the group's work is essential. The documents created during this phase of the team's interactions will be referenced throughout the quality improvement process as the agreed on guiding principles, rules, and accountabilities each team member holds.

Several forms or documents can be found to document the team's expectations. At a minimum, the team will want to identify the team leader, the secretary (responsible for documenting and distributing meeting minutes and agendas), and the responsibilities of each team member. Attendance requirements, frequency of meetings, length of meetings, and commitment to completing work between meetings are the focal points of discussion between the team members.

Searching the Internet for sample team charters provides a wealth of templates or formats for teams to consider if the organization does not have a preferred or approved template. A charter is a written agreement defining what a team is going to accomplish and how success will be measured. The charter focuses the team's efforts and documents the expectations that team members have of one another. By using a team charter, discussion between multidisciplinary team members can be guided to include key focal points in team dynamics and important issues can be agreed on before the team engages in change. A signed charter indicates the formal beginning of a project and a commitment to one another.

Most professionals hold common beliefs about group process and goal attainment, but ground rules provide the boundaries for how team members will interact. Many organizations have established ground rules for team interactions based on their mission and shared values. Although these ground rules provide basic tenets for group interactions, it is important to offer team members the chance to modify rules to reflect what they believe the guiding principles should be. Common content for ground rules includes valuing each person and their input; anticipating unique contributions from all team members; courteous, honest, and respectful communication; and the agreement that each member will represent the work of the team in a positive manner.

CNLs are positioned to monitor the improvement activities from the team leader position as a coordinator and manager of care through teaching, guidance, mentoring, and leveraging the language of the improvement process. Effective use of team tools can set expectations and provide elements that document activities and progress that lead to the attainment of project goals.

Linking Quality Improvement to the Clinical Immersion Experience and the Daily Life of a CNL

Embedded in the CNL role are expectations of accountability for patient-centered, cost-effective care across practice settings and measurable outcomes that demonstrate improved safety, quality, and EBP. The CNL curriculum supports the development of clinical leaders who can manage change by leading members of the interdisciplinary team in complex care environments (AACN, 2007; Rusch & Bakewell-Sachs, 2007).

All CNLs are required to complete 400 to 500 clinical hours throughout their educational experience, with 300 to 400 hours devoted to a clinical immersion experience. During the clinical immersion experience, the student enacts the CNL role and competencies in an organization (AACN, 2007; Rusch & Bakewell-Sachs, 2007). Quality improvement may be offered as a separate course in the curriculum or threaded throughout the educational experience in several courses, but the culmination of the CNL clinical immersion experience is grounded in principles demonstrated through quality improvement projects. As members of the nursing profession, CNLs will be expected to identify areas for improvement within the care delivery system, assess and plan meaningful change at the microsystem level, and measure clinical and financial outcomes to demonstrate improved outcomes that align with strategic organizational goals aimed at improving cost, quality, and safety.

As clinical leaders and members of the nursing profession, CNLs are also expected to participate in self-evaluation and reflective thinking (AACN, 2007). This includes examining individually held assumptions, values, and beliefs with an open mind, supported by the use of critical thinking skills to explore different per-spectives, solutions, and options offered by members of the interdisciplinary team or the literature. The clinical immersion experience offers CNL students a venue to share the outcomes of quality improvement activities, as well as the reflective practice, learning, and insights gained related to leading teams, evaluating practice and implementing EBPs, and guiding or mentoring others in quality improvement processes aimed at patient safety and improved care delivery. Documents assembled during the quality improvement process can then become a part of the students' clinical immersion portfolio.

After completion of the clinical immersion experience in their formal educa-tion, CNLs are expected to replicate elements of the clinical immersion in daily practice. Often, organizations rely on the CNL to bring quality improvement strat-egies into a microsystem to support organizational change and performance. This means working within the microsystem culture to implement change without the educational process as a guide. The scope and anticipated duration of an improve-ment project may be less than the 15-week semester, but the elements of the clin-ical immersion experience can be replicated to map the process steps required when leading a microsystem quality improvement. The discipline of documenting process steps, gaining consensus around the problem, establishing ground rules, engaging interdisciplinary team members, and using quality and sustainability tools is unchanged. A common pitfall experienced by graduate CNLs is the omission of different steps in the process (believed to be academic exercises), which leads to frustration and delays in achieving desired results.

Journaling as a Reflective Practice to Gather Insights

Many CNLs complete clinical journals during their course work, but growing evidence suggests that personal journaling is also an effective reflective practice to gather insights into our own thoughts and behaviors. Journaling is a vehicle to promote personal growth and learning (Hiemstra, 2001). Journals are not time or experience logs but rather a place for reflection, introspection, development of personal and professional awareness, and recording what has been learned. The reflective journal serves several purposes, including a place to record one's thoughts about and reactions to clinical situations, events, professional activities, and insights. According to Lasater and Nielson (2009), guided reflective journals offer professional nurses views of a situation from multiple perspectives, a search for alternative explanations of events, and the use of evidence to support or evaluate a decision or position.

Reflective journaling requires thought and introspection. A reflective journal is not a diary, resource book, or log of daily activities. It is a place to record experiences, ideas, and insights to build greater self-awareness and allow an introspective view of the team dynamics, clinical leader responsibilities, and progress toward goals. A journal chronicles self-assessment, self-evaluation, and evolving perspective.

Principles of reflective writing identified by Hecker and colleagues include:

- An opening to explore what we can become without being judged. Stories are a gift to ourselves and others and express the uniqueness of individuals and their circumstance as well as the common ground they share.
- What we bring to an experience is essential to our understanding of what occurs. This is influenced by our past, our future, and our present world views.
- A deeper understanding enables us to integrate former learning with experiences, to form relationships between parts of knowledge, and to search for meaning.

- We reflect because issues that need consideration arise both before and after we act. As nurses, we are agents of history for ourselves and others.
- Critical reflection promotes an understanding of diversity in beliefs, values, behavior, and social structures. Any claims to a universal truth or total certainty are questioned. The more we share our thoughts and feelings, the more we challenge accepted views of traditions and myths, which have kept alternate interpretations from becoming possibilities.
- Reflection is not a political act.
- Because reflective writing is a personal journey, students are to write only what they feel comfortable sharing.
- Journal writings are not right or wrong, simply places to discuss movement in thinking.
- Journal entries are reflections, which often evoke more questions than answers. The purpose of forming questions is to help focus on personal meaning and interpretation in the reflective moment.
- Journals are confidential between the student and the instructor.
- Change is the only constant, and writing reflectively offers a way to examine the meaning of change. (Hecker, Amon, & Nickoli, n.d.)

The following list offers a starting point for reflective journaling content:

- Explore questions for inquiry that are important to you
- Record significant experiences, including associated feelings and thoughts
- Analyze patterns and relationships
- Appreciate learning and celebrate success
- Respond to new ideas
- Examine your assumptions, beliefs, and values
- Consider alternative perspectives
- Develop personal theories
- Take thoughtful action

Thoughtful reflection is an ongoing process. Insights are often gained because the fear of judgment by others is removed as thoughts are written freely. Studies have identified that journaling daily allows individuals to problem solve and appreciate insights, leading to a sense of empowerment and opportunities to choose actions or celebrate actions that are uncovered when written. A journal is not a showpiece. Like learning, it will always be a work in progress. It should be approached with curiosity and openness.

Conclusion

With increasing national demands from regulators, payers, and consumers to support effectiveness of interventions to improve patient safety and quality of care, change efforts formed by quality improvement initiatives provide a systematic, disciplined, and reliable process to support decision making and measurement aimed to improve patient care quality in the healthcare delivery system. Developing a data-driven, outcomes-oriented structure grounded in role accountability will be essential. The CNL is well positioned to lead multidisciplinary teams in their efforts to implement quality improvement at the microsystem level.

Summary

- As coordinators of care with a system of care focus, the CNL has a responsibility to lead interdisciplinary teams in quality improvement initiatives.
- Irrespective of the quality methods employed in an organization, quality improvement relies on a systematic and disciplined approach to understanding care processes.
- Evidence-based practices inform the selection of appropriate interventions and inform quality improvement to support quality care and data-driven outcomes.
- Scanning the environment for individual and system risks is an important responsibility of CNLs.

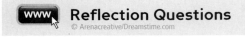

Reflection Questions

© Arenacreative/Dreamstime.com

1.   What part of the quality improvement process do you feel most prepared for? What part do you feel least prepared for?
2.   What resources are available in your organization to assist you with quality improvement?

3. How do you see the CNL interacting with other members of the clinical team to advance quality improvement, risk anticipation, and evidence-based practices?

4. Identify a process in your microsystem that could benefit from an interdisciplinary team effort. Talk to members of your team to create an action plan.

WWW Learning Activities
© Arenacreative/Dreamstime.com

1. Interview a member of your organization's quality improvement department. Identify the quality methods, tools, and measurement techniques used in the organization.

2. Meet with a member of your risk management team. Explore the tools and reports they create for members of the senior leadership team. Explain the CNL role and inquire about the risks this person believes a CNL could address in his or her microsystem.

3. Locate the quality reports and metrics that are distributed to leaders throughout the organization. Identify three metrics that you believe the CNL could impact.

4. Outline the steps you would take if you were going to develop a quality improvement plan to address a metric CNLs could address.

References

American Association of Colleges of Nursing. (2007). *White paper on the role of the clinical nurse leader*. Retrieved from http://www.aacn.nche.edu/cnl

American Society for Healthcare Risk Management Monographs Taskforce. (2005). *Enterprise risk management part one: Defining the concept, recognizing its value*. Retrieved from http://www.ashrm.org/ashrm/education/development/monographs/ERMmonograph.pdf

Bakken, S., Cimino, J., & Hripcsak, G. (2004). Promoting patient safety and enabling evidence-based practice through informatics. *Medical Care, 42*(2), II, 49–56.

Berwick, D., Nolan, T., & Whittington J. (2008). The triple aim: Care, health, and cost. *Health Affairs, 27*(3), 759–769.

Bowcutt, M., Wall, J., & Goolsby, M. (2006). The clinical nurse leader: Promoting patient-centered outcomes. *Nursing Administration Quarterly, 30*(2), 156–161.

CHUBB HealthCcare. (2004). *Effective health care risk management programs: Components for success*. Retrieved from http://www.chubb.com/businesses/csi/chubb1148.pdf

Department of Health and Human Services. (2009). Evidence-based care/performance measurement. Retrieved from http://www.hhs.gov/secretary/about/goal1.html

Haase-Herrick, K. (2005). The opportunities of stewardship. *Nursing Administration Quarterly, 29*(2), 115–118.

Hecker, T., Amon, J., & Nickoli, E. (n.d.). *Reflective writing in nursing.* Retrieved from http://www.tru.ca/disciplines/eng309/nursing/nursing.htm

Hedges, C. (2006). Research, evidence-based practice, and quality improvement: The 3-legged stool. *AACN Advanced Critical Care, 17*(4), 457–459.

Hiemstra, R. (2001). *Uses and benefits of journal writing.* In L. M. English & M. A. Gillen (Eds.), *Promoting journal writing in adult education* (pp. 19–26). San Francisco, CA: Jossey-Bass.

Hwang, R., & Herndon, J. (2007). The business case for patient safety. *Clinical Orthopaedics and Related Research, 457,* 21–34.

Institute of Medicine. (1999). *To err is human: Building a safer health system.* Washington, DC: National Academies Press.

Institute of Medicine. (2001). *Crossing the quality chasm: A new health system for the 21st century.* Washington, DC: National Academies Press.

Institute of Medicine. (2003). Health professions education: A bridge to quality. Retrieved from http://www.iom.edu/Reports/2003/Health-Professions-Education-A-Bridge-to-Quality.aspx

The Joint Commission. (2008). *Health care at the crossroads: Guiding principles for the development of the hospital of the future.* Retrieved from http://www.jointcommission.org/assets/1/18/Hosptal_Future.pdf

Lasater, K., & Nielson, A. (2009). Reflective journaling for clinical judgment development and evaluation. *Journal of Nursing Education, 48*(1), 40–44.

Lohr, K. (1990). *Medicare: A strategy for quality assurance.* Washington, DC: National Academy Press.

McLaughlin, C., & Kaluzny, A. (2005). *Continuous quality improvement in health care: Theory, implementations, and applications* (3rd ed.). Sudbury, MA: Jones and Bartlett.

Nelson, E., Batalden, P., & Godfrey, M. (2007). *Quality by design. A clinical microsystems approach.* San Francisco, CA: Jossey-Bass.

Newhouse, R. (2006). Selecting measures for safety and quality improvement initiatives. *Journal of Nursing Administration, 36*(3), 109–113.

Newhouse, R. (2007). Diffusing confusion among evidence-based practice, quality improvement, and research. *Journal of Nursing Administration, 37*(10), 432–435.

Rusch, L., & Bakewell-Sachs, S. (2007). The CNL: A gateway to better care. *Nursing Management.* doi: 10.1097/01.NUMA.0000266719.94334.96

Shaw, P., Elliott, C., Isaacson, P., & Murphy, E. (2003). *Quality and performance improvement in healthcare: A tool for programmed learning* (2nd ed.). Chicago, IL: American Health Information Management Association.

Thompson, P., & Lulham, K. (2007). Clinical nurse leader and clinical nurse specialist role delineation in the acute care setting. *Journal of Nursing Administration, 37*(10), 429–431.

Tornabeni, J., Stanhope, M., & Wiggins, M. (2008). The CNL vision. *Journal of Nursing Administration, 36*(3), 103–108.

Wiggins, M. (2008). The partnership care delivery model: An examination of the core concept and the need for a new model of care. *Journal of Nursing Management, 16,* 629–638.

Suggested Readings

AHRQ. *Tools and strategies for quality improvement and patient safety*
www.ahrq.gov/legacy/qual/nurseshdbk/docs/HughesR_QMBMP.pdf
Institute for Healthcare Improvement
http://ihi.org
National Quality Forum
www.qualityforum.org
The Joint Commission
www.jointcommission.org/
Centers for Medicare and Medicaid Services
www.cms.gov
AHRQ. *Sustaining and spreading quality improvement: A conversation with Julie Kliger, MPA, BSN, director, integrated nurse leadership program*
http://innovations.ahrq.gov/content.aspx?id=3433
ASHRM—Advocacy, health reform
http://www.ashrm.org/ashrm/advocacy/healthcare_reform/index.shtml
AHRQ—Getting safer care
http://www.ahrq.gov/consumer/safety.html
Introduction to the future of healthcare risk management
http://www.mshrm.org/programs/online-documents/2011/05%20-%20
Future%20of%20Risk%20Management.pdf
GAO. Improving medicare program management
http://www.gao.gov/highrisk/agency/hhs/improving-medicare-management
.php

Transformation and Quality Improvement in the Delivery Model

■ Elizabeth Triezenberg and Lauran Hardin

Hospital consumer assessment of healthcare providers and systems (HCAHPS) pain satisfaction scores for orthopedics were in the 50th percentile and identified as a first priority for intervention.

The orthopedic CNL and the pain management CNL collaborated to uncover the root cause of pain dissatisfaction. Rounding with surgeons, staff, and patients revealed gaps in education and communication. Pain was managed using a reactive approach with little communication between surgeon, nurse, and patient.

Using the systems analyst role of the CNL, pain satisfaction was looked at across the continuum of care—from the orthopedic surgeon's office to care at home after surgery. Initial intervention focused on education. The preoperative total joint class was redesigned to better prepare patients to partner in managing their pain. A multidisciplinary collaborative process was engaged with the surgeon's office, preadmission testing, surgery, and inpatient staff to redesign patient education, screening, and pain management on discharge.

An evidence-based process was created to assess and treat pain during hospitalization. The orthopedic CNL rounded on patients daily and mentored staff in how to create a plan for pain management. Mentoring and modeling best practice care in the moment resulted in nurses rapidly developing the skills to differentiate types of pain and the appropriate medication, partner with patients for a pain plan, and communicate the plan across disciplines.

Patients who have had a total joint replacement are now able to verbalize their need for pain medications as well as the plan they are using to manage pain during hospitalization and at discharge. Staff nurses are discussing the patients' pain plans not only with the patients but with the other nurses and the surgeon. Most importantly, patients are stating their pain is better controlled and that staff are doing what they can to control their pain. HCAHPS scores improved from the 50th percentile to the 90th percentile.

Partnerships for Patient Quality and Safety

Kevin Hengeveld and Lauran Hardin

In 2010, over 50% of psychiatric medical unit admissions were dementia patients needing treatment for behavior control. Assessment completed by the CNL revealed staff injuries, staff fear and lack of knowledge, extended length of stay, and patient deaths.

With mentoring, the staff unit-based council developed an evidence-based guideline for care. Advanced dementia patients cannot self-report pain, fear, or bowel, bladder, and environmental concerns. The guideline taught staff how to treat and anticipate needs in this vulnerable population, increasing their confidence in care and decreasing injuries from patient agitation.

CNLs then collaborated to assess the root cause of outcomes involving psychiatry, medicine, and palliative care. Families of dementia patients are challenged with making complex end-of-life decisions regarding code status and feeding tubes. A process was developed to trigger the integration of palliative care for decision-making support from the day of admission, giving families time to develop relationships and struggle through complex issues. Complex issues were solved sooner, patients were transferred to the appropriate setting in less time, and average length of stay (ALOS) decreased from 14 to 10 days.

Analysis of deaths found that some patients did not really need to be admitted to the unit in the first place. Hospice patients and near end-of-life patients were not best served in a locked psychiatric unit. The act of transferring the patient was often traumatic near the end of life. A collaborative process between CNLs was engaged to create risk assessment at entry points to the hospital (intake coordinators and the emergency department). Clinical support was offered to get patients the services they needed in the setting they were already in. CNLs partnered with hospices from the community to improve outcomes for the population. These combined efforts decreased dementia deaths in the unit to zero. Data for the unit is shown in the figure.

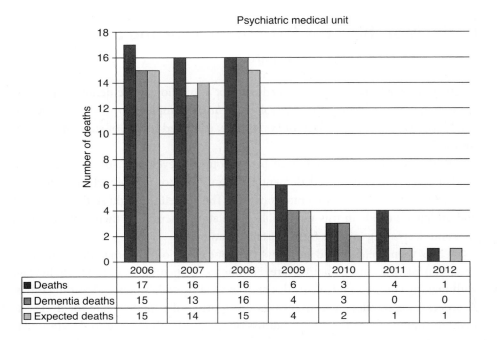

Psychiatric medical unit

	2006	2007	2008	2009	2010	2011	2012
Deaths	17	16	16	6	3	4	1
Dementia deaths	15	13	16	4	3	0	0
Expected deaths	15	14	15	4	2	1	1

Quality of Care: Improving Transitions to Home in Elderly Veterans After Hospitalizations

Mary E. Mathers
South Texas Veterans Health Care System

Falls are a common adverse event and are more frequently reported than medication errors, equipment-related incidents, and documentation errors. The devastating impacts of falls on the elderly can be catastrophic. Falls are the leading cause of death-related injury; 50% of older adults never regain prior functional status after a hip fracture, and 30% will die within 6 months of a hip fracture. After 3 days in the hospital, all patients, no matter what age, are at risk for a fall posthospitalization due to deconditioning, but the elderly are especially at risk. Studies have shown that 20% of people fall in the first month after discharge from the hospital. Calls were made to patients of the geriatric evaluation and management clinic 48 to 72 hours posthospitalization. The literature indicated that patients typically do not express themselves appropriately to describe inadequate self-care tasks. The questions were then scripted to capture the pertinent details of a safe transition to home. The questions were:

1. Since your discharge have you had any difficulty standing, transferring, or changing position in bed?
2. Since your discharge are you able to toilet and bathe yourself?
3. Since your discharge have you experienced any dizziness or unsteadiness?
4. Do you know when your discharge follow-up appointment is scheduled?

When these questions elicited a positive response, further planning for home care was initiated.

A daily afternoon briefing was held to discuss discharges. The interprofessional team, composed of the physician (medical director), CNL, social worker, and pharmacist, would discuss what plan of care was appropriate for the patient. During our first year of this process improvement there was a 75% reduction of falls posthospitalization and a readmission reduction of 10%; an estimated cost savings of $100,000.

Impact of an Educational Program for Nurses to Prevent Central Line–Associated Blood Stream Infections: CNL Student Quality Improvement Project

Lissy Joseph

The central line–associated blood stream infection (CLABSI) rate remained consistently high for several months compared to the national benchmark, as noted by the Veterans Health system in a southwestern state. Noncompliance with current practices and lack of proper documentation was evident after monitoring the patients with central lines for 1 month. The clinical guideline for intravenous therapy was reviewed and compared with the guidelines from accrediting agencies such as The Joint Commission and the Centers for Disease Control and Prevention. A PowerPoint presentation was developed in consultation with the infection control department and intravenous therapy team manager. Multiple educational sessions were held with a pretest and posttest to measure the knowledge level of the nurses in the unit. To increase the compliance rate of weekly dressing change, a specific day of the week was selected by the nurses. Every nurse in the unit was verified for competency using a check-off list. Monitoring of every central line in the unit for compliance with dressing change and intravenous tubing change for 1 month was done.

An improvement in dressing change compliance rate of 80% was observed after the first month. Noncompliant staff were given one-on-one attention and encouraged to check the status of the dressing during shift change report. At the end of the second month, the compliance rate increased to 92%. No CLABSI was reported during these 2 months. The CLABSI rate was reduced by 40% in 2 months. Though a 100% compliance in dressing change could not be attained in 2 months, significant improvement and a continous downward trend of CLABSI rate was noted. Senior leaders in the system noticed the improvement in the step-down unit and hospital-wide mandatory educational sessions were initiated. Tremendous decrease in the infection rate (35%) was observed in the facility within 6 months.

Rapid Response Improvement at University of South Alabama Medical Center

Sheri Salas
Nurse Educator, University of South Alabama College of Nursing

Lisa Mestas
Asst. Administrator of Clinical Services/CNO, University of South Alabama Medical Center

Problem Statement

Patients who are discharged from the intensive care units (ICU) to medical–surgical floors before they are stable are at risk for deterioration and readmission to the ICU. Early discharge from the ICU can increase the likelihood of ICU readmission and postdischarge unanticipated death if patients are discharged before they are stable (Badawi & Breslow, 2012). There are many negative implications related to readmission to the ICU. Readmission to the ICU is associated with worse outcomes and increased cost. ICU readmissions are not only attributable to patient-related factors but also to discharge and transition processes (Daniel et al., 2012). Many patients who have been prematurely discharged from the ICU have rapid response (RR) events and are readmitted to the ICU within 24 hours of the transfer. The purpose of this project is to improve the transition process of patients at the University of South Alabama Medical Center (USAMC) from a higher level of care to medical–surgical floors in an effort to reduce RR events and bounce back transfers within 24 hours of moving to the floor by creating an assessment tool that assigns patients a risk score prior to transfer.

Gap Analysis

The sixth floor at USAMC had 60 RR events from March to August 2012. Thirty-five percent (21) of those RRs took place within 24 hours of transfer from a higher level of care, and 13 of those patients had to transfer back to a higher level of care (bounce backs). Sixty-two percent of patients who had an RR event within 24 hours of transfer out of the ICU bounced back. The average length of stay in the ICU after readmission to the ICU was 4.5 days. The cost of 4.5 ICU days for 13 patients was $68,191. The cost for one extra day in the ICU prior to the original transfer to the floor was $13,697. The cost avoidance for monitoring patients based on an assessment tool for 1 more day is $54,494.

Data and assessment of past RRs has shown that patients could be transferred to the floor with high acuity levels at risk for adverse events on the medical–surgical units. No standard assessment tool is in place to ensure patients are stable to transfer to the floors. RR events take floor nurses away from the bedsides of other patients, and the ICU is interrupted with a declining patient when an RR results in a bounce back transfer. Continuity of care is compromised in these events, and length of stay is increased when a patient has complications after an RR event. An RR event raises the cost of the hospital stay by adding ICU days due to ICU readmission.

Project Goals

The following goals for this project are based on the Institute of Medicine's Six Aims for Improvement (Greene, 2007):

- Safety: Ensure that patients are stable enough to transfer to the medical–surgical floors from the ICU

- Effectiveness: Implement an assessment tool with indicators that are based on reliable research and develop a score predictive for the USAMC population based on data collected from sixth floor and ICU transfers
- Patient-Centered Care: Use the individual patient's data to develop a risk score and involve the patient/family in the process of notifying the nurse of sudden changes
- Timeliness: Ensure that the assessment tool does not slow down the transfer process by piloting it on recent transfers before moving it to the ICU
- Efficiency: Decrease bounce back transfers, which increase costs for hospital stays and increase lengths of stay
- Equality: All transferring patients will be scored by the same assessment tool to determine stability for the medical surgical floors

Process

The process of this project will follow the plan-do-study-act (PDSA) model (NHS Institute, 2008):

- Plan: There will be an adult risk assessment tool created to assess patients prior to transferring from the ICU to the floor at USAMC in an effort to decrease the number of bounce back transfers to the ICU. This tool will be tested on the sixth floor among patients received from the surgical trauma intensive care unit (STICUs).
- Do: The patients transferring to the sixth floor from ICU settings will be assessed by the tool and given risk scores based on their status at transfer, and patients in STICU ready for transfer will be scored prior to leaving the ICU.
- Study: The data collected from transfers will be used to determine risk scores predictive to the USAMC patient population.
- Act: The tool will be implemented on patients who are transferring from STICU to the sixth floor at USAMC. If RR events and bounce back transfers have decreased among patients who have transferred from a higher level of care within 24 hours, the tool will be adopted throughout the hospital.

Evaluation and Outcomes

The project will be evaluated by comparing the RR data after implementation of the risk assessment tool to the RR data prior to the tool. If this information shows a decrease in the number of RR events and readmissions to the ICU within 24 hours of transfer to the floor, then the tool will have had a positive impact on patient safety at USAMC.

References

Badawi, O., & Breslow, M. (2012). Readmissions and death after ICU discharge: Development and validation of two predictive models. *Plos One, 7*(11). Retrieved from http://www.plosone.org/article/info%3Adoi%2F10.1371%2Fjournal.pone.0048758

Daniels, C., Farmer, C., Gajic., O., Kashyap., R., Ofoma., U., & Pickering, B. (2012). Does implementation of a previously validated prediction tool reduce readmission rates into a medical intensive care unit? *Chest, 142*(4). Retrieved from http://journal.publications.chestnet.org/article.aspx?articleid=1376124

Greene, B. (2007). Tracking the six aims of the IOM report: Crossing the quality chasm—Healthcare in the 21st century. *Journal of Ambulatory Care Management, 30*(4), 281–282. Retrieved from http://www.nursingcenter.com/Inc/JournalArticle?ID=741559&JournalID=54005&IssueID=741596

NHS Institute for Innovation and Improvement. (2008). Plan, do, study, act. Retrieved from http://www.institute.nhs.uk/quality_and_service_improvement_tools/quality_and_service_improvement_tools/plan_do_study_act.html

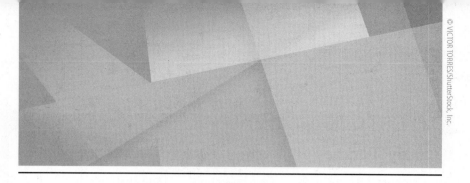

TWELVE

Analyzing and Managing Data: The Clinical Nurse Leader's Role

James M. Smith

 Learning Objectives
© Arenacreative/Dreamstime.com

- Define a problem in terms of objective and measurable data and a desired target or goal
- Determine the information that needs to be collected to explore solutions
- Consider possible problem solutions, select an intervention, and design an evaluation study
- Identify and describe tools for displaying data and converting them into meaningful information

> It is a capital mistake to theorize before one has data.
>
> **Sherlock Holmes**

Key Terms

Problem identification   Data collection   Data analysis
Data display and dissemination

CNL Roles

Advocate   Catalyst   Integrator
Broker   Risk averter

CNL Professional Values

Accountability   Outcome management   Quality improvement
Interprofessional teams   Integrity   Financial stewardship
Social justice

CNL Core Competencies

Data analysis   Design/management/coordination of care
Critical thinking   Ethical decision making   Communication
Assessment   Information and healthcare technologies
Resource management

Introduction

One of the roles of the clinical nurse leader (CNL) is to pursue clinical scholarship in the application of research to the clinical setting and the resolution of clinical problems. In this role, the CNL has accountability for the evaluation and improvement of outcomes, which includes not only using evidence-based practices but also striving to solve ad-hoc problems as they arise in the point-of-care setting. The keys to solving problems are knowing how to (1) identify and document problems, (2) analyze processes to derive possible solutions, (3) design intervention strategies, and (4) collect and analyze outcome data. These tasks require a comfort level with data, quality improvement methodology, and statistical concepts, as noted in the Clinical Nurse Leader Curriculum Framework Addendum to the American Association of Colleges of Nursing's (AACN's) *White Paper on the Role of the Clinical Nurse Leader* (AACN, 2007).

However, the task does not stop there; dissemination of findings in an informative and user-friendly format is essential. Among the CNL's tasks are the education of healthcare team members and "practical experience in the dissemination of clinical knowledge such as grand rounds, case presentations, and journal clubs" (AACN, 2007, p. 8). Sometimes the successful presentation and dissemination of information to other team members and to the organization at large (in charts, reports, posters, and presentations) can be the determining factor in whether or not these results impact practices at the program and organizational level.

Three aspects of data are critical to the improvement process: (1) data to document the existence of a problem, (2) data on the processes that result in the problematic outcome, and (3) data to demonstrate that an improvement initiative resulted in actual improvement.

Let's Improve . . . And Let's Do It Now!

It is a given that the CNL and other staff in a hospital or healthcare setting want to improve care. Not only do staff want to improve care, but they want to improve it as soon as possible. Although this intention is laudable, it often leads to problems that can impede the process of improvement, if not derail it altogether.

How often have you heard someone define a problem in phrases like this: "Housekeeping needs to do a better job!" This may sound like a fine problem statement—after all, lack of cleanliness in healthcare facilities is not only aesthetically displeasing but also represents a serious risk of patient harm. Other versions of this type of problem statement are common in other areas as well: "The Administration needs to build more parking!" or "The patients need to learn that they cannot miss their clinic appointments!"

This type of problem formulation arises from staff's laudable desire to fix problems, but, if one thinks about the problem statement "Housekeeping needs to do a better job," it becomes apparent that it is actually a proposed solution to a perceived problem, not a problem statement. Often when staff perceive a problem, they immediately think of a way to solve it and then state the problem as not having implemented their perceived solution, which may or may not be the most effective and efficient solution. Perhaps housekeeping needs to do a better job, or perhaps staff and visitors need clearer cleanliness reminders/guidelines, or perhaps there should be more obvious and plentiful places to put trash.

In addition, these "solution-type" problem statements usually impute blame to someone for the problem. In the given examples, it is housekeeping's fault that the facility is not clean, or the administration's fault that there is not enough parking, or the patients' fault for missing their appointments. "Let's work together to solve this problem by acknowledging up front that it's your fault" is not exactly the best way to start. Blame has no place in problem solving.

There are two steps in problem identification. The first is to collect objective and measureable data on the problem. What observations led to the conclusion that the facility is not as clean as it should be? Does the completion of periodic observational checklists reveal that ward floors are not clean, that bathrooms have paper towels on the floor, or that the cafeteria has used dishes remaining on the tables? Obtaining observable and measurable data on a possible problem often requires the collaborative skills of the CNL, working together with staff from many different areas of the facility (e.g., ward, quality improvement, administrative, business office).

Once objective and measurable data on the problem have been obtained, the CNL must ask, "Compared to what?" In addition to objective and measurable data, all problem statements should have a clearly stated desired solution level, namely a target or goal. This target can be based on national standards, accreditation requirements, organizational performance goals, or the desires of the program leader or chief executive officer. The target needs to be stated clearly and explicitly. If the current state does not meet the target, a problem exists. The decision about whether to address this or not relates to how great the deviation is from the desired target and how great the impact is on patient care or facility operations.

Causes of Problems

In a classic article published in *The New England Journal of Medicine*, Donald Berwick pointed out the folly of trying to improve an organization by eliminating incompetent or unmotivated workers from the workforce (Berwick, 1989). The vast majority of problem outcomes are not caused by poor employees (the so-called "bad apples"). Directing all improvement efforts at ridding the organization of these employees will not create significant improvement, and indeed will induce many coping behaviors that actually degrade performance (e.g., by employees distorting data). The vast majority of problematic outcomes are caused by deficiencies that occur in the sequence of processes that lead to the problematic outcome. This is as true of healthcare facilities as it is of automobile manufacturers or insurance companies, or even the local supermarket. Berwick notes that the most important investments in quality improvement are to study the complex production processes used in health care, noting that "we must understand them before we can improve them" (Berwick, 1989, p. 55).

The good news is that a business degree is not needed to find a possible solution—all that it takes is a detailed study to determine which process(es) contribute most to a problem outcome. In fact, in many instances, the solution will be readily apparent after studying the facts. It is reported that Willie Sutton, the famous bank robber, once said that he robbed banks "because that's where the money is!" Following Willie's example, the best strategy is to determine where the biggest bang for the buck is in the chain of processes that lead to a problematic outcome. Put another way, what are the specific point(s) in this process chain which, when changed, will produce the most dramatic improvement in outcome? Collect data on the processes, and the data will actually lead to a solution.

Study the Process: Find the Solution

There are various ways for the CNL to study processes (e.g., flow charts, fishbone diagrams, etc.), and many books have been written on processes and tools of improvement, some specifically tailored to healthcare settings (Brassard & Ritter, 2008; Graban, 2011).

Here is an example of a problem resolution that illustrates the importance of focusing on the most critical elements of a process. The authors of this study were interested in reducing delays in coronary thrombolysis for acute myocardial infarction patients in a 10-bed intensive care unit (ICU; Bonetti, Waeckerlin, Schuepfer, & Frutiger, 2000). In a sample of 16 consecutively measured patients (patients 1–16), these delays averaged 57 minutes, as compared to a generally accepted standard of 30 minutes. To determine how to improve this process, staff carefully monitored the next five admissions requiring thrombolysis (patients 17–21) and also met as an interprofessional team to discuss the specific causes of delays that each had personally experienced. This monitoring and discussion revealed a total of 22 different causes of delays that were listed on a fishbone diagram. The most noteworthy of these causes were a lack of communication and cumbersome/inadequate guidelines for handling this type of patient.

After implementing new communication and practice guidelines, door-to-needle time was tracked for the next 16 patients who required thrombolysis (patients 22–37); the results were a dramatic reduction in door-to-needle time. From a baseline intervention average time of 57 minutes (+/– 25.4), the postintervention time fell to an average of 32 minutes (+/– 9.0). This change was statistically significant ($p < 0.002$). In the baseline, 0 of 16 patients met the 30-minute standard, whereas in the postintervention phase, 10 of 16 patients met the standard.

The improvement in this ICU project is exactly what is desired from a quality improvement initiative—an overall better level of performance and less variability. This dramatic improvement was achieved by addressing a critical handful of the 22 causes of delay identified by the team in its process analysis.

A very simple test of whether or not an intervention introduced a statistically significant improvement over time is the run chart. The Institute for Healthcare Improvement has a brief but excellent online resource on run charts, which includes an Excel template as well as instructions for interpretation (Institute for Healthcare Improvement, 2011). Control charts can also be used to test the significance of interventions over time (Carey & Lloyd, 2001; Kelley, 1999).

One of the things the CNL should keep in mind in collecting data on process(es) is to collect the most detailed (granular) data that time and resources allow. For example, one facility had a problem with the system of escorts who took long-term care patients to clinics in the "main" hospital. There were complaints that escorts were late or sometimes did not arrive at all, and there was a feeling that a possible cause was that there were too many appointments in the afternoon. Had tallies of morning and afternoon appointments been kept, an increase in demand in the afternoon, but not a very dramatic one, would have been evident (see **Figure 12-1**).

Fortunately, much more detailed (granular) information was collected on the exact times that escorts were requested, so a much finer analysis of the process could occur. **Figure 12-2**, drawn from exactly the same data but plotted for every half-hour interval of the day, shows a much more detailed and informative picture of the fluctuation in demand for escorts.

By collecting data at this granular level, the facility was able to understand the process much more fully. These data, combined with additional analyses by day of week and the names of the specific clinics requiring escorts allowed the facility to intervene in this process in a very strategic way, by leveling out peak demands, increasing supply during peak periods, or a combination of both. That is the value of granular data.

Figure 12-1   Number of escorts in morning and afternoon.

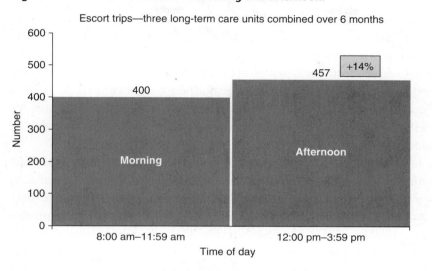

Escort trips—three long-term care units combined over 6 months

Figure 12-2   Number of escorts for every half hour during the day.

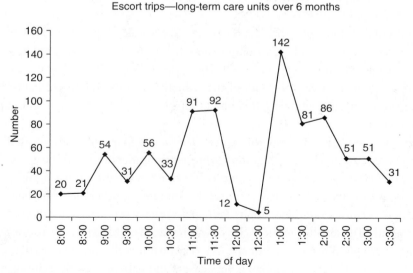

Escort trips—long-term care units over 6 months

Time of day = 30-minute period starting with the time listed.

Something Else

The need for data on the current status of the problem and data on the process steps that are involved in producing a problematic outcome was previously discussed. Following is a discussion of a third use of data—data collected to determine whether an intervention produced a real change in the outcome. However, before collecting outcome data one of the most important questions the CNL should ask is, "If I find after analyzing the results that a real change occurred (i.e., one most likely not due to chance) can I be sure that the results are due to my intervention, or could they be due to something else?"

Say, for example, that based on patient feedback, a CNL is planning a small improvement project to assess the effectiveness of telephone reminders in reducing the percentage of missed appointments. Parenthetically, many companies, both large and small, evaluate "small bets" such as this before implementing an initiative on a larger scale (Sims, 2011). The project involved (1) collecting baseline data for a month, (2) introducing telephone reminders, and (3) collecting follow-up data after the introduction of the telephone reminders. This was a one-group pretest–posttest design. Although this type of design is classified as "preexperimental" or "nonexperimental" because of the many problems associated with it (Campbell & Stanley, 1963; Heffner, 2004; Lennon-Dearing & Neeley-Barnes, 2012), it is nonetheless very frequently used in applied settings (as opposed to research settings) often due to forces requiring rapid responses.

The results of this study indicated that the percentage of missed appointments was reduced after the introduction of the reminders, and that the results were very unlikely to be due to chance (i.e., they were statistically significant). Could the CNL conclude that telephone reminders were the cause of the reduction in missed appointments? Most poster presentations employing this one-group pretest–posttest design would draw that conclusion.

Here are a few more details about the project. The facility in question was located in the northeastern United States, the month without reminders was February, and the month with reminders was March. Is it possible that a reduction in the number of missed appointments in March was caused by something other than the telephone reminders? How about the weather? Perhaps February was a particularly cold and snowy month. The director of these clinics was replaced on March 1. The former director was a very good physician, but she was very business-like and not particularly patient friendly. The new physician is very casual and patient friendly. Is it possible that the new and more patient-friendly director was the cause of the reduced number of missed appointments in March? The possible effects of the weather and the new director are considered threats to internal validity, namely, threats to the validity of conclusions a researcher may draw about an intervention. Other threats to the design relate to its external validity, namely, threats to the generalizability of its findings to other settings. The point of this example is to show that even if statistically significant results exist, a poor design choice can leave the conclusion in doubt.

Could the design of this small project have been improved? Definitely. The most dramatic improvement would have been to randomly assign patients either to a "no reminder group" or a "reminder group" and then collect data for both groups over the entire 2 months. Both groups would be influenced by the weather factor and the new director factor (as well as all other factors, some of which may be unknown). Randomization, given a sufficient number of cases, is the great equalizer. If a researcher has limited knowledge about this method and thus must employ the one-group pretest–posttest design, could it be improved? Yes—by doing all that can be done to avoid confounding factors. For example, scheduling an evaluation during a period when the weather would not be expected to have such a dramatic effect on missed appointments, and by scheduling it during a period in which the clinics would not be undergoing any dramatic changes (in leadership, clinic location, etc.). This approach would not rule out any other factors (e.g., an unexpected reduction in co-pay starting in March), but it would at least reduce the possible effect of known or anticipated confounding factors (e.g., the weather and the appointment of a new director).

How to choose the best design for an evaluation is a topic unto itself. Succinct descriptions of a number of basic design options (preexperimental, quasi-experimental, and true experimental designs) may be found in several sources (Campbell & Stanley, 1963; Heffner, 2004; Lennon-Dearing & Neeley-Barnes, 2012).

Analyzing Data: Tests of Statistical Significance

In statistics, a basic distinction is made between "descriptive statistics" (mean, mode, median, correlation, etc.) and "inferential statistics" (those that lead to $p < 0.05$ type conclusions). Consider this scene that illustrates the latter—a father and his young daughter meet a friend whom they have not seen in a few years, and the following brief interaction ensues:

Father: "You remember my daughter, Maggie?"
Friend: "My, she's gotten big. What grade is she in? The third?"

Why would the friend guess the third grade? Probably because of the child's size (primarily her height). The friend probably has a small database in his head of children he knows who are third graders (his own children, relatives, neighbors, etc.) and he compared this child to that database to make an educated guess (an inference) that she is in the third grade based on his recollection of the average height of third graders (mean) and the fact that all third graders are not exactly the same height (deviations from the mean). Could he be wrong? Certainly. Despite the fact that an educated guess based on height might place her in the third grade, she could actually be a tall second grader or a short fourth grader.

Inferences like this are made often. Consider this statement, "I think I can leave work on time, stop for pizza, and still get Bobby to his soccer game on time to play." This inference is based on data that have been accumulated over the course of time, data on how likely it is that a person will be able to leave work on time, how long it takes to drive to the pizza store, how long it takes to cook the pizza, how long it takes to drive home and eat, how long it takes to drive to the soccer game, and whether the coach will allow Bobby to play even if he arrives a few minutes late. This line of thinking requires making a series of educated guesses, actually quite a complicated series, with the distinct possibility that these guesses could be wrong; that is exactly what inferences are—making decisions under conditions of uncertainty.

Now take the previous example of the daughter, father, and friend, and suppose that the friend did not know any third graders; instead, someone gave him data on the heights of third graders. But instead of being given the heights of just a few third graders, he was given the heights of hundreds of third graders. Could an educated guess be made in this case? Yes, but there would be too much data to calculate in his head.

Recall also the previous example of telephone reminders. An intervention (telephone reminders) was introduced, and then the evaluation was designed to preclude the results being due to factors other than the reminders (e.g., weather or organizational or personnel changes). The evaluation was completed and the percentage of missed appointments for the period before reminders and the period after reminders was calculated. There was a reduction in the percent of missed appointments for the period after reminders. Can it be concluded that the reminders did in fact reduce missed appointments? Not just yet.

If data had been collected on missed appointments for each of the 2 months without introducing any change, and the average for each month was found, would these averages be exactly the same? This is highly unlikely, so the question remains,

"Is the difference observed due to an intervention or is it due to the natural variability in the process?" Inferential statistics helps answer the question, "How likely is it that chance (the natural variability of the process) caused the difference we observed?"

The majority of inferential statistics are built on a model of the normal curve, illustrated in **Figure 12-3** with hypothetical data on the height of third-grade girls with a mean of 50.0 inches and a standard deviation (SD) of 3.0 inches. As indicated, given these parameters, 68% of third graders would fall within +/–1 SD of the mean (i.e., from 47 to 53 inches), whereas 95% of third graders would fall within +/–2 SD of the mean (i.e., from 44 inches to 56 inches).

An educated guess about whether a girl of a certain height is likely to be in the third grade can be made based on the normal distribution of heights shown in Figure 12-3. If the height is more than 2 SD above or below the mean, the probability of not being a third grader is high. Similarly, an educated guess about whether the difference between two means is indicative of a real difference can be made by comparing this difference to a normal distribution of mean differences with a mean of 0.0 and the standard error of the difference between two means (SE$_{\text{mean difference}}$, comparable to the SD in the third-grade example). If the obtained difference between means is more than 2 SE$_{\text{mean differences}}$ from the mean of 0.0, it is possible to conclude that the difference between the two means is a real difference, not one due to the natural variability of the process.

One of the tests commonly employed to assess the likelihood that chance accounts for results is known as the student's t-test, which is an example of statistical inference. There are two types of t-tests—one that tests between groups composed of the same subjects tested before and after an intervention (known as a dependent

Figure 12-3   Hypothetical normal curve distribution for the height of third-grade girls.

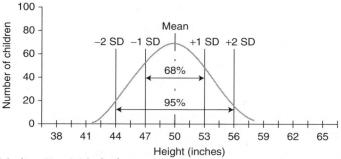

(Mean = 50.0 inches; SD = 3.0 inches)

t-test) and another that tests between two separate groups, one of which receives the intervention and one of which does not receive the intervention or that has the standard intervention (known as an independent t-test). Computing a t-test in Excel is easy; there are a number of books and websites that illustrate the process (Goldwater, 2007; Schmuller, 2009).

The Excel t-test results include the computed t-value and the exact probability of the result (i.e., the difference found between means) being due to chance. The values labeled as "two-tailed" should be used. Usually the chance (null) hypothesis is rejected if the exact probably of the result being a chance occurrence is less 5 in 100 times (usually denoted as $p < 0.05$). In this instance, an educated guess would be that the result is not due to chance, but rather due to something else, presumably the intervention if it is designed well.

There are many other tests of statistical significance based on the normal curve that are appropriate in varying situations (e.g., when comparing means of more than two groups). In addition, some inferential tests are not based on the normal curve (e.g., when the data consist of counts or rankings). These "nonparametric" tests are simpler to compute than those based on the normal curve, are nearly as powerful in detecting differences, and in many instances can be done merely with a calculator and a set of reference tables. The classic and very practical text on nonparametric statistics, *Nonparametric Statistics for the Behavioral Sciences*, is still available (Siegel, 1956).

There are two areas of caution in inferential statistics. First, the conclusions are always probability statements. If it is more likely that the result was due to an intervention than to the natural chance variation of the process (the probability of the latter being 0.05 or less), there is still the possibility, remote though it may be, that the result was due to chance. For statisticians, conclusions become more firmly established by confirming results from multiple studies (i.e., from replications). Second, inferential statistics allows us to draw conclusions about whether the intervention produced a real effect but cannot indicate whether this effect is important. Statistical significance is not the same as real world importance.

Suppose, for example, that statistical analysis indicated that telephone reminders did indeed reduce missed appointments, from 14.7% in the "no reminder group" to 13.5% in the "reminder group"; this is an actual reduction of 1.2% and is statistically significant ($p < 0.05$). Now also suppose that the reminder system costs $10,000 per month to operate. Even though there is a reduction in missed appointments as a result of the reminder system, a manager must decide whether the reduction of 1.2% is worth the expenditure of $10,000 per month. Or suppose that a new medication is more effective in reducing hypertension than other medications ($p < 0.05$) but is much more expensive or has a much more problematic side effect profile. The physician, in collaboration with the patient, must decide whether the more effective reduction in hypertension outweighs the cost and side effects. Inferential statistics does not make decisions for us; decisions are made based on a variety of factors.

Analyzing Data: Correlations

Sometimes evaluation studies done in applied settings involve correlations between two sets of data, for example, ratings by two different raters on the same scale for the same patients, blood values on split samples analyzed by older and newer blood analyzers, or the amount of fish oil supplements consumed and cardiovascular risk score. Note that in all these examples the scores in the two sets of data are "paired"— by patient, by blood sample, or by consumer.

Correlation, most commonly the Pearson product moment (linear) correlation, is a measure of the association between two sets of numbers (arrays). Correlations may range from +1.00 (high positive) to –1.00 (high negative). But what does a correlation really mean? If a new piece of laboratory equipment correlates 0.98 with the old piece of equipment, is it safe to replace the old equipment with the new equipment? If the ratings of two raters are highly correlated, is it fine to use them interchangeably?

Begin by noting that the biggest driver of the size of a correlation is the relative positions of values in the two arrays. The highest positive correlations result when the highest values in one array are closely aligned (i.e., paired) with the highest values in the other array, and lowest with lowest. If these values are plotted in a scatter plot that has values for one array on the x-axis and values for the other array on the y-axis, the resulting scatter plot will be close to a straight line, sloping up from the lower left to the upper right (see **Figure 12-4**, scatter plot A). Conversely, the highest negative correlations result when the highest values in one array are closely aligned with the lowest values in the other array and, conversely, the lowest with the highest. If these values are plotted in a scatter plot that has values for one array on the x-axis and values for the other array on the y-axis, the resulting scatter plot will be close to a straight line, sloping down from the upper left to the lower right (Figure 12-4, scatter plot B).

Figure 12-4   Scatter plots illustrating a high positive correlation (scatter plot A) and a high negative correlation (scatter plot B).

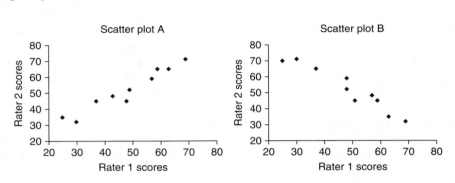

In interpreting correlations, the size of the correlation is most important (see **Table 12-1**). A note of caution—sometimes large sample sizes can produce statistically significant correlations that are so low as to be practically meaningless.

Computing a correlation in Excel is very easy. Follow these steps:

1. Open an Excel spreadsheet and enter 10 values in two adjacent columns.
2. Select any empty cell on a sheet (somewhere below the two arrays is fine) and type in "=correl(."
3. Click and drag down the first column of numbers (dotted lines will now enclose the first array) and type in a comma.
4. Click and drag down the second column of numbers (dotted lines will now enclose the second array).
5. Finish by typing a closed parenthesis sign and hit "Enter."

Your correlation will appear. Keep this spreadsheet open to use it again.

Table 12-1   Interpretative Guidelines for Size of Correlations

Size of Correlation	Interpretation
0.9–1.0	Very highly correlated
0.7–0.9	Highly correlated
0.5–0.7	Moderately correlated
0.3 – 0.5	Low correlation
< 0.3	Little if any correlation

In addition to its simplicity, another nice feature of computing correlations in Excel is that if there are data sets with missing data (one data value or the other or both have data values missing), the correlation as computed in the listed steps automatically eliminates any data pair where one or the other or both data values are missing. There is no need to sort the data to get complete data set pairs.

There are two major cautions that should be kept in mind in interpreting correlations. First, a correlation, even a high correlation, explains nothing—nothing whatsoever—about the comparability of the means of the two groups. Try this in the spreadsheet you created. Note the correlation previously computed. Now add 100 to each of the values in the second set of numbers. Although the means are now dramatically different, with one mean being exactly 100 points higher with the addition of the constant, the correlation stayed exactly the same. That is because in adding a constant no change was made in the relative positions of values in the two arrays in reference to each other—if the original correlation was relatively high, high scores on one are still associated with high scores on the other and low scores on one are still associated with low scores on the other. That is why, for example, a high correlation between readings on two pieces of laboratory equipment does not signify that they produce comparable values. Even though values on split blood samples for the two machines may be highly correlated, the new machine may be giving triglyceride levels that are two or three (or who knows how many) times higher than the old equipment. A second, and very important, caution about correlations is that a high correlation does not mean that one variable (*A*) causes the other variable (*B*). Correlation does not mean causation. *A* may cause *B*, or *B* may cause *A*, or they both may be caused by some other factor.

An example of drawing erroneous conclusions occurred in correlation studies of hormone replacement therapy and the risk of developing coronary heart disease (CHD). This 1991 meta-analysis of multiple epidemiological studies of women taking postmenopausal estrogens concluded that there was a reduced risk of CHD, which was "unlikely to be explained by confounding factors." Based on this finding, the Food and Drug Administration approved a label change, which included the prevention of heart disease as an indication for hormone replacement therapy (Lawlor, Smith, & Ebrahim, 2004). However, subsequent to these correlational studies, two large randomized trials found either no effect on CHD or a slightly increased risk (Hulley et al., 1998; Rossouw et al., 2002), and many have speculated on the possible confounding factors in the earlier epidemiological studies (Barrett-Connor, 2004; Kuller, 2004; Petitti, 2004; Lawlor et al., 2004;

Vandenbroucke, 2004). Despite problems associated with epidemiological (cor-relational) studies, they remain a valuable tool in identifying possible areas for more controlled trials.

Presenting Data

Although narratives and tables can be very useful in conveying results, charts are one of the most effective means of communicating, if they are selected with care and designed properly. As Roam (2011) notes in a broader context, "the mechanism for making good verbal communication great is to add the visual" (p. 51). It is not uncommon to see posters of improvement projects that were well designed and well executed with truly meaningful results that were hindered in the exposition by the use of poorly drawn charts.

Microsoft Office 2007 offers a dazzling array of chart choices; there are 11 types of charts and numerous variations of each. The challenge is to pick the correct chart for the data from among this vast array of 73 chart types/variations. Naomi Robins suggests a simple rule for selecting the most effective chart, "One graph is more effective than another if its quantitative information can be decoded more quickly or more easily by most observers" (Robbins, 2005, p. 6). The good news is that when this rule is applied to data that are typically presented in a hospital or other health-care setting, only a handful of the 73 chart types/variations meet the criterion of being able to convey information quickly and easily to most observers.

The first step in choosing a chart type is to select and format a chart that conveys the information that (the subject matter expert deems) is most important. It is not good practice to simply give raw data to an expert in chart design and delegate this decision to the expert. Consider the example of a CNL in a hypothetical South Beach Clinic who was concerned about declining patient satisfaction. The CNL desired to know whether this was affecting the number of patients enrolling and dropping out of the clinic (enrollees and attrition), so the CNL asked the data person to construct a chart of monthly data on enrollees and attrition over the past year. The data are presented in **Figure 12-5**. What conclusion can be drawn from this chart? How con-vincing is the conclusion?

Now suppose that instead of asking for a chart of enrollees and attrition the data person was told that the information of most interest was whether the clinic was gaining or losing patients each month (i.e., enrollees minus attrition). This data

Figure 12-5   South Beach Clinic: Enrollees and attrition by month.

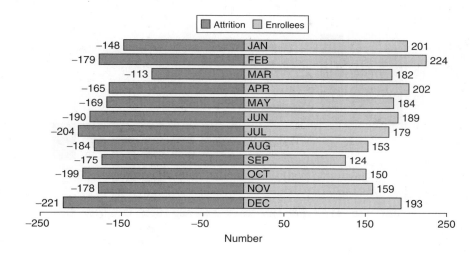

is presented in **Figure 12-6**. What conclusion could be drawn? How convincing is the conclusion? Both charts were drawn from exactly the same data; Figure 12-5 presents data, and Figure 12-6 presents information of value to management.

Other pitfalls in chart design to be avoided are poor title(s) for charts or axes (vague or incomplete), chart junk (e.g., distracting or space-wasting pictures or templates, shading/color for no purpose), and the use of the third dimension (e.g., depth of field effects in columns, bars, line, or pie charts), which conveys no information and makes the chart much more difficult to read and interpret (Smith, 2012).

Types of Charts

Here are some guidelines for different types of charts:

1. *Column (vertical) and bar (horizontal) charts.* These are ideal for showing values for independent categories on the *x*-axis, for example, different hospitals, different departments, and the like. Column charts (but not bar charts) can also be used to show a trend over time (e.g., years, months) but should not be used to convey a trend over long time intervals (more than

Figure 12-6 **South Beach Clinic: Net change by month.**

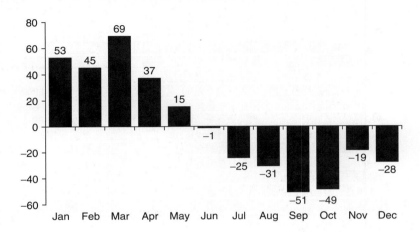

approximately eight time intervals). Never truncate the *y*-axis (the value axis) in a column or bar chart. Bar charts are particularly useful when the *x*-axis labels (categories) are lengthy.

2. *Line charts.* Line charts are ideally suited to showing trends over time for either short- or long-term intervals. The value axis (*y*-axis) of line charts may be truncated. Stacked lines are difficult to interpret by most observers and should be avoided.

3. *Pie charts.* Despite the widespread use of these charts, most experts in chart design agree that they should not be used. Observers cannot easily compare angular quantities in a pie chart, much less compare angles in a group of pie charts. Tufte (1983) wrote, "A table is nearly always better than a dumb pie chart; the only worse design than a pie chart is several of them, for then the viewer is asked to compare quantities located in spatial disarray both within and between pies . . ." (p. 178). Few (2007) wrote that, "Of all the graphs that play major roles in the lexicon of quantitative communication . . . the pie chart is by far the least effective. Its colorful voice is often heard, but rarely understood. It mumbles when it talks" (p. 1). If the goal is to show the distribution of data from numerous categories adding up to a total number or percentage (the typical use of a pie chart), use a column or bar chart, preferably arranged

in a Pareto format (highest value first progressing to the lowest value). If one absolutely must use a pie chart (e.g., your supervisor really, really likes them), it is possible to improve it somewhat by arranging the segments in increasing or decreasing order of magnitude.

4. *Scatter charts.* These are used when both the *x*-axis and the *y*-axis are composed of continuous values (e.g., scores 0 through 100 or 5.0 through 45.0). These are typically used to show a relationship between two sets of continuous variables. Use the "scatter with only markers" chart; do not use scatter charts with lines.

In general, area, stock, surface, donut, or bubble charts are of limited utility in most applications in a healthcare setting. Radar charts may be effective in certain instances, for example in showing performance on a number of variables in relation to targets that are different for each of the variables. There are a number of books on chart design; basic texts include those by Zelazny (2001) and Robbins (2005). The book by Few (2009) is of value for those desiring a more technical and comprehensive treatment.

Summary

- The vast majority of problems result from issues in work processes that result in a problematic outcome. Poor employee performance accounts for only a small percentage of these problems.
- Before attempting to find and implement a solution, objective and measurable data should be obtained on current performance. This data should be compared to a clear and an explicit desired target or goal.
- Data on the processes that produce problematic outcomes are the key to solutions. If you study these processes well, along with data, in many cases the solution will be readily apparent.
- Designing an evaluation strategy to assess a proposed solution requires care to ensure that the results of the evaluation are as unambiguous as possible.
- Dissemination of findings in an informative and user-friendly format is essential and can be the determining factor in whether these results impact practices at the program and organizational level. Charts are one of the most useful formats for presenting data, but it is essential that the correct chart be selected to ensure that the most critical information is clearly displayed.

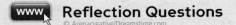

Reflection Questions

© Arenacreative/Dreamstime.com

1. How open is your organization to identifying problems? How willing is it to commit time and energy to solving them?
2. If you saw a problematic outcome, how would you approach getting your team involved in finding a solution? How would you respond to a staff member who said that this was always the way it had been and that things could not be improved?

Learning Activities

© Arenacreative/Dreamstime.com

1. Consider a problem outcome that occurs frequently or from time to time in your work setting. List the processes involved in producing this outcome and consider how you could collect data on these process steps.
2. Examine a published evaluation study. What design was used? What are the risks of this design? Did the authors adequately address them?
3. Select five published evaluation/research articles that used charts to display findings. Were the findings presented clearly so that they could be understood immediately? Was the correct chart selected for the data presented? Did these charts avoid the basic pitfalls of chart design?

References

American Association of Colleges of Nursing. (2007). *White paper on the role of the clinical nurse leader*. Washington, DC: Author. Retrieved from http://www.aacn.nche.edu/Publications /WhitePapers/ClinicalNurseLeader07.pdf

Barratt-Connor, E. (2004). Commentary: Observation versus intervention—what's different? *International Journal of Epidemiology, 33*(3), 457–459.

Berwick, D. M. (1989). Continuous improvement as an ideal in healthcare. *New England Journal of Medicine, 320*(1), 53–56.

Bonetti, P. O., Waeckerlin, A., Schuepfer, G., & Frutiger, A. (2000). Improving time-sensitive processes in the intensive care unit: The example of 'door to needle time' in acute myocardial infarction. *International Journal for Quality in Healthcare, 12*(4), 311–317.

Brassard, M., & Ritter, D. (2008). *The memory jogger II: Healthcare edition*. Salem, NH: Goal/QPC.

Campbell, D. T., & Stanley, J. C. (1963). *Experimental and quasi-experimental designs for research*. Chicago, IL: Rand McNally.

Carey, R. G., & Lloyd, R. C. (2001). *Measuring quality improvement in healthcare: A guide to statistical process control applications.* Milwaukee, WI: ASQ Quality Press.

Few, S. (2007, August). Save the pies for dessert. *Visual Business Intelligence Newsletter,* 1–14.

Few, S. (2009). *Now you see it: Simple visualization techniques for quantitative analysis.* Oakland, CA: Analytics Press.

Goldwater, E. (2007) *Using Excel for statistical data analysis—caveats.* Retrieved from http://people.umass.edu/evagold/excel.html

Graban, M. (2011). *Lean hospitals: Improving quality, patient safety, and employee engagement* (2nd ed.). Boca Raton, FL: CRC Press.

Heffner, C. L. (2004). Research methods, Chapter 5: Experimental design. Retrieved from http://allpsych.com/researchmethods/experimentaldesign.html

Hulley, S., Grady, D., Bush, T., Furberg, C., Herrington, D., Riggs, B., & Vittinghoff, E. (1998). Randomized trial of estrogen plus progestin for secondary prevention of coronary heart disease in postmenopausal women. Heart and Estrogen/progestin Replacement Study (HERS) Research Group. *JAMA, 280*(7), 605–613.

Institute for Healthcare Improvement. (2011). Run chart tool. Retrieved from http://www.ihi.org/knowledge/pages/tools/runchart.aspx

Kelley, D. L. (1999). *How to use control charts for healthcare.* Milwaukee, WI: ASQ Quality Press.

Kuller, L. H. (2004). Commentary: Hazards of studying women: The oestrogen oestrogen/progesterone dilemma. *International Journal of Epidemiology, 33*(3), 459–460.

Lawlor, D. A., Smith, G. D., & Ebrahim, S. (2004). Commentary: The hormone replacement-coronary heart disease conundrum: Is this the death of observational epidemiology? *International Journal of Epidemiology, 33*(3), 464–467.

Lennon-Dearing, R., & Neeley-Barnes, S. L. (2012). Quantitative research. In H. R. Hall & L. A. Roussel (Eds.), *Evidence-based practice: An integrative approach to research, administration and practice* (pp. 3–21). Burlington, MA: Jones & Bartlett Learning.

Petitti, D. (2004). Commentary: Hormone replacement therapy and coronary heart disease: Four lessons. *International Journal of Epidemiology, 33*(3), 461–463.

Roam, D. (2011). *Blah, blah, blah: What to do when words don't work.* New York, NY: Penguin Group.

Robbins, N. B. (2005). *Creating more effective graphs.* Hoboken, NJ: John Wiley & Sons.

Rossouw, J. E., Anderson, G. L., Prentice, R. L., LaCroix, A. Z., Kooperberg, C., Stefanik, M. L., … Ockgene, J. (2002). Writing Group for the Women's Health Initiative Investigators. Risks and benefits of estrogen plus progestin in healthy postmenopausal women: Principal results from the Women's Health Initiative randomized controlled trial. *JAMA, 288*(3), 321–333.

Schmuller, J. (2009). *Statistical analysis with Excel for dummies.* Hoboken, NJ: Wiley Publishing, Inc.

Siegel, S. (1956). *Nonparametric statistics for the behavioral sciences.* New York, NY: McGraw-Hill.

Sims, P. (2011). *Little bets: How breakthrough ideas emerge from small discoveries.* New York, NY: Free Press.

Smith, J. M. (2012). Problems with 3D charts. Retrieved from http://blog.indezine.com/2012/08/problems-with-3d-charts-by-james-m-smith.html

Stampfer, M. J., & Colditz, G. A. (1991). Estrogen replacement therapy and coronary heart disease: A quantitative assessment of the epidemiologic evidence. *Preventive Medicine, 20*(1), 47–63.

Tufte, E. R. (1983). *The visual display of quantitative information.* Cheshire, CT: Graphics Press.

Vandenbroucke, J. P. (2004). Commentary: The HRT story: Vindication of old epidemiological theory. *International Journal of Epidemiology, 33*(3), 456 –457.

Zelazny, G. (2001). *Say it with charts: The executive's guide to visual communication.* New York, NY: McGraw-Hill.

Transferring Patient Care—Continuity Between Organizations: The Psychiatric Patient Care Experience

Laurie A. Schwartz and Susan E. Koons

Pine Rest Christian Mental Health Services (PRCMHS) is a 150-bed freestanding psychiatric hospital located 10 miles from Saint Mary's Health Care (SMHC), a Trinity Health Organization. Psychiatric patients requiring medical assessment, treatment, or emergency services are frequently transferred to SMHC when medical situations arise. Following the emergency department (ED) evaluation, the patients are returned to PRCMHS or admitted to SMHC. The transfer process lacked standardization, causing communication gaps and prolonged patient ED stays, and was reflected in patient outcomes, unmet expectations, and increased staff dissatisfaction for both organizations. In response, the CNLs, at the direction of risk management and senior leadership at their respective facilities, partnered to lead a process improvement project.

Utilizing a Lean process improvement methodology, the CNLs directed a 15-member team of various disciplines from the two organizations through the project. Through deliberate collaboration, the team identified barriers, obstacles, and process gaps and developed and initiated a detailed action plan to improve the patient transfer experience to the ED.

Process flow improvements and tools were identified and developed at each organization. An improved patient transfer process flow, including collaborative design of a prearrival form (PAF) tool with telephone communication scripting and a patient transfer packet and checklist, improved the handoffs between the organizations. Internal process improvements at PRCMHS included an ambulance call system, psychiatric sitter guidelines, and an after-hour call tool for the psychiatric nurse communicating with the on call medical team. At SMHC, whiteboards and hourly rounding with the psychiatric sitter have improved the communication flow and resulting communication to PRCMHS.

Initial outcome data, including staff surveys, indicate 100% completion and resulting satisfaction with the PAF, which alerts the ED to the incoming psychiatric patient. The after-hour general information to medical (GIM) tool, designed in a situation, background, assessment, recommendation (SBAR) format, is a guideline to equip nursing in providing accurate, pertinent information to after-hour on-call medical providers. With the use of the GIM tool, during a 3-month monitoring period, the average number of after-hour calls decreased by 55%. GIM tool usage increased from 5% to 90%. The average number of inappropriate, nonurgent, after-hour calls decreased by 50%. Patient length of stay in the ED and subsequent sitter time decreased by 1 hour for this patient population. Overall staff satisfaction improved by a rate of 50%, which was the stated outcome goal.

This collaborative effort was led by CNLs who have expertise in risk assessment and microsystem analyses in psychiatric and emergency nursing care. Implementation of this process improvement has generated additional systemwide awareness, produced impetus for ongoing change processes, and generated transfer process revisions for programs and transfers to other facilities. Ultimately, it has improved relationships between two organizations, created an understanding of shared experiences, and improved the transfer process of a complex patient.

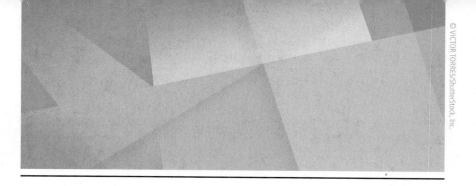

THIRTEEN

The Role of Informatics and Decision Support in Advancing Clinical Nurse Leader Practice

Julia Stocker-Schneider

Learning Objectives

- Discuss the role of informatics in decision support
- Identify how information and decision support can guide clinical nurse leaders' practice
- Discuss the relevance and importance of database management and asking and answering clinical questions

> Imagination is more than knowledge.
>
> **Albert Einstein**

Introduction

The need to improve the safety and quality of health care in the United States has been evident over the last decade and has led to a call for significant transformation of our healthcare system (Institute of Medicine [IOM], 1999,

Key Terms

Informatics	Decision support	Database management
Consumer informatics	Health literacy	

Health Insurance Portability and Accountability Act (HIPAA)

CNL Roles

Information manager	Outcomes manager	Member of a profession
Team member	Systems analyst and risk anticipator	
Client advocate	Educator	

CNL Professional Values

Altruism	Integrity	Social justice
Accountability	Human dignity	

CNL Core Competencies

Data analysis	Design/manage/coordinate care
Critical thinking	Ethical decision making
Communication	Assessment
Information and healthcare technologies	Resource management

2001). Major national strategies have been identified to support the goals of safe, effective, patient-centered, timely, efficient, and equitable care. One such initiative includes the broad use of informatics and technology in health care and the creation of a national health information infrastructure that will support safe, reliable, and high-quality healthcare (IOM, 2004b). Recognized potential benefits of the widespread adoption of electronic health record (EHR) systems include improved safety, disease prevention, chronic disease management, and efficiency in healthcare delivery; potential savings resulting from these gains are projected at more than $81 billion annually (Hillestad et al., 2005).

Although recognition of the essential nature of informatics in health care and nursing has grown, significant efforts were required to remove barriers to implementation by health systems and health providers. The recent Health Information Technology for Economic and Clinical Health (HITECH) Act contained in the American Recovery and Reinvestment Act (2009) provided for unprecedented investment in and expansion of health information technology in the United States and included provisions to incentivize hospitals and providers who demonstrate "meaningful use" of EHRs (Blumenthal & Tavenner, 2010). According to the Office of the National Coordinator for Health Information Technology (ONC, 2012), 35% of all nonfederal acute care hospitals reported using basic EHRs in 2011, which represents a doubling of hospital adoption of EHRs since 2009. Further, the ONC reports that 85% of hospitals intend to adopt EHRs according to the provisions set forth in the HITECH Act.

The clinical nurse leader (CNL) role was conceived to meet the need for high-quality graduates prepared for clinical leadership, implement outcomes-based practice and quality improvement strategies, practice at the full scope of education and ability, and create and manage microsystems of care that are responsive to the needs of individuals and families (American Association of Colleges of Nursing [AACN], 2007). The use of informatics and technology are necessary for the achievement of the goals of the CNL role.

Given the gains to be achieved from the use of healthcare and nursing informatics, the increasingly widespread availability of health information technology, and the primacy of informatics to the role of the CNL, informatics should be fully incorporated into the day-to-day work of the CNL. Information management and clinical decision support are primary ways a CNL can leverage informatics to achieve desired outcomes.

Healthcare and Nursing Informatics

Healthcare informatics is a multidisciplinary science that involves the integration of healthcare science, computer science, information science, and cognitive science to support the management of healthcare information (Hunter & Bickford, 2011). Nursing informatics is a subset of healthcare informatics; it is a nursing specialty that integrates nursing science, computer science, and information science to manage and communicate data, information, knowledge, and wisdom in nursing practice (American Nurses Association [ANA], 2008).

Nursing informatics is concerned with data, information, knowledge, and wisdom. These metaparadigm concepts of the specialty build on one another. Data are defined as discrete entities that are objectively described without interpretation. Information refers to data that are interpreted, organized, or structured; knowledge is the synthesis of information that leads to the identification and formalization of relationships. Wisdom is the use of knowledge to manage and solve human problems. The goal of nursing informatics is to support nurses, patients, and other care providers in their decision making in all roles and across various settings (ANA, 2008).

Informatics Competencies in Nursing and in the CNL Role

As informatics has become more integrated into the delivery of health care, in recent years much attention has been given to the growing need for nurses and other health-care providers to demonstrate informatics competence. Nursing informatics competencies were conceptualized by Staggers, Gassert, and Curran (2002) as including computer skills, informatics knowledge, and informatics skills. The major categories of informatics competencies identified in the research include the following:

- *Computer Skills:* Administration, communication, data access, decision support, documentation, education, monitoring, basic desktop software, systems, quality improvement, research, CASE (computer-aided software engineering tools), project management, simulation
- *Informatics Knowledge:* Data, impact, privacy/security, systems, education, research, usability and ergonomics, regulations
- *Informatics Skills:* Evaluation, role, analysis, data structures, design/development, fiscal management, implementation, management, privacy/security, programming, requirements, system maintenance, system selection, testing, research, training, education (Staggers, Gassert, & Curran, 2001)

This list includes all identified categories for the four levels of nursing informatics practice; competencies were delineated for beginning nurses, experienced nurses, informatics specialists, and informatics innovators. Beginning nurse competency was heavily focused on categories related to computer skills and some informatics knowledge, with no informatics skills. Experienced nurse informatics competencies include mostly computer skills and informatics knowledge, with the addition of a few select information skills. Informatics specialist competencies include high-level computer skills, all categories of informatics knowledge, and the majority of the informatics skills categories. Informatics innovators possess advanced competencies in computer skills, informatics knowledge, and informatics skills and are distinguished from the other levels largely by the extent of their informatics skills and knowledge (Staggers et al., 2001).

Informatics and the CNL Role

Of the 10 assumptions outlined in the AACN's white paper on the CNL role, the following 4 are fundamentally connected to informatics:

1. Client care outcomes are the measure of quality practice.
2. Practice guidelines are based on evidence.
3. Information will maximize self-care and client decision making.
4. Communication technology will facilitate the continuity and comprehensiveness of care. (AACN, 2007, pp. 6–10)

Building a practice that focuses on outcomes measurement and quality improvement is best accomplished using informatics tools and skills that support collection and analysis of outcomes. Informatics integration can support the identification of evidence, which is the basis for formulating guidelines that support the transformation of data into information, knowledge, and wisdom. Further, information technology can incorporate guidelines and decision support that lead to improved practice guideline adherence and the routine use of evidence in clinical decisions. The capacity of information technology to support decision making by patients and families also assists CNLs in promoting self-care and informed decision making that leads to improved outcomes, particularly for those individuals with chronic disease.

The AACN's white paper (2007) identified 17 fundamental aspects of the role of the CNL. Of these, 15 are best accomplished through the use of informatics. Specific key aspects of the CNL role linked to the use of informatics include the following:

- Design and provision of health promotion and risk reduction services for diverse populations
- Provision of evidence-based practice

- Population-appropriate health care to individuals, clinical groups/units, and communities
- Clinical decision making
- Design and implementation of plans of care
- Risk anticipation
- Participation in identification and collection of care outcomes
- Accountability for evaluation and improvement of point of care outcomes
- Mass customization of care
- Education and information management
- Delegation and oversight of care delivery and outcomes
- Team management and collaboration with other health professional team members
- Development and leveraging of human, environmental, and material resources
- Management and use of client-care and information technology
- Lateral integration of care for a specialized group of patients (AACN, 2007, pp. 10–11)

CNL Core Informatics Competencies

Core CNL competencies that require informatics knowledge and skills include the following:

- *Critical Thinking:* CNLs should incorporate the use of data, decision support, and evidence to think critically about practice problems and solutions, evaluate outcomes of patient care, and design and improve client care.
- *Communication:* The exchange of information between the CNL and all members of the microsystem is vital and should include electronic communication, documentation, and communication within the EHR; the access and use of data and information from many sources; and the ability to support self-care and the education of clients and families using electronic means.
- *Nursing Technology and Resource Management:* CNLs should demonstrate knowledge of the system lifecycle, including the acquisition, use, and evaluation of technology to support patient care. Additionally, they should understand usability factors that reflect the human–computer interaction.

- *Health Promotion, Risk Reduction, and Disease Prevention:* CNLs should use database query methods to identify clients at risk and adopt electronic strategies that support health promotion and disease prevention.
- *Illness and Disease Management:* Data, information, knowledge, and wisdom should be used by the CNL to support illness and disease management activities, including managing risk and illness progression, as well as promoting the use of personal health tools to support clients and their families in self-care activities.
- *Information and Healthcare Technologies:* The CNL should be a leader and role model within the microsystem in the use of informatics to support care delivery. The CNL should support the use of informatics to generate information, knowledge, and wisdom about client outcomes. Further, the effectiveness of microsystems processes that contribute to outcomes achievement can best be understood and improved on by using informatics. The CNL should consistently advocate for the use of decision support to promote evidence-based practice. The CNL should also provide a leadership role throughout the systems lifecycle as new technologies and information management systems are incorporated into practice.
- *Ethics:* Protected patient information should be made secure in all information technologies (including handheld devices and smartphones) as outlined in the Health Insurance Portability and Accountability Act (HIPAA); CNLs should advocate for the judicious and secure use of protected patient information only by those who require it.
- *Healthcare Systems and Policy:* CNLs should be knowledgeable about policies and regulations pertaining to the use of informatics (such as HIPAA, the HITECH Act, and the "meaningful use" regulation)
- *Providing and Managing Care:* Best practices for the management of patient care for clients and populations requires the use of informatics, including use of databases to generate information, knowledge, and wisdom, and decision support for microsystem providers and clients and families.
- *Designing/Managing/Coordinating Care:* The CNL should incorporate informatics practices in all aspects of the design, management, and coordination of patient care. Knowledge generated from information systems should be used to continually improve care for individual clients and for the entire microsystem.

CNL Informatics End-of-Program Competencies

The AACN's (2007) white paper on the CNL identifies the following end of CNL master's degree education program competencies that relate to the use of informatics:

- Uses information systems and point of care technology to improve patient outcomes
- Effective communication (including electronically) to achieve quality client outcomes and lateral care integration for a patient population
- Identifies clinical and cost outcomes (that may be analyzed using the EHR or other organization data) that improve safety, effectiveness, timeliness, efficiency, quality, and the degree to which they are client centered
- Participates in systems review (including identification of appropriate EHR and organizational data) to critically evaluate and anticipate risks to client safety to improve quality of client care delivery
- Assumes accountability for healthcare outcomes for a specific group of clients within a unit or setting (relying on informatics to accomplish), recognizing the influence of the meso- and macrosystems on the microsystem
- Assimilates and applies research-based information (using decision support as appropriate) to design, implement, and evaluate client plans of care
- Uses appropriate teaching/learning principles and strategies (including consumer decision support, as well as current information, materials, and technologies) to facilitate the learning of clients, groups, and other healthcare professionals.

The Impact of Informatics on Care Delivery

Numerous benefits of the use of informatics in health care have been identified, including:

- Access to secure, timely, pertinent patient information where and when it is needed
- The means to record and manage episodic and longitudinal patient information
- Support for planning and delivery of evidence-based care to individuals and groups
- Streamlining clinical work flow

- Supporting the collection of data for quality improvement, outcomes reporting, billing, resource planning, and performance management (Hebda & Czar, 2013).

These benefits translate into improvements in client care that result from information control features that support patient safety, clinical decision support, improved communication among care providers, and the building of information and knowledge through aggregation of data that provides for pattern recognition, decision support, and microsystem processes and outcomes knowledge for use in quality improvement.

The Electronic Health Record

The EHR generally serves as the centerpiece in leveraging information technology. It is known as an enterprise solution because it incorporates the management of clinical functions with business functions. An EHR is a longitudinal electronic record of patient health information generated during one or more encounters in any care setting. Information contained in an EHR includes patient demographics, medical history, problems, medications, immunizations, vital signs, progress notes, and laboratory and radiology reports. The EHR automates clinical information and streamlines the clinician's workflow. It serves as the complete record of a patient's clinical encounters (HIMSS, 2012).

Clinical Decision Support

Clinical decision support (CDS) refers to the process of enhancing health-related decisions and actions through the use of relevant, organized clinical knowledge and patient information to improve health and healthcare quality and outcomes (Osheroff et al., 2012). This broad definition is useful in that it captures the spectrum of CDS, from EHRs that match patient information and clinical knowledge for clinicians in real time, to the manual use of clinical knowledge to support decisions. Common forms of CDS include the use of charts to simplify complex information (e.g., growth charts), EHR templates, medication prescribing and administration alerts and reminders, medication formularies, clinical guidelines, and health literature databases (e.g., CINAHL; Berner & LaLande, 2007; Dowding et al., 2009). The three key purposes of CDS are to:

1. Assist in problem solving with semistructured problems
2. Support (rather than replace) the judgment of a manager or clinician
3. Improve the effectiveness of the decision-making process

A clinical decision support system (CDSS) is a computerized system that provides clinicians or patients with pertinent clinical knowledge and patient-related information in a timely manner that enhances patient care (Androwich & Ross Kraft, 2011).

As noted previously, essential aspects of CDS include the process of using organized clinical knowledge and patient information for the purpose of improving patient care. As such, CDS, through data analysis and data mining, is useful, although this form of retrospective review is not considered a CDSS (Berner & LaLande, 2007). Regardless of the sophistication of the CDS approach, CDS is associated with the use of informatics. The process of decision support relies on turning practice data into information, knowledge, and wisdom, which serve as the very basis of nursing informatics. Despite the desire to move toward CDSSs, vendors have been slow to include significant CDSS features. Dramatic growth in the availability of enhanced CDSS features in EHRs has been evident since passage of the HITECH Act, as the "meaningful use" regulation supporting the act requires the use of CDSS by providers in order to be eligible for "meaningful use" incentives (Harrison & Lyerla, 2012).

Using Databases to Generate Information, Knowledge, and Wisdom

Databases are capable of generating information and knowledge for CDS through the use of query and reporting techniques. Data, or discrete objective entities (e.g., pulse rate 88 bpm) are generally entered into databases using forms that are typically visible to the user in an EHR. A database is a collection of related objects, including tables, forms, queries, and reports. Once data are entered, they are organized into tables so that they can be stored and retrieved in an organized way. The tables are connected by identical key fields that relate them to one another. A query is the mechanism that is used to ask questions of the data from one or more related tables. Reports are used to display information generated from the query (Sewell & Thede, 2013). Through the query process, desired data are aggregated and organized in a way that generates information. Interpretation of information in the context of clinical practice by clinicians turns information into knowledge. The application of knowledge to the provision of care by the clinician or nurse creates and involves wisdom.

Querying the Data

Given the role of the CNL as outlined earlier in this chapter, it is clear that CNLs should be knowledgeable regarding the overall process of generating information from database analysis using the query process. Generally, the CNL may not be the one directly querying the data. However, possessing a clear understanding of the process and the requirements for running queries will greatly enhance the likelihood of success in a querying effort. The following is a general outline of steps that should be taken by the CNL in collaboration with the available informatics expert in the system (e.g., the nurse informaticist, systems analyst, etc.) to query client and microsystem data:

1. *Determine the question you want to ask of the data:* Identify what it is you wish to learn about from the data (e.g., risk factors for certain outcomes, etc.).
2. *Understand what data are available:* Queries may only be made of available data. Think about data that you know are entered in your EHR or in other places in your organization using other information technology solutions.
3. *Determine which of the available data would best answer your question:* List all of the data elements you require (including time frame). Make sure to adhere to HIPAA standards. Whenever possible, data should be "scrubbed" to remove patient identifiers.
4. *Evaluate the integrity of the data:* Consult with your organization's informatics specialist to identify any known problems with the quality of the data (e.g., missing, inaccurate, not retrievable, etc.) (Hebda & Czar, 2013).
5. *Determine if the data are standardized:* Data collected in a standardized format (e.g., via dropdown or radio button) are much more easily aggregated and queried than other forms of data. Data entered in text fields cannot be aggregated unless they are converted to data using Natural Language Processing. If data are being aggregated across databases and vendors, the vendors must adhere to data vocabulary and content standards in order to be interoperable (Francisco, 2011; Sensmeier, 2011).
6. *Investigate the EHR's capacity to run basic queries:* Most EHRs have the capacity to generate report "pick lists" that can be customized and run by certain groups

of authorized users. If you can run your query this way, seek information technology (IT) support as needed to run and analyze the report.

7. *Ask for a custom query to be run:* If the data elements you wish to query cannot be run through a "pick list," follow your organization's procedure to request the required query. Consult with your informatics nurse or systems analyst to assist you with interpretation of the query.

Data Mining and Analytics

The term used to describe the process of selecting, storing, and modeling large volumes of data to discover unknown patterns and relationships of use is known as data mining (Bellazzi & Zupan, 2008). Although data mining (also known as knowledge discovery) has been around since the 1990s, the process is just beginning to be widely used due to the dramatic increase in the availability of "big" data, advances in technology that have enabled data to be more retrievable, improved use of standards that promote interoperability, and technological advances that have led to the development of better query methods and tools. Analysis of big data has followed trends in other industries and has increasingly been referred to as analytics (Hasson, 2012). Data analytics may be helpful to CNLs in improving understanding of risk, client outcomes, and microsystem processes and outcomes. Generally, this type of analysis requires the support of a systems analyst or nurse informaticist.

Clinical Decision Support Systems

As mentioned previously, CDSSs have become increasingly available and serve as beneficial tools to support clinical decisions in real time. Although wide variability exists across CDSSs, most contain these three major parts:

1. *Knowledge Base:* Consists of compiled information, often in the form of if–then rules (e.g., *if* a nurse attempts to administer a PRN medication sooner than the ordered frequency, *then* a warning or stop will be presented).

2. *Inference or Reasoning Engine:* Contains the formulas for combining the associations or rules in the knowledge base to the patient data.

3. *Mechanism to Communicate with the User:* Involves the input of patient data into the system and the output message to the user who will be making the decision.

Variability in CDSSs is related to the following factors:

- *Standalone or Integrated:* Such as a knowledge lookup engine contained in a smartphone or knowledge integration into an EHR.
- *Active or Passive:* Does the system provide active alerts, or does it passively respond to data that are entered?
- *Knowledge Based or Predictive:* Is the support provided by connecting the user to pertinent knowledge contained in the system, or does it recognize patterns in the data to make predictions based on the trajectory of previous such occurrences in the database? (Berner & LaLande, 2007)

Integrating CDS to Improve Outcomes

The desired result of CDS is to improve outcomes, a major role for the CNL. As a microsystems leader, the CNL is well poised to lead efforts to implement CDS solutions for improving client and microsystem outcomes. Osheroff and colleagues (2012) recommend use of the Five Rights Framework for CDS to guide the process. According to the framework, the "rights" to be considered include the following:

1. *The Right Information (What):* What information will be communicated to the user to support decision making?
2. *The Right Person (Who):* The care team members who are the desired targets for the information must be identified.
3. *The Right CDS Intervention Format (How):* The intervention types and circumstances must be determined; use care to select the right tool for the job.
4. *The Right Channel (Where):* The delivery location for the information must be determined (e.g., the EHR). For CDS interventions that do involve the EHR, a nurse informaticist or systems analyst should be involved to determine what interventions are feasible within the system. Vendor products typically contain a range of CDS functions, though additions and changes generally can be made. The healthcare organization's IT staff may need to work with the vendor to accomplish certain CDS interventions.
5. *The Right Time in the Workflow (When):* The effectiveness of CDS is timing dependent. If the information is not delivered at the right time in the user workflow, the desired impact will not be achieved.

Keys to Success in CDS Intervention

Successful implementation of a CDS intervention involves using a change approach within the microsystem. Considerations for developing a CDS plan should include the following:

- *Involve the Right Stakeholders:* Make sure end users and other key participants are part of the planning and development process for the CDS.
- *Determine Goals:* Clearly define what you are trying to accomplish as a microsystem through use of the CDS intervention.
- *Plan the CDS:* Use the "Five Rights" framework to determine what, who, how, where, and when you plan to deliver.
- *Understand Capabilities:* CDS interventions may be limited by what the organization's EHR can do, so careful involvement of the organization's IT staff and consultation with the vendor as needed is essential.
- *Communicate:* As with the introduction of any change, communication is essential to gain buy-in for the CDS intervention.
- *Evaluate:* Plan for how you will monitor the effectiveness of the program and provide mechanisms for improvement.

Improving Outcomes with Clinical Decision Support: An Implementer's Guide (Osheroff et al., 2012) serves as an excellent guide for a more detailed approach to implementing CDS.

Consumer Decision Support

The assumptions underlying the CNL role specifically identify the role of information as maximizing self-care and client decision making. Thus, consumer decision support is a tool that should be used in CNL practice. Consumer decision support can take many forms, including:

- *Health Information Seeking:* Many electronic resources are available for clients who are seeking health information, including Internet sources and mobile device applications.
- *Communication and Support:* Email, online support groups, and social media are available.

- *Personal Health Records:* Personal health records that allow patients to retain personal health information (such as health and medication history) and to generate recordings to support self-care are increasingly available and may eventually be interoperable with EHRs.

Regardless of the form of decision support, health literacy should be considered. Health literacy is defined as the extent to which individuals have the ability to obtain, process, and understand basic health information needed to make appropriate health decisions (IOM, 2004a). Access to electronic forms of CDS by clients and family members should be assessed, and their ability to locate and assess the quality of health information should also be taken into account (Alpay, Verhoef, Xie, Te'eni, & Zwetsloot-Schonk, 2009). These challenges notwithstanding, CNLs should incorporate the use of consumer decision support into practice in clinical microsystems as a mechanism to improve patient outcomes (Zielstorff & Frink, 2011).

Summary

- Informatics is a valuable tool that should be well incorporated into the CNL role.
- The use of informatics supports quality and efficiency in care delivery in the microsystem.
- CDS is a powerful and increasingly available component that relies on and is often delivered by informatics solutions.
- CDS can be leveraged by CNLs through data queries, data mining and analytics, and the use of CDSSs.

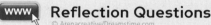 **Reflection Questions**
© Arenacreative/Dreamstime.com

1. Evaluate your level of competence with informatics. What areas do you need to learn more about, and how can you gain the necessary knowledge?
2. What client outcomes or microsystems issues are you aware of that could be ameliorated by using CDS? Formulate a question that can be asked of the data and determine the data elements you would likely need to answer the question.

3. How well do you manage information within your microsystem? Identify ways that you might more fully leverage informatics in your microsystem to support quality, safe, and efficient care.

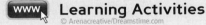

Learning Activities

1. Speak with your organization's nurse informaticist, systems analyst, or IT department to find out what reports can be generated from your EHR. Discuss which queries you can run yourself and the steps required to run them. Inquire about the possibility of running additional reports and what your organization's process is to request these queries.
2. Determine the types of CDS that your organization currently uses in its microsystem. Identify areas that might benefit from a CDS intervention.
3. Review your EHR for CDSS functions. Talk with your organization's nurse informaticist, systems analyst, or IT department to determine the feasibility of expanding the CDSS in your current system.

References

Alpay, L., Verhoef, J., Xie, B., Te'eni, D., & Zwetsloot-Schonk, J. H. M. (2009). Current challenge in consumer health informatics: Bridging the gap between access to information and information understanding. *Biomedical Informatics Insights*, *2*(1), 1–10.

American Association of Colleges of Nursing. (2007). *White paper on the role of the clinical nurse leader*. Washington, DC: Author. Retrieved from http://www.aacn.nche.edu/publications /white-papers/cnl

American Nurses Association. (2008). *Nursing informatics: Scope and standards of practice*. Silver Spring, MD: Author.

Androwich, I. M., & Ross Kraft, M. (2011). Incorporating evidence: Use of computer-based clinical decision support systems for health professionals. In V. K. Saba & K. A. McCormick (Eds.), *Essentials of nursing informatics* (5th ed., pp. 427–436). New York, NY: McGraw Hill.

Bellazzi, R., & Zupan, B. (2008). Predictive data mining in clinical medicine: Current issues and guidelines. *International Journal of Medical Informatics*, *77*(2), 81–97. doi:10.1016/j .ijmedinf.2006.11.006

Berner, E. S., & LaLande, T. J. (2007). Overview of clinical decision support systems. In E. S. Berner (Ed.), *Clinical decision support systems* (Vol. 6, pp. 463–477). New York, NY: Springer.

Blumenthal, D., & Tavenner, M. (2010). The "meaningful use" regulation for electronic health records. *The New England Journal of Medicine, 363*(6), 501–504.

Dowding, D., Randell, R., Mitchell, N., Foster, R., Lattimer, V., & Thompson, C. (2009). Clinical decision support systems in nursing. In B. Staudinger, V. Höß, & H. Ostermann (Eds.), *Nursing and clinical informatics: Socio-technical approaches* (pp. 26–40). Hershey, PA: IGI Global.

Francisco, P. (2011). The quest for quality: Turning data into information. *Nursing economic$, 29*(2), 101–104.

Harrison, R. L., & Lyerla, F. (2012). Using nursing clinical decision support systems to achieve meaningful use. *Computers, Informatics, Nursing, 30*(7), 380–385. doi:10.1097/NCN.0b013e31823eb813

Hasson, J. (2012). VA harnesses big data for broader impact. *Aol Government.* Retrieved from http://gov.aol.com/2012/08/23/va-harnesses-big-data-for-broader-impact/?icid=apb1#page1

Hebda, T., & Czar, P. (2013). *Handbook of informatics for nurses and healthcare professionals* (5th ed.). Boston, MA: Pearson.

Hillestad, R., Bigelow, J., Bower, A., Girosi, F., Meili, R., Scoville, R., & Taylor, R. (2005). Can electronic medical record systems transform health care? Potential health benefits, savings, and costs. *Health Affairs (Project Hope), 24*(5), 1103–1117. doi:10.1377/hlthaff.24.5.1103

HIMSS. (2012). Electronic health record (EHR). Retrieved from http://www.himss.org/ASP/topics_ehr.asp

Hunter, K. M., & Bickford, C. J. (2011). The practice specialty of nursing informatics. In V. K. Saba & K. A. McCormick (Eds.), *Essentials of nursing informatics* (5th ed., pp. 171–189). New York, NY: McGraw Hill.

Institute of Medicine. (1999). *To err is human: Building a safer health system.* Washington, DC: National Academies Press.

Institute of Medicine. (2001). *Crossing the quality chasm: A new health system for the 21st century.* Washington, DC: National Academies Press.

Institute of Medicine. (2004a). *Health literacy: A prescription to end confusion.* Washington, DC: National Academies Press.

Institute of Medicine. (2004b). *Patient safety: Achieving a new standard for care.* Washington, DC: National Academies Press.

Office of the National Coordinator of Health for Health Information Technology. (2012). Electronic health record systems and intent to attest to meaningful use among non-federal acute care hospitals in the United States: 2008–2011. *ONC Data Brief, 1*, 1–7.

Osheroff, J. A., Teich, J. M., Levick, D., Saldana, L., Velasco, F. T., Sittig, D. F., . . . Jenders, R. A. (2012). *Improving outcomes with clinical decision support: An implementer's guide* (2nd ed.). Chicago, IL: HIMSS.

Sensmeier, J. (2011). Health data standards: Development, harmonization, and interoperability. In V. K. Saba & K. A. McCormick (Eds.), *Essentials of nursing informatics* (5th ed., pp. 233–45). New York, NY: McGraw Hill.

Sewell, J., & Thede, L. (2013). Databases: Creating information from data. *Informatics and nursing: Opportunities and challenges* (4th ed., pp. 155–80). Philidelphia, PA: Walters Kluwer Health/ Lippincott Williams & Wilkins.

Staggers, N., Gassert, C. A., & Curran, C. (2001). Informatics competencies for nurses at four levels of practice. *Journal of Nursing Education, 40*(7), 303–316.

Staggers, N., Gassert, C. A., & Curran, C. (2002). A Delphi study to determine informatics competencies for nurses at four levels of practice. *Nursing Research, 51*(6), 383–90. Retrieved from http://www.ncbi.nlm.nih.gov/pubmed/12464758

Zielstorff, R. D., & Frink, B. B. (2011). Consumer and patient use of computers for health. In V. K. Saba & K. A. McCormick (Eds.), *Essentials of nursing informatics* (5th ed., pp. 577–601). New York, NY: McGraw Hill.

FOURTEEN

Using Evidence to Guide CNL Practice Outcomes

■ Clista Clanton

www. Learning Objectives

- ■ Describe the clinical nurse leader's role as an information and outcomes manager
- ■ Identify the clinical nurse leader's use of information systems and the technology and skills needed to synthesize data, information, and knowledge in evaluating and improving patient outcomes
- ■ Discuss some of the core competencies that have been identified for the master's level prepared nurse for evidence-based practice
- ■ Describe critical appraisal tools for evaluating quantitative and qualitative research evidence
- ■ Discuss reference management software programs that are useful in the collection and organization of information sources and the formatting of in-text citations and bibliographies

Key Terms

Evidence-based practice   Information management
Outcomes management
Critical appraisal tools   Reference management
Core competencies for evidence-based practice

CNL Roles

Clinician   Client advocate   Educator
Information manager   Life-long learner   Member of a profession
Outcomes manager

CNL Professional Values

Accountability   Genuineness   Integrity

CNL Core Competencies

Information and healthcare technologies   Critical thinking
Nursing technology and resource management   Communication

Introduction

The first definition of evidence-based medicine (EBM) involved the integration of individual clinical expertise with the best available external clinical evidence from systematic research (Sackett, Rosenberg, Gray, Haynes, & Richardson, 1996), with later evolutions adding patient values and preferences regarding treatment. As EBM spread and was adopted by other healthcare disciplines, several notable evidence-based practice (EBP) models, such as the ACE star model of knowledge transformation (Stevens, 2005) and the Iowa model of evidence-based practice to promote quality care (Titler, 2007), evolved in nursing to help guide practice. Regardless of the model or approach used to implement research in practice, certain

> We may have a perfectly adequate way of doing something, but that does not mean there cannot be a better way. So we set out to find an alternative way. This is the basis of any improvement that is not fault correction or problem solving.
>
> Edward De Bono, Six Thinking Hats

skills are necessary to locate, appraise, and use information. The clinical nurse leader (CNL) has been tasked with both an information management and outcomes manager role that requires using information systems and technology and synthesizing data, information, and knowledge in order to evaluate and improve patient outcomes (American Association of Colleges of Nursing [AACN], 2007).

Developed by the AACN in 2000, the newness of the CNL role means that there are very few published accounts of how CNLs approach or use evidence in their practice. One doctor of nursing practice project did report that recent CNL program graduates with less than 5 years of nursing experience continued to use their CNL competencies as they gained experience in a clinical environment (Klich-Heartt, 2010). Encouragingly, over two-thirds ($n = 35$) of the survey respondents reported that they were able to assimilate research-based evidence to improve their unit outcomes. Given the limited published data on CNLs in practice, we can also look at nursing in general or those in roles such as the clinical nurse specialist (CNS) for examples of how nurses have selected and used evidence to improve their practice. CNSs access written evidence from a variety of sources, most often using literature tailored to their specialty or clinical practice, clinical practice guidelines, Internet use at work, nursing literature, and medical literature. However, at least one study showed that they "never to rarely" conducted their own computerized literature searches using databases. Interestingly, they also "never to rarely" used search services or librarians, nor did they use the affiliated libraries at their university, college, or health institution. Information is sought frequently from people-based evidence sources and include personal experience, what has worked for years, physicians, clinical experience on a previous or current unit, or other nurses working in their clinical setting (Profetto-McGrath, Negrin, Hugo, & Smith, 2010). For routine clinical nursing practice, preferred knowledge sources were personal interactions with coworkers or patients and personal experience (Estabrooks, Chong, Brigidear, & Profetto-McGrath, 2005).

Another study conducted in a critical care setting showed that nurses preferred information from colleagues over text and electronic information sources to support clinical decisions (Marshall, West, & Aitken, 2011). In fact, relying on evidence from the research literature to support decisions in clinical practice was viewed as problematic by both the bedside and senior nurse clinicians. Reasons for this included the volume of available information and the expertise needed to locate and critically appraise research articles, classic obstacles that have been cited by health professionals for as long as implementing evidence into practice has been emphasized in health care (Cook, Mulrow, & Haynes, 1997; Sackett, 1997; Shorten & Wallace, 1997). It is apparent that there are still real and perceived obstacles that need to be overcome in accessing and using the research literature in everyday nursing practice, at both the general and specialist levels, and indeed nurses estimate that less than half of their current practices are evidence based (Melnyk et al., 2004).

Interestingly, nurses with the highest level of capability beliefs reported that they used research findings in clinical practice more than twice as often as those with lower levels of capability beliefs. They also participated in the implementation of evidence seven times more often (Wallin, Boström, & Gustavsson, 2012). Originating out of the social cognitive psychology field, capability beliefs are also known as self-efficacy beliefs; they have been defined as a person's belief in his or her ability to succeed in specific situations (Bandura, 1997). Self-efficacy is also linked to competency, as opposed to being an intrinsic individual characteristic. Given that EBP can be used as an approach to solving problems, familiarity with and competence in the steps necessary to form clinical questions, search for and appraise clinical evidence, and apply that evidence in the CNL's practice domain should reinforce feelings of self-efficacy and strengthen capability beliefs.

It may be useful to discuss some of the core competencies that have been identified for the master's level prepared nurse for evidence-based practice (Stevens, 2005). This is by no means an exhaustive list of the competencies, but it does include those that are integral to the CNL's information and outcomes manager roles:

- Conduct searches for locating primary research studies in multiple databases
- From multiple sources, locate evidence summary reports for practice implications in the context of EBP
- Using existing standards, critically appraise evidence summaries for practice implications in the context of EBP

- Assemble evidence resources from multiple sources on selected topics into reference management software
- Assemble clinical practice guidelines from various sources

Given that one of the reasons for creating the CNL role was to promote patient safety, here is a core competency developed for patient safety research that elegantly summarizes some of the key elements of the EBP core competencies:

> Able to find, appraise and synthesize the evidence, to translate research findings into concrete changes, to communicate effectively to a variety of audiences, to employ change management techniques, and to take a leadership role in promoting patient safety within an organization. (Andermann et al., 2011)

EBP Core Competency: Conduct Searches to Locate Primary Research Studies in Multiple Databases/ EBP Core Competency: Assemble Clinical Practice Guidelines from Various Sources

There are many different information sources that can be used in EBP. The sheer volume can lead to a sense of frustration and uncertainty about which resource to use, or an overdependence on resources that are familiar but not always appropriate. To efficiently retrieve high-quality evidence to support decisions, it is important to know what resource to use with different questions. A useful classification model for information sources is the 6S model, which arranges evidence sources into a six-layer pyramid (DiCenso, Bayley, & Haynes, 2009). In the 6S model, the goal is to start with the highest level of information resources and work downward to locate evidence to answer questions. Higher-level databases consist of resources that have some type of value-added process included, such as critically appraised synopses of research by diseases or condition. These type of resources are designed to save time and help with the difficulty in accessing and assimilating large amounts of research findings from the primary journal literature, which are commonly cited obstacles to implementing EBP (Cook et al., 1997; Sackett, 1997). See **Figure 14-1** for a visual representation of the 6S model.

The lowest level of the 6S pyramid contains original studies from the journal literature, which are indexed in databases such as PubMed, OVID Medline, CINAHL, Scopus, and PsychINFO. These databases provide a way to do topic searches; each

Figure 14-1 The 6S hierarchy of preappraised evidence.

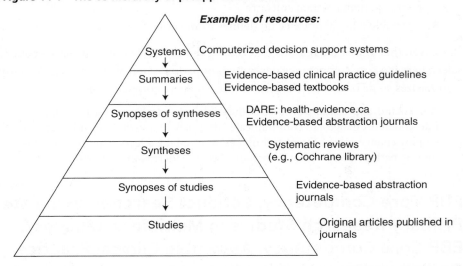

Examples of resources:

Systems — Computerized decision support systems

Summaries — Evidence-based clinical practice guidelines / Evidence-based textbooks

Synopses of syntheses — DARE; health-evidence.ca / Evidence-based abstraction journals

Syntheses — Systematic reviews (e.g., Cochrane library)

Synopses of studies — Evidence-based abstraction journals

Studies — Original articles published in journals

Source: DiCenso, A., Bayley, L., & Haynes, R. B. (2009). Accessing pre-appraised evidence: Fine-tuning the 5S model into a 6S model. *Evidence Based Nursing, 12*(4), 99–101. doi:10.1136/ebn.12.4.99-b

database has its own search interface, indexing or classification system, and ways to limit search results.

Although search engines like Google are not listed in the 6S hierarchy of resources, it is naïve to think that Google or other Internet search engines are not being used by health professionals when they need information. Google does index PubMed, so it is possible to bring up pertinent health science–related articles when doing a topic search. Using Google Scholar (http://scholar.google.com/) is a better option for EBP information, as it weeds out nonscholarly content such as blogs, personal websites, and advertisements. Ironically, if you do not know the URL for Google Scholar, the easiest way to locate it is to "Google" it, as direct links to the Scholar version are not prominent among the Google suite of links for its products. A Google search for "pain management patient satisfaction scores" returned 8,500,000 hits, whereas Google Scholar returned 104,000. In contrast, PubMed returned 550 articles. For focused searches that retrieve high-quality and relevant articles, citation databases such as PubMed, CINAHL, and Scopus are a better option due to their more sophisticated search and limitation capabilities. However, Google Scholar can be a good option to complement searches in citation databases, especially when comprehensiveness of the search is important. There is also the issue of access to the full text of journal articles to consider, although Google Scholar does have the capability to link out to the full text content of institutions via "Library links" in the Scholar Settings section.

EBP Core Competency: From Multiple Sources, . Locate Evidence Summary Reports for Practice Implications in Context of EBP

Evidence summary reports are useful in that they can identify relevant research on a particular topic and usually include some sort of critical appraisal of the studies reviewed. In the 6S hierarchy of resources (DiCenso et al., 2009), evidence summaries are the second level of the pyramid, right under the systems level. Summaries draw from the lower level information sources such as systematic reviews and single research studies that are indexed in databases such as PubMed, CINAHL, and Scopus, but they then synthesize that information to provide a full range of evidence concerning the management of particular diseases or conditions. In this category, you find databases such as Dynamed, UptoDate, ACP PIER, and clinical practice guidelines. Databases at this level are ideal for use at the point of care, as they are designed to locate the best available evidence quickly to inform patient care decisions. See **Table 14-1** for specific resources by category.

EBP Core Competency: Using Existing Standards, Critically Appraise Evidence Summaries for Practice Implications in the Context of EBP

There are multiple resources available to aid in critically appraising the health science literature. The American Medical Association (AMA) has a comprehensive guide designed to help a scholar learn how to distinguish solid evidence, devise strong search strategies for clinical questions, critically appraise the medical literature, and then optimally apply that evidence-based information for patient care; it is called *The User's Guide to Medical Literature: A Manual for Evidence-Based Clinical Practice* (Guyatt, Rennie, Meade, & Cook, 2008). Originally published in the *Journal of the American Medical Association (JAMA)* as separate articles, they are

Table 14-1 6S Hierarchy of Information Resources

Haynes' Pyramid Levels	Free Resources	Subscription Resources
Systems	None	Institutional electronic health records with decision support link out to evidence-based resources
Summaries	National Guideline Clearinghouse http://www.guideline.gov/ Trip Database www.tripdatabase.com/	ACP PIER pier.acponline.org BMJ Best Practice bestpractice.bmj.com Clinical Evidence clinicalevidence.bmj.com Dynamed dynamed.ebscohost.com FirstConsult http://www.firstconsult.com/php /410824135-20/home.html JBI + Ovid http://www.joannabriggs.edu.au/JBI%20 and%20OVID Mosby's Nursing Consult http://www.elsevier.com/electronic-products/mosbys-nursing-consult UptoDate http://www.uptodate.com/home
Synopses of syntheses	Database of Reviews of Effects (DARE) www.crd.york.ac.uk/CRDWeb/ Evidence Updates plus.mcmaster.ca/evidenceupdates/	ACP Journal Club acpjc.acponline.org/ Evidence-Based Nursing ebn.bmj.com/ Evidence-Based Mental Health ebmh.bmj.com Evidence-Based Medicine ebm.bmj.com

Table 14-1 6S Hierarchy of Information Resources (continued)

Haynes' Pyramid Levels	Free Resources	Subscription Resources
Syntheses	AHRQ Evidence Reports http://www.ahrq.gov/research/findings /evidence-based-reports/ Best Evidence for Nursing + plus.mcmaster.ca/NP/ Database of Reviews of Effects (DARE) www.crd.york.ac.uk/CRDWeb/ PubMed Clinical Queries for Systematic Reviews www.ncbi.nlm.nih.gov/pubmed/clinical Trip Database www.tripdatabase.com/	Clinical Evidence clinicalevidence.bmj.com Cochrane Database of Systematic Reviews www.thecochranelibrary.com JBI + Ovid http://www.joannabriggs.edu.au/JBI%20 and%20OVID
Synopses of single studies	Evidence Updates http://plus.mcmaster.ca/evidenceupdates/ PubMed Clinical Queries www.ncbi.nlm.nih.gov/pubmed/clinical Trip Database www.tripdatabase.com/	ACP Journal Club acpjc.acponline.org/ Evidence-Based Nursing ebn.bmj.com/ Evidence-Based Mental Health ebmh.bmj.com Evidence-Based Medicine ebm.bmj.com
Studies	PubMed www.ncbi.nlm.nih.gov/pubmed Trip Database www.tripdatabase.com/	CINAHL www.ebscohost.com/cinahl/ PsycINFO www.apa.org/psycinfo/ Scopus www.scopus.com/home.url

now updated and compiled in a single edition. There is also the "The How to Read a Paper" series, authored by Trisha Greenhalgh and published by the *British Medical Journal (BMJ)*, which explains how to read and interpret different kinds of research papers; the series includes helpful articles on topics such as statistics for the nonstatistician (Greenhalgh, n.d.).

There are also specific instruments and methods that have been developed to aid in critically appraising clinical practice guidelines. Clinical practice guidelines are systematically developed statements that assist practitioners and patients in making decisions about appropriate health care for specific clinical circumstances (Grossman, Field, & Lohr, 1990). The Appraisal of Guidelines Research and Evaluation II (AGREE II) instrument provides a framework to assess the quality of clinical practice guidelines, as well as providing a methodological strategy for developing guidelines and informing what information should be reported and how it should be reported. The AGREE II instrument replaces the original AGREE instrument, which was developed in 2003 by a group of international guideline developers and researchers (AGREE Collaboration, 2003). Composed of 23 items that cover 6 domains, AGREE II allows developers or reviewers a way to assign numeric values to a guideline's scope and purpose, stakeholder involvement, rigor of development, clarity of presentation, applicability, and editorial independence. The AGREE II instrument and a user's manual can be downloaded from http://www.agreetrust.org/.

The GuideLine Implementability Appraisal v.2.0 (GLIA) is another tool that can help those trying to implement guidelines to address identified barriers. The developers of GLIA define implementability as a set of characteristics that predict the relative ease of implementing guideline recommendations, and indicators of implementability focus on the ease and accuracy of translation of guidelines into healthcare systems (Shiffman et al., 2005). The tool consists of 30 questions, and GLIA users should prepare to use the instrument by selecting those recommendations within a specific guideline for which implementation is planned. GLIA is free with registration and can be downloaded from http://gem.med.yale.edu/glia/login.htm.

The Preferred Reporting Items for Systematic Reviews and Meta-Analyses, also known as the PRISMA Statement, is an evidence-based minimum set of items for reporting in systematic reviews and meta-analyses (see **Table 14-2**). Although it was designed for developers, the 27-item checklist provides a comprehensive overview of items that are useful in evaluating systematic reviews and meta-analyses (Liberati et al., 2009). Going through the checklist to see if items are included or were reported

Table 14-2   Preferred Reporting Items for Systematic Reviews and Meta-Analyses (PRISMA)

Section/Topic	#	Checklist Item	Reported on Page #
TITLE			
Title	1	Identify the report as a systematic review, meta-analysis, or both.	
ABSTRACT			
Structured summary	2	Provide a structured summary including, as applicable: background; objectives; data sources; study eligibility criteria, participants, and interventions; study appraisal and synthesis methods; results; limitations; conclusions and implications of key findings; systematic review registration number.	
INTRODUCTION			
Rationale	3	Describe the rationale for the review in the context of what is already known	
Objectives	4	Provide an explicit statement of questions being addressed with reference to participants, interventions, comparisons, outcomes, and study design (PICOS).	
METHODS			
Protocol and registration	5	Indicate if a review protocol exists, if and where it can be accessed (e.g., web address), and, if available, provide registration information including registration number.	
Eligibility criteria	6	Specify study characteristics (e.g., PICOS, length of follow-up) and report characteristics (e.g., years considered, language, publication status) used as criteria for eligibility, giving rationale.	
Information sources	7	Describe all information sources (e.g., databases with dates of coverage, contact with study authors to identify additional studies) in the search and date last searched.	
Search	8	Present full electronic search strategy for at least one database, including any limits used, such that it could be repeated.	
Study selection	9	State the process for selecting studies (e.g., screening, eligibility, included in systematic review, and, if applicable, included in the meta-analysis).	

(continues)

Table 14-2 **Preferred Reporting Items for Systematic Reviews and Meta-Analyses (PRISMA) (continued)**

Section/Topic	#	Checklist Item	Reported on Page #
Data collection process	10	Describe method of data extraction from reports (e.g., piloted forms, independently, in duplicate) and any processes for obtaining and confirming data from investigators.	
Data items	11	List and define all variables for which data were sought (e.g., PICOS, funding sources) and any assumptions and simplifications made.	
Risk of bias in individual studies	12	Describe methods used for assessing risk of bias of individual studies (including specification of whether this was done at the study or outcome level), and how this information is to be used in any data synthesis.	
Summary measures	13	State the principal summary measures (e.g., risk ratio, difference in means).	
Synthesis of results	14	Describe the methods of handling data and combining results of studies, if done, including measures of consistency (e.g., I2) for each meta-analysis.	
Risk of bias across studies	15	Specify any assessment of risk of bias that may affect the cumulative evidence (e.g., publication bias, selective reporting within studies).	
Additional analyses	16	Describe methods of additional analyses (e.g., sensitivity or subgroup analyses, meta-regression), if done, indicating which were prespecified.	
RESULTS			
Study selection	17	Give numbers of studies screened, assessed for eligibility, and included in the review, with reasons for exclusions at each stage, ideally with a flow diagram.	
Study characteristics	18	For each study, present characteristics for which data were extracted (e.g., study size, PICOS, follow-up period) and provide the citations.	
Risk of bias within studies	19	Present data on risk of bias of each study and, if available, any outcome level assessment (see Item 12).	
Results of individual studies	20	For all outcomes considered (benefits or harms), present, for each study: (a) simple summary data for each intervention group and (b) effect estimates and confidence intervals, ideally with a forest plot.	

Table 14-2   Preferred Reporting Items for Systematic Reviews and Meta-Analyses (PRISMA) (continued)

Section/Topic	#	Checklist Item	Reported on Page #
Synthesis of results	21	Present results of each meta-analysis done, including confidence intervals and measures of consistency.	
Risk of bias across studies	22	Present results of any assessment of risk of bias across studies (see Item 15).	
Additional analysis	23	Give results of additional analyses, if done (e.g., sensitivity or subgroup analyses, meta-regression [see Item 16]).	
DISCUSSION			
Summary of evidence	24	Summarize the main findings including the strength of evidence for each main outcome; consider their relevance to key groups (e.g., healthcare providers, users, and policy makers).	
Limitations	25	Discuss limitations at study and outcome level (e.g., risk of bias), and at review level (e.g., incomplete retrieval of identified research, reporting bias).	
Conclusions	26	Provide a general interpretation of the results in the context of other evidence and implications for future research.	
FUNDING			
Funding	27	Describe sources of funding for the systematic review and other support (e.g., supply of data); role of funders for the systematic review.	

Source: Moher, D., Liberati, A., Tetzlaff, J., Altman, D. G., & The PRISMA Group. (2009). Preferred reporting items for systematic reviews and meta-analyses: The PRISMA statement. *PLoS Med, 6*(6), e1000097. doi:10.1371/journal.pmed1000097

correctly can help to determine the quality of the systematic review or meta-analysis if no other synopsis is available. More information and downloads are available at http://www.prisma-statement.org/.

For those in clinical practice who may want to carry out a more rapid appraisal of a systematic review, there is the 11-question AMSTAR (Assessment of Multiple SysTemAtic Reviews; see **Table 14-3**). This validated tool was developed by building on empirical data collected from previously developed tools and expert opinion. It

Table 14-3 The AMSTAR Measurement Tool

1. Was an "a priori" design provided? The research question and inclusion criteria should be established before the conduct of the review.	❑ Yes ❑ No ❑ Can't answer ❑ Not applicable
2. Was there duplicate study selection and data extraction? There should be at least two independent data extractors, and a consensus procedure for disagreements should be in place.	❑ Yes ❑ No ❑ Can't answer ❑ Not applicable
3. Was a comprehensive literature search performed? At least two electronic sources should be searched. The report must include years and databases used (e.g., Central, EMBASE, and MEDLINE). Key words and/or MESH terms must be stated, and where feasible, the search strategy should be provided. All searches should be supplemented by consulting current contents, reviews, textbooks, specialized registers, or experts in the particular field of study, and by reviewing the references in the studies found.	❑ Yes ❑ No ❑ Can't answer ❑ Not applicable
4. Was the status of publication (i.e., grey literature) used as an inclusion criterion? The authors should state that they searched for reports regardless of their publication type. The authors should state whether or not they excluded any reports (from the systematic review), based on their publication status, language, etc.	❑ Yes ❑ No ❑ Can't answer ❑ Not applicable
5. Was a list of studies (included and excluded) provided? A list of included and excluded studies should be provided.	❑ Yes ❑ No ❑ Can't answer ❑ Not applicable
6. Were the characteristics of the included studies provided? In an aggregated form such as a table, data from the original studies should be provided on the participants, interventions, and outcomes. The ranges of characteristics in all the studies analyzed (e.g., age, race, sex, relevant socioeconomic data, disease status, duration, severity, or other diseases) should be reported.	❑ Yes ❑ No ❑ Can't answer ❑ Not applicable
7. Was the scientific quality of the included studies assessed and documented? "A priori" methods of assessment should be provided (e.g., for effectiveness studies if the author(s) chose to include only randomized, double-blind, placebo controlled studies, or allocation concealment as inclusion criteria); for other types of studies alternative items will be relevant.	❑ Yes ❑ No ❑ Can't answer ❑ Not applicable
8. Was the scientific quality of the included studies used appropriately in formulating conclusions? The results of the methodological rigor and scientific quality should be considered in the analysis and the conclusions of the review and explicitly stated in formulating recommendations.	❑ Yes ❑ No ❑ Can't answer ❑ Not applicable

Table 14-3   The AMSTAR Measurement Tool (continued)

9. Were the methods used to combine the findings of studies appropriate? For the pooled results, a test should be done to ensure the studies were combinable, to assess their homogeneity (i.e., Chi-squared test for homogeneity, I2). If heterogeneity exists, a random effects model should be used and/or the clinical appropriateness of combining should be taken into consideration (i.e., is it sensible to combine?).	❏ Yes ❏ No ❏ Can't answer ❏ Not applicable
10. Was the likelihood of publication bias assessed? An assessment of publication bias should include a combination of graphical aids (e.g., funnel plot, other available tests) and/or statistical tests (e.g., Egger regression test).	❏ Yes ❏ No ❏ Can't answer ❏ Not applicable
11. Was the conflict of interest stated? Potential sources of support should be clearly acknowledged in both the systematic review and the included studies.	❏ Yes ❏ No ❏ Can't answer ❏ Not applicable

Reprinted from: Shea, B. J., Hamel, C., Wells, G. A., Bouter, L. M., Kristjansson, E., Grimshaw, J., ... Boers, M. (2009). AMSTAR is a reliable and valid measurement tool to assess the methodological quality of systematic reviews. *Journal of clinical epidemiology, 62*(10), 1013–1020. doi:10.1016/j.jclinepi.2008.10.009. Used with permission from Elsevier.

is designed to take about 15 minutes to administer and has good interrater reliability (Shea et al., 2009).

The tools mentioned thus far are for quantitative research, but what about tools that appraise qualitative research? When complex, multicomponent interventions are introduced into equally complex healthcare systems, both quantitative and qualitative research methods will be needed in order to effectively evaluate success (Berwick, 2008). Qualitative research is deeply rooted in descriptive modes of research and has the goal of uncovering truths that exist while developing an understanding of reality and how individuals perceive what is real (Williamson, 2009). Qualitative research serves as more of an umbrella term that covers different approaches arising out of the fields of anthropology, sociology, and psychology. Some of the commonly used study methods for health science research are ethnography, phenomenology, and grounded theory. Consequently, a consensus regarding quality criteria for qualitative research has yet to be determined. There are several published tools to help in critically appraising qualitative research (Duffy, 2005; Melnyk & Fineout-Overholt, 2011; Polit & Beck, 2011). In addition, a recent literature review identified six questions to help guide the evaluation of qualitative research articles (Jeanfreau & Jack, 2010):

1. Did the qualitative research describe an important practice-related problem addressed in a clearly formulated research question?
2. Was the qualitative approach appropriate?
3. How were the participants selected?
4. What were the researchers' roles in conducting the study, and have they been taken into account?
5. What methods did the researcher use for collecting data, and are they described in appropriate detail?
6. What methods did the researcher use to analyze the data, and what measures were used to ensure that scientific rigor was maintained?

EBP Competency: Assemble Evidence Resources from Multiple Sources on Selected Topics into Reference Management Software

Early on in the evidence-based movement, competencies regarding the management of information were being discussed and recommendations made.

> All professional decision-makers should have a system for storing the knowledge and evidence that is essential to their practice in a way which can be retrieved whatever the reason for the search; they should:
>
> have, or have access to, a computerized reference management system
>
> be able to input individual records to that system
>
> be able to download the results of a search to their system
>
> be able to perform searches on their system using more than one search item (Gray, 1997, p. 67)

Reference management software can help with the collection and organization of information sources and the formatting of in-text citations and bibliographies. (See **Figure 14-2** for an example of a screen in one of these programs.) Some commercial reference management software packages available are EndNote, RefWorks, and Procite. Free reference management applications include Zotero and Mendeley.

Figure 14-2   Zotero reference manager.

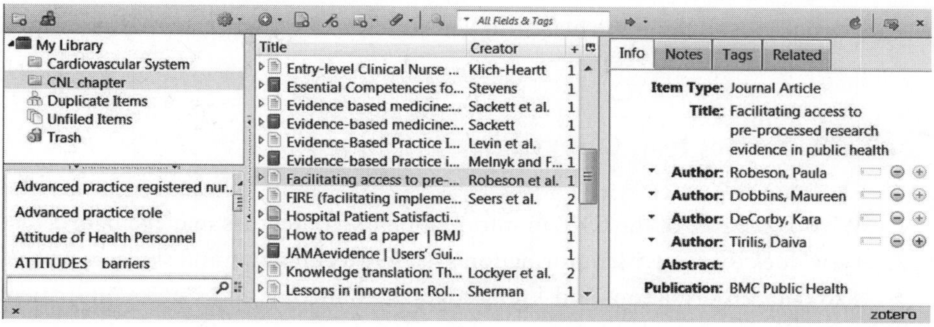

Source: Zotero.

Regardless of which reference management option chosen, perhaps one of the more important things to emphasize is to use the software from the beginning of the information-gathering phase, as doing so will allow for organizing information into collections that can be easily accessed when the information needs to be used or formatted into some sort of finished product.

Summary

- Good information management skills are integral to implementing evidence in practice. The ability to locate relevant research to answer clinical questions and other information needs involves knowing what information resources will best answer your questions quickly and efficiently.
- Using higher level information resources that contain critically appraised summaries is ideal, but when the answers are not located in those resources, understanding what tools are available to help in the critical appraisal process of individual research studies, systematic reviews, meta-analyses, and clinical practice guidelines will be necessary.
- Organizing that information so that it is easily managed and accessible will also help to save time and allow for the sharing and dissemination of information among colleagues.

- Strengthening skills in these information management core competency areas will then ideally lead to stronger feelings of self-efficacy and capability beliefs, resulting in the better implementation of evidence from the research into practice.

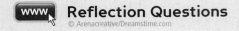

Reflection Questions

1. What is the role of the CNL in information and outcomes management?
2. How does the CNL use information systems, technology, and skills to synthesize data, information, and knowledge in evaluating and improving patient outcomes?
3. What are the core competencies that have been identified for the master's level prepared nurse for evidence-based practice?

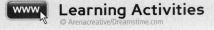

Learning Activities

1. With a group of peers (e.g., classmates, fellow nurses) select a systematic review and critically appraise the research evidence using one of the tools described in this chapter.
2. Select evidence-based guidelines (e.g., National Clearinghouse Guidelines), and with your peers, critically appraise them.

References

AGREE Collaboration. (2003). Development and validation of an international appraisal instrument for assessing the quality of clinical practice guidelines: The AGREE project. *Quality & Safety in Health Care, 12*(1), 18–23.

American Association of Colleges of Nursing. (2007). White paper on the role of the clinical nurse leader. Retrieved from http://www.aacn.nche.edu/publications/white-papers/cnl

Andermann, A., Ginsburg, L., Norton, P., Arora, N., Bates, D., Wu, A., & Larizgoitia, I. (2011). Core competencies for patient safety research: A cornerstone for global capacity strengthening. *BMJ Quality & Safety in Health Care, 20*(1), 96–101. doi:10.1136/bmjqs.2010.041814

Bandura, A. (1997). *Self-efficacy: The exercise of control.* New York, NY: Macmillan Publishers.

Berwick, D. M. (2008). The science of improvement. *JAMA, 299*(10), 1182–1184. doi:10.1001/jama.299.10.1182

Cook, D. J., Mulrow, C. D., & Haynes, R. B. (1997). Systematic reviews: Synthesis of best evidence for clinical decisions. *Annals of Internal Medicine, 126*(5), 376–380 doi:10.7326 /0003-4819-126-5-199703010-00006

DiCenso, A., Bayley, L., & Haynes, R. B. (2009). Accessing pre-appraised evidence: Fine-tuning the 5S model into a 6S model. *Evidence Based Nursing, 12*(4), 99–101. doi:10.1136/ebn.12.4.99-b

Duffy, J. R. (2005), Critically appraising quantitative research. Nursing & Health Sciences, *7,* 281–283. doi: 10.1111/j.1442-2018.2005.00248.x

Estabrooks, C. A., Chong, H., Brigidear, K., & Profetto-McGrath, J. (2005). Profiling Canadian nurses' preferred knowledge sources for clinical practice. *The Canadian Journal of Nursing Research, 37*(2), 118–140.

Gray, J. A. (1997). Evidence-based public health—what level of competence is required? *Journal of Public Health Medicine, 19*(1), 65–68.

Greenhalgh, T., for BMJ. (n.d.). How to read a paper. Retrieved from http://www.bmj.com /about-bmj/resources-readers/publications/how-read-paper

Grossman, J. H., Field, M. J., & Lohr, K. N. (Eds); Committee to Advise the Public Health Service on Clinical Practice Guidelines, Institute of Medicine. (1990). *Clinical practice guidelines: Directions for a new program*. Washington, DC: National Academy Press.

Guyatt, G., Rennie, D., Meade, M., & Cook, D. (2008). *Users' guides to the medical literature: Essentials of evidence-based clinical practice* (2nd ed.). New York, NY: McGraw Hill Professional.

Jeanfreau, S. G., & Jack, L., Jr. (2010). Appraising qualitative research in health education: Guidelines for public health educators. *Health Promotion Practice, 11*(5), 612–617. doi:10.1177/1524839910363537

Klich-Heartt, E. (2010). Entry-level clinical nurse leader: Evaluation of practice. Doctor of nursing practice (DNP) projects. Retrieved from http://repository.usfca.edu/dnp/5

Liberati, A., Altman, D. G., Tetzlaff, J., Mulrow, C., Gøtzsche, P. C., Ioannidis, J. P. A., ... Moher, D. (2009). The PRISMA statement for reporting systematic reviews and meta-analyses of studies that evaluate health care interventions: Explanation and elaboration. *Annals of Internal Medicine, 151*(4), W–65. doi:10.7326/0003-4819-151-4-200908180-00136

Marshall, A. P., West, S. H., & Aitken, L. M. (2011). Preferred information sources for clinical decision making: Critical care nurses' perceptions of information accessibility and usefulness. *Worldviews on Evidence-Based Nursing, 8*(4), 224–235. doi:10.1111/j.1741-6787.2011.00221.x

Melynk, B. M., & Fineout-Overholt, E. (2011). *Evidence-based practice in nursing and healthcare* (2nd ed.).Philadelphia, PA: Wolters Kluwer; Lippincott Williams, Wilkins.

Melnyk, B. M., Fineout-Overholt, E., Fischbeck Feinstein, N., Li, H., Small, L., Wilcox, L., & Kraus, R. (2004). Nurses' perceived knowledge, beliefs, skills, and needs regarding evidence-based practice: Implications for accelerating the paradigm shift. *Worldviews on Evidence-Based Nursing, 1*(3), 185–193. doi:10.1111/j.1524-475X.2004.04024.x

Polit, D. F., & Beck, C. T. (2011). *Nursing research: Generating and assessing evidence for nursing practice*. Philidelphia, PA: Wolters Kluwer; Lippincott Williams, Wilkins.

Profetto-McGrath, J., Negrin, K. A., Hugo, K., & Smith, K. B. (2010). Clinical nurse specialists' approaches in selecting and using evidence to improve practice. *Worldviews on Evidence-Based Nursing, 7*(1), 36–50. doi:10.1111/j.1741-6787.2009.00164.x

Sackett, D. L. (1997). *Evidence-based medicine: How to practice and teach EBM.* London, England: Churchill Livingstone.

Sackett, D. L., Rosenberg, W. M., Gray, J. A., Haynes, R. B., & Richardson, W. S. (1996). Evidence based medicine: What it is and what it isn't. *British Medical Journal, 312*(7023), 71–72.

Shea, B. J., Hamel, C., Wells, G. A., Bouter, L. M., Kristjansson, E., Grimshaw, J., ... Boers, M. (2009). AMSTAR is a reliable and valid measurement tool to assess the methodological quality of systematic reviews. *Journal of Clinical Epidemiology, 62*(10), 1013–1020. doi:10.1016/j.jclinepi.2008.10.009

Shiffman, R. N., Dixon, J., Brandt, C., Essaihi, A., Hsiao, A., Michel, G., & O'Connell, R. (2005). The GuideLine Implementability Appraisal (GLIA): Development of an instrument to identify obstacles to guideline implementation. *BMC Medical Informatics & Decision Making, 5*(1), 23–28.

Shorten, A., & Wallace, M. (1997). Evidence-based practice. When quality counts. *Australian Nursing Journal, 4*(11), 26–27.

Stevens, K. R. (2005). *Essential competencies for evidence-based practice in nursing.* San Antonio: Academic Center for Evidence-Based Practice, University of Texas Health Science Center.

Titler, M. (2007). Translating research into practice. *American Journal of Nursing, 107*(Supple.), 26–33. doi:10.1097/01.NAJ.0000277823.51806.10

Wallin, L., Boström, A. M., & Gustavsson, J. P. (2012). Capability beliefs regarding evidence-based practice are associated with application of EBP and research use: Validation of a new measure. *Worldviews on Evidence-Based Nursing, 9*(3), 139–148. doi:10.1111/j.1741-6787.2012.00248.x

Williamson, K. M. (2009). Evidence-based practice: Critical appraisal of qualitative evidence. *Journal of the American Psychiatric Nurses Association, 15*(3), 202–207. doi:10.1177/1078390309338733

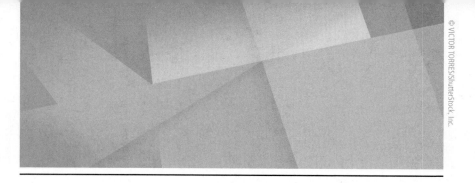

FIFTEEN

Engaging in Evidence-Based Practice to Guide Clinical Nurse Leader Practice Outcomes

 Beverly A. Priefer, Melissa V. Taylor, and Anna C. Alt-White

WWW Learning Objectives

- Define evidence-based practice and related key concepts
- Describe how evidence-based practice contributes to quality outcomes and patient-centered care
- Describe how clinical nurse leaders use evidence to guide practice
- Identify and discuss tools that distinguish evidence-based practice from other change activities

Introduction

A vital role of the clinical nurse leader (CNL) is to facilitate an evidence-based practice environment in which the best available evidence, clinical expertise, and patient preferences are integrated at the point of care with the goal of improved patient outcomes. Much of the evidence-based practice literature

Key Terms

Evidence-based practice	Quality outcomes	Evidence
Research	Quality improvement	

CNL Roles

Clinician	Advocate	Information manager
Life-long learner	Member of a profession	Outcomes manager
Educator		

CNL Professional Values

Advocacy	Altruism	Human dignity
Accountability	Integrity	

CNL Core Competencies

Critical thinking	Ethics	Health and systems policy
Communication	Diversity	Information and technologies
Design/management/coordination of care		

focuses on the process used to identify the interventions that comprise the evidence component of this definition, with little discussion of the clinical expertise and patient preferences components. Evidence-based practices, although certainly important, do not guarantee improved patient outcomes. This is illustrated in the two scenarios, *Flu Season* and *A Restless Night*, later in this chapter. Despite the fact that the nurses in these two scenarios knew the best evidence-based intervention for their patients' situations—flu shot and intermittent pneumatic compression device—the patients' personal decisions trumped both best available evidence and the nurses' clinical expertise. The immediate outcomes were that neither patient chose to receive evidence-based interventions.

Definitions

Current definitions of evidence-based practice evolved from evidence-based medicine (EBM; Oxman, Sackett, & Guyatt, 1993). Over time, the definition of evidence-based practice expanded, first to include clinical expertise (Sackett, Rosenberg, Gray, Haynes, & Richardson, 1996) and later to include patient preferences (Straus, Richardson, Glasziou & Haynes, 2005). In 2007, Sigma Theta Tau International (STTI) defined evidence-based practice as a "process of shared decision-making between practitioner, patient, and others significant to them based on research evidence, the patient's experiences, and preferences, clinical expertise or know-how and other available robust sources of information" (STTI, 2008, p. 57). Similarly, other contemporary definitions of evidence-based practice (Dearholt & Dang, 2012; Houser & Oman, 2010; Melnyk & Fineout-Overholt, 2011; Titler, 2010) also include the integration of best available evidence, clinical expertise, and patient preferences.

> It is a capital mistake to theorize before you have all the evidence. It biases the judgment.
>
> Sir Arthur Conan Doyle

This chapter's focus is to move the CNL beyond process to practice, that is, to the dynamic interaction between the nurse and patient at the point of care where this integration of evidence, clinical expertise, and patient preferences comes alive. The EBP process is the means by which evidence is identified and translated into evidence-based practices. During these dynamic interactions, decisions are made by the nurse and the patient that affect both the care rendered and the patient outcomes. **Figure 15-1** illustrates this integration of best available evidence (evidence-based practices), clinical expertise, and patient preferences. This dynamic interaction occurs within and is influenced by the microsystem and the overall organizational context.

Key Evidence-Based Practice Concepts

This section discusses each of the evidence-based practice components in more detail.

Best Available Evidence

In the clinical setting, evidence is information that is used to make decisions about therapeutic interventions; these interventions are synonymous with evidence-based

Figure 15-1   Integration of the best available evidence, clinical expertise, and patient preferences.

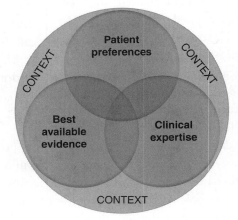

practices. The evidence-based practice process is a systematic process or methodology used to identify the best available evidence and translate that evidence into interventions (i.e., evidence-based practices; Melnyk, Fineout-Overholt, Stillwell, & Williamson, 2010). It is critical to understand this process because it is the means by which interventions are identified. This process is described in numerous texts and articles (Dearholt & Dang, 2012; Houser & Oman, 2010; Melnyk & Fineout-Overholt, 2011; Titler, 2010) and includes a series of steps: asking a question, acquiring the evidence, appraising and synthesizing the evidence, applying the evidence, and assessing the outcomes (EBBP, n.d.).

Working through this process to identify evidence-based practices or interventions requires a team of individuals that may be referred to as the evidence-based practice project team. Those who might be affected by potential changes in practice need to be involved in evaluating the evidence, deciding whether the evidence supports a practice change, and implementing and assessing that change. Prior to beginning this process, it is important for the project team to meet with leadership to ensure that any potential practice changes will be supported and necessary resources provided.

Asking a Question

To engage in an evidence-based practice requires an understanding of the therapeutic interventions performed at the point of care. Such an understanding begins by asking questions about practice, such as:

- Why are we engaging in this practice?
- Is there a better way?
- Does this practice benefit our patients?
- Should we do something different?

Questioning is fundamental to practice and frequently occurs in response to clinical problems or issues raised by nurses at the point of care. What these clinical questions are really asking is whether there is evidence either to support a current practice or suggest a new or different practice. There are several formats that can be used to write a clinical question (Moseley, 2012). The chosen format is not as important as the understanding that the purpose of a format is to focus the clinical question and provide the key terms for searching the databases. One of the common formats for writing clinical questions is the PICO or PICOT format, which is an acronym:

Patient population or problem
Intervention
Comparison
Outcome
Time frame

For example, in the flu scenario, the PICO components are easily identified in the following practice question: Is there evidence to suggest that in older adults (**P**opulation) influenza vaccination (**I**ntervention) compared with no vaccination (**C**omparison) results in decreased incidence of influenza (**O**utcome)? The key terms "older adult," "influenza vaccine," and "influence incidence" would be entered into a database search.

Acquiring the Evidence

Not all evidence is equal in its ability to inform practice. Finding the best evidence to answer the clinical question requires an understanding of how information is categorized. Historically, categories of evidence have been described using a multilayered pyramid illustration, with each layer corresponding to a different category of evidence. There are over 20 different evidence pyramids, all depicting slightly different categories or shapes. See **Figure 15-2** for an example of such a pyramid. The highest levels in the pyramid generally correspond to systematic reviews and meta-analyses and provide the most robust, credible evidence to answer clinical questions. The next level is categories of research designs used in studies, and the lower levels of the pyramid correspond to nonresearch sources of evidence such as case reports, quality

Figure 15-2   University of Illinois levels of evidence pyramid.

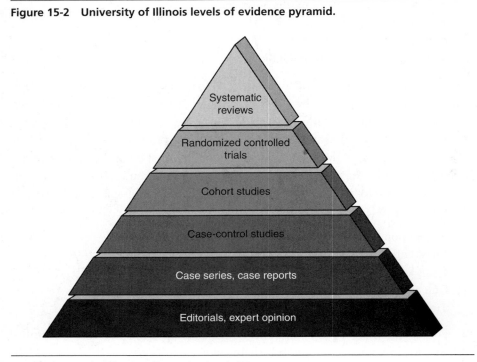

Source: http://ebp.lib.uic.edu/nursing/node/12

improvement data, textbooks, and consensus (Dearholt & Dang, 2012; Houser & Oman, 2010; Melnyk & Fineout-Overholt, 2011; Titler, 2010).

These pyramids have evolved from clinical questions related to the efficacy of interventions and the belief that the randomized controlled trial (RCT) is the best way to answer such questions (Kroke, Boeing, Rossnagel, & Willich, 2003). The implication of these hierarchies is that some types of categories of evidence will provide more credible information to answer clinical questions, with the research designs near the top of the pyramid providing the most robust, credible evidence to answer clinical questions.

An RCT, often described as the "gold standard" research design, is a robust design for answering research questions about intervention effectiveness such as, "Is there evidence to suggest that saline is as effective as heparin for maintaining IV patency?"

It is important to remember that not all research questions can be answered using an RCT design. An RCT is unlikely to answer a clinical question such as, "Is there evidence to suggest that removal of scatter rugs will prevent in-home falls?" because ethical and practical considerations would make such a study unrealistic. Even when RCTs are available as sources of evidence to inform practice, good quality RCTs are conducted under rigorous conditions with ideal subjects that meet strict inclusion and exclusion criteria; these ideal subjects may be very different depending on practice areas and the patient population. Furthermore, because RCT interventions are tested in a controlled manner, these interventions may not translate to the patient population and the clinical environment.

Although evidence pyramids are likely to persist, it is important to remember that these diagrams are representations of the different types of research and nonresearch that serve as the evidence to answer clinical questions. There are no bad research designs; one design may simply be better able to answer a research question than another (Kroke et al., 2003).

A simplified way to approach searching for evidence is to think about evidence in one of two broad categories: research evidence or nonresearch evidence. Research evidence includes systematic reviews, evidence-based guidelines, and quantitative and qualitative research studies. Nonresearch evidence is published opinion articles, case studies, and quality improvement data.

It is best to begin searching for evidence by looking for published systematic reviews, meta-analyses, and evidence-based guidelines. If none are available, next search for published research. Working with a biomedical librarian or a colleague with expertise in searching databases will facilitate the searching process.

Common databases used to search for evidence are MEDLINE, Cumulative Index for Nursing and Allied Health Literature (CINAHL), and the Cochrane Library. MEDLINE can be accessed free through PubMed (www.pubmed.gov), and the PubMed website provides several tutorials on how to search this database. CINAHL and the Cochrane Library require subscriptions. It is important to record each database search strategy so that anyone can replicate the search at a later date. EBP textbooks (Dearholt & Dang, 2012; Melnyk & Fineout-Overholt, 2011) provide step-by-step guidance on searching these databases.

Appraising the Evidence
The next step in the EBP process is to determine whether the gathered evidence will answer the clinical question. Evidence alone does not direct interventions;

Flu Season

The following dialogue takes place between a nurse and a patient who is reluctant to receive a flu shot.

Nurse: "Mary, it is fall and now is the time the clinic starts giving flu shots. We have received our first shipment of flu shots, and based on good evidence and my personal experience in caring for those who have developed influenza, I would like to give you a flu shot today."

Mary: "Thanks for the offer, but I do not want a flu shot. The only time I ever got the flu shot I got sick and I know someone who knows someone who knows someone who also got sick when she got the flu shot."

Nurse: "Do you remember in what way you got sick when you had the flu shot?"

Mary: "I had a headache."

Nurse: "I know that some people think that the flu shot can give them the flu. But the viruses in the flu shot are killed so the vaccine itself cannot cause the flu. Sometimes people do have a sore arm or some redness around the injection site. The headache you experienced was likely due to something other than the flu shot. Let me ask you—are you around children frequently?"

Mary: "Yes, I take care of my grandchildren one day a week."

Nurse: "Children are susceptible to influenza and can get quite sick if they develop it. If you develop influenza, you might pass it onto your grandchildren."

Mary: "If I do not feel well, I just call my daughter and tell her I cannot take care of the kids."

Nurse: "That is a very wise decision because it is certainly difficult to take care of children when you do not feel well and I know you would not want to pass on any illness to your grandchildren.

"Well, it is still relatively early in the season and you do have time to change your decision. I would like to give you this pamphlet on the flu shot. There are some good suggestions about healthy living during flu season, such as suggestions for food to eat, a recommendation for the amount of sleep to get, how to cover your coughs and sneezes, and how to avoid contact with those who might have the flu.

"I will share your decision with the rest of our staff by documenting your decision in our records. I do see you have another appointment in 1 month. Would it be okay for us to ask you at that time if you have changed your mind about the flu shot?"

Mary: "Sure, you can ask, but I will not change my mind."

Nurse: "Thank you for agreeing that we may ask you again. It's been a pleasure seeing you today. Goodbye."

A Restless Night

The following dialogue takes place between a nurse and a patient who has recently undergone surgery.

Nurse: "Mr. Johnson, I see that you don't have your IPCDs on."

Mr. Johnson: "What is an IP—whatever?"

Nurse: "I apologize—IPCD is our short-cut way of saying sequential compression device or these leg wraps that are lying in your bed."

Mr. Johnson: "I told my wife to remove them, I cannot stand them."

Nurse: "I am not sure if anyone has told you the reason for these stockings. They have been ordered for you because, given the type of orthopedic surgery you had, these stockings, along with a type of heparin, are recommended to prevent blood clots. If the stockings bother you, maybe I can readjust them."

Mr. Johnson: "Do not bother; I am not going to wear them. Here, you take them." (*He gives them to the nurse.*)

Nurse: "Can you tell me a little more about your decision—is there a reason you can share about why you do not want to wear them?"

Mr. Johnson: "Yeah, when I was in 'Nam I was a prisoner of war and I was tied down at night, and I cannot stand having anything constricting me. So you might as well take these away."

(*continues*)

A Restless Night (continued)

Nurse: "Is it only at night that it bothers you to have anything tight on your body?"

Mr. Johnson: "I think so, well, I guess I don't know."

Nurse: "Well, the guidelines for using these stockings with the type of surgery you had recommend that they be on at least 18 hours a day. Perhaps we could keep them off 6 hours during the night—we could leave them off until morning, reapply them, and see how it goes."

Mr. Johnson: "Well, ask me again in the morning. Maybe I will give it a try."

Nurse: "I understand your reluctance to wear the stockings at night and I am going to communicate this to the staff by documenting this in your chart and on your plan of care. In the morning I will talk with your nurse and remind her to ask you about trying the stockings in the morning. If that does not work, the staff tomorrow will think about some other options as an alternative to the stockings, as our primary concern is to prevent you from developing blood clots."

rather, it is the appraisal and synthesis of the evidence that contributes to decisions about whether to implement practice changes. Appraisal and synthesis consist of two stages. In the first stage, each individual piece of evidence is read and evaluated by at least two project team members to determine the level (category) of evidence (RCT, systematic review, observational study, expert opinion, etc.) and the quality of the evidence. Evidence quality refers to the credibility of the evidence—are the results believable? For research studies, this means the extent to which bias has been minimized through the precision and implementation of the study design and the rigor of the analysis.

There are many different strategies for evaluating and rating the quality of individual studies (some examples of these are available in the texts referenced at the end of the chapter). Examples of rating scales are "good-fair-poor" (Houser & Oman, 2010) and "high quality-good quality-low quality" (Dearholt & Dang, 2012). After evaluating each individual source of evidence, the project team will decide whether to eliminate any evidence sources rated as poor or low quality. Those sources of evidence that remain are referred to as the "keepers" (Fineout-Overholt, Melynk, Stillwell, & Williamson, 2010a).

During the second stage, the collective evidence, often referred to as the "body of evidence" (Fineout-Overholt, Melynk, Stillwell, & Williamson, 2010c), is evaluated for overall quality (e.g., Are the majority of evidence sources of good quality?), quantity of evidence (e.g., number of published articles or nonpublished sources of evidence), and consistency of outcome measures of interest (e.g., Do all studies report a decrease in falls?). The evidence synthesis is facilitated by creating an evidence table that helps to organize the quality, quantity, and outcomes of each source of evidence. Examples of evidence tables are found in Melnyk and Fineout-Overholt's text (2011) and Dearholt and Dang's text (2012). Using the evidence table, the team will return to the original question and ask whether there is evidence to answer the clinical question and, if so, if the overall strength of that evidence is strong enough to recommend a practice change.

When the evidence synthesis reveals a strong body of evidence to answer a clinical question—several good quality research articles or systematic reviews that report similar outcomes—the team can feel confident about considering a practice change. If the level of evidence is somewhat weak, it is important to remember that evidence is only one component of EBP, and in some circumstances, clinical expertise and patient preferences may weigh more heavily in point-of-care practice decisions. **Figure 15-3** illustrates the two stages of the appraisal and synthesis process in the process of reaching a final decision about the overall strength of evidence.

Applying the Evidence

The decision about whether to apply the evidence to initiate a practice change requires the team to consider the overall strength of evidence supporting the practice change, the context in which the practice change will be implemented, and patient factors that might affect achieving anticipated outcomes from the change. All who are involved in implementation or who are affected by the practice change need to understand the following: why the change is necessary, the strength of evidence supporting the practice change, the likely consequences of not making the change, and the anticipated benefits of doing so. CNLs are often the leaders of these teams.

All practice change is contextual; that is, any change occurs within an environment supported by human and material resources. Organizations differ in shared

Figure 15-3   Evidence appraisal process.

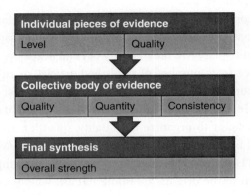

governance structures for reviewing and approving proposed practice changes. Upon receiving approval to proceed with implementation, the team will need to answer the following questions about the proposed intervention:

- Who will implement the intervention and when?
- What is the procedure for implementing the intervention?
- What is the training, and who will provide the training?
- How will performance be monitored?
- How will staff be rewarded for successful and sustained implementation?

Implementing a practice intervention is challenging, as any change introduces uncertainty and often requires learning new skills or modifying old ones. Much of the daily work of health care is habitual (Nilsen, Roback, Brostrom, & Ellstrom, 2012); for nurses, this habitual work includes many repetitive behaviors such as daily shift handoffs, patient assessment, medication administration, and documentation in the electronic medical record. Understanding the nurses' current workflow patterns and including them in implementation planning will help to minimize the disruption in daily routines when introducing a new practice change.

A practice change would be easy if it could be accomplished by simply educating staff and demonstrating new skills. However, education and demonstration alone do not produce sustained change, as shown by the continued challenge of getting healthcare workers to comply with hand hygiene interventions (Pincock, Bernstein, Warthman, & Holst, 2012). There is an entire field of research—implementation research—that investigates "strategies to increase the rate and extent of adoption and sustainability of EBP by individuals and organizations to improve clinical and operational decision making" (Adams & Titler, 2009, p. 330). Various frameworks used by implementation researchers include the promoting action on research implementation in health services (PARIHS) framework, diffusion of innovations theory, the translation research model, and the knowledge transfer framework.

Recently, Cullen and Adams (2012) published a practice guide that is an organizing framework to assist the project team in selecting implementation strategies to "move clinical practice recommendations into routine workflow in practice" (p. 223). Cullen and Adams identified four phases of implementation—(1) creating awareness and interest, (2) building knowledge and commitment, (3) promoting action and adoption, and (4) pursuing integration and sustaining use. The action items listed within each implementation phase focus both on those individuals who are likely to either engage in the new practice change or be affected by the change and on building an organization support system. Although this practice guide provides a comprehensive list of implementation strategies, there is little discussion about to how to incorporate patient preferences into these strategies so that proposed practice changes are appropriate for the patient population and acceptable to patients.

Clearly, implementation requires a team of individuals who understand the evidence supporting the practice change and who are committed to that change. The implementation team may consist of the same individuals who were part of the project team that gathered and assessed the evidence or may include members who have skills in championing change, education, or marketing. The team may decide to test the practice change for a limited time to identify procedure or process problems that need to be rectified.

It is important to carefully evaluate the potential benefit of a practice change relative to unintended consequences to the patient or burden for the nurse. This is especially true when the evidence is weak, limited, or inconclusive.

Assessing the Evidence

The goal of any evidence-based practice change is to improve outcomes. To assess whether these outcomes actually occur requires a formal, objective evaluation. This evaluation consists of three phases. In the first phase, the team evaluates the fidelity of the intervention, that is, whether the practice change was implemented as intended. Information is collected about how the change is being implemented, the frequency of implementation, and problems executing the intervention. The second phase of the evaluation assesses knowledge improvement and can be assessed through administration of pre- and posttest evaluations to determine whether staff understand the "why and how" of the practice change. In the third phase of evaluation, the team collects data to measure anticipated outcomes. Sometimes these outcomes will be quantifiable, such as the number of patients served per day in a clinic, the average waiting time for clients, the hospital-acquired pressure ulcer rate, or the percentage of patients who received influenza vaccine. Other times, outcomes may be qualitative, such as nurses' perceptions about patient and family satisfaction. When assessing outcomes, it is important to use credible measures, such as a carefully constructed survey, to collect the information.

When an objective assessment indicates that an evidence-based practice change has been successfully implemented, additional effort is required to sustain the evidence-based practice. A successfully sustained practice change requires a shared understanding among nurses and other healthcare professionals in the organization about the value of the practice change. Value can be conveyed through formal policies and by the organization directing resources to develop training materials and to offer periodic retraining. Finally, the implementation team needs to address the issue of how long to monitor the evaluation plan. The valuable information about sustainability provided by ongoing evaluation must be weighed against the burden of time and resources associated with conducting this evaluation.

This section discussed the evidence component of an evidence-based practice and described the process used to identify and implement evidence-based practices. It is through understanding this process that nurses come to understand the logic underlying those evidence-based interventions they bring to the patient at the point of care.

Patient Preferences

Although evidence-based interventions are critical to offering patients a standard of care with a scientific basis, the scenarios at the beginning of the chapter demonstrate that ultimately patients control the acceptance or rejection of interventions, and their decisions will likely affect anticipated outcomes. Patients' rejections of interventions may cause healthcare providers to experience some internal tension, especially when the rejected interventions relate to outcomes that are measured and are critical in assessing the hospital or clinic's overall performance.

Healthcare providers who approach patients armed with evidence-based interventions may be stunned when patients do not embrace offered interventions because they generally have greater knowledge of the evidence that supports interventions than the patient. In the first scenario, the nurse probably did not expect that the patient would refuse a flu shot given the widely publicized evidence that flu vaccination decreases the incidence of influenza. In the second scenario, the nurse likely was puzzled by the patient's refusal to accept an intervention designed to protect him from developing postoperative blood clots. The challenge for both of these nurses was to understand the perspective and emotions underlying their patients' responses to the interventions (flu shot and intermittent sequential compression devices). What the nurses learned through probing questions initiated a new conversation that conveyed respect for each patient's decision and afforded an opportunity to provide additional information and suggestions for modifying the intervention.

How patients decide what interventions to accept completely, accept with modifications, or reject depends on many factors such as knowledge about the intervention, values, personal goals, fears, social support, and cost. There is a growing body of literature on shared decision making between healthcare workers and patients, and there are many different types of decision aids designed to assist with patient decision making (O'Connor, Stacey, Tugwell, & Guyatt, 2005). However, many of these decisions aids are time consuming and may be impractical to apply in busy care settings.

Given that evidence-based practice occurs at the point of care, the "tools" that the nurse uses to assist patients in making care decisions are those qualities that comprise the nurse's clinical expertise. These will be discussed in the next section.

Clinical Expertise

Clinical expertise is the proficiency, judgment, critical reasoning, and wisdom acquired through professional and educational experiences (Benner, Hughes, & Sutphen, 2008; DiCenso, Ciliska, & Guyatt, 2005). Benner and Leonard (2011) identify two organizing principles of thought and action that underlie the development of clinical expertise. "Clinical grasp" describes the fundamental process of clinical inquiry—understanding how each unique patient fits within known patterns of health and illness, and disease processes and trajectories. "Clinical forethought" is the habitual application of the logic of nursing. It involves a thoughtful anticipation of the consequences of nursing decisions—anticipating the needs of patients and attuning to the unexpected. A key component of clinical forethought is "future think," which, according to Benner and Leonard, "captures the way judgment is suspended in a predictive net of thoughtful planning ahead and preparing the environment for likely eventualities" (p. 181).

Clinical expertise is also grounded in commitment to life-long learning and evolves as nursing's knowledge base grows. New knowledge and evidence may conflict with what was considered previous expertise in the field of nursing and must be understood though the lens of current and past experiences. The usefulness and applicability of new evidence is contextual to the area in which nursing care is provided. Engaging in life-long learning underpins a profession grounded in new knowledge and expertise, rather than tasks alone. The clinical inquiry mind-set that drives the continual quest for nursing expertise is the perfect segue into cultivating an evidence-based practice mind-set. Translating best evidence into the practice setting is where EBP begins to take shape in improving nursing care outcomes in the context of the clinical setting. A CNL who routinely practices with clinical grasp and forethought is perfectly positioned to understand how new evidence fits, how it can be used to improve current nursing practice, and how it can be spread to multiple care settings.

EBP does not, however, stop with the process. A knowledgeable and experienced nurse will see how evidence applies to the unique clinical needs of each patient, and will, in turn, communicate with that patient how the evidence applies to a particular situation. It is an obvious point, but one worth reiterating, that at the core of "integrating" best available evidence with patient preferences is the ability to communicate the evidence in a way that the patient can understand it and use it to make healthcare decisions. As illustrated in the preceding scenarios, the nurse communicated the evidence in an effective way for the patient, and consistent with the EBP paradigm, patient preferences drove the outcome decision. In these cases, it is vital that the nurse draws on clinical expertise in the area of ethics and "future think" and continues to provide opportunities for the patient to reconsider personal healthcare decisions.

Successful integration of the best available evidence and patient preferences hinges on knowledge of the evidence and the patient. Without knowledge of the best available evidence, nursing's practice becomes, at best, outdated, and, at worst, potentially harmful. The knowledge acquired through the EBP steps becomes meaningful when an attuned nurse uses clinical expertise to take patient preferences into account. Such a nurse will understand how new information relates to clinical issues as they are experienced by a particular patient.

The Importance of Evidence-Based Practice

Three Institute of Medicine (IOM) reports underscore evidence-based practice as a core competency (2003), the need to create an infrastructure to support EBP (2001), and the need to prepare the workforce to better serve patients in a world of expanding knowledge and rapid change (2011). Nurses, particularly CNLs, are well positioned to be the role model on their units for evidence-based practice, thereby influencing the quality and outcomes of care.

Posa, Harrison, and Vollman (2006) described the value of an evidence-based intervention for preventing central line–associated blood stream infections (CLA-BSI). Outcomes improved, with only one CLA-BSI in 6 months, and measurable cost savings. In this example and other interventions, EBP shapes the organization through a favorable return on the investment and enhanced retention and recruitment of staff. Other advantages from a nursing perspective include cultivating an environment of inquiry, enhancing critical thinking, evaluating nursing contributions to outcomes, realizing cost savings, increasing staff satisfaction, and improving quality of care.

The presence of evidence-based nursing practices impacts others and promotes interprofessional collaboration. Collaboration supports life-long learning for patients, families, and staff. The result is the presence of a stimulating and energizing milieu for attracting and retaining the next generation of healthcare providers and leaders.

Evidence-Based Practice and Other Change Activities

Nurses are increasingly engaged in a variety of activities to improve patient care. These include research, evidence-based practice, quality improvement, and systems redesign. There is some confusion about these activities, and the differences are not always clear. The "common rule" defines research as "a systematic investigation, including research development, testing and evaluation, designed to develop or contribute to generalizable knowledge" (U.S. Department of Health and Human Services, 2005). Under this definition, those activities that involve patient interactions or that collect identifiable patient information constitute research from an institutional review board (IRB) perspective. Evidence-based practice integrates the best available evidence, clinical expertise, and patient preferences at the point of care, with the goal of improved patient outcomes. Evidence-based practice considers influences on practice—internal and external—and encourages critical thinking when applying evidence to the care of patients.

Quality improvement focuses on creating improvements in practice and outcomes of care (Centers for Medicare and Medicaid Services, 2003) by reducing errors and needless mortality and morbidity (Sullivan, Gleason, Rooney, Groszek, & Bernard, 2005). Systems redesign is a systematic approach using a set of tools to increase the reliability of processes by eliminating barriers and identifying opportunities to vary practices within a system (Hagg et al., n.d.)

Research generates new knowledge that serves as the foundation to support the interventions of an evidence-based practice. Quality improvement and systems redesign focus on the processes for implementing intervention. A local IRB can assist in determining which of the earlier referenced activities require oversight.

Summary

- A vital role of the CNL is to facilitate and role model an evidence-based practice.
- Evidence-based practice integrates the best available evidence, clinical expertise, and patient preferences at the point of care with the goal of improved patient outcomes.
- Evidence-based practices are not the same as an evidence-based practice.
- The EBP process is the means by which evidence is identified and translated into evidence-based practices.
- The EBP process is a team sport.
- Evidence-based practices decrease variability by providing a scientific basis for interventions.

Reflection Questions

© Arenacreative/Dreamstime.com

Think about your daily interaction with patients and the interventions that you perform at the point of care:

1. Do you know the evidence basis for these interventions?
2. How do you share the evidence base information with patients and other team members?

3. Have you been in a situation where a patient refused any treatment, medication, or therapy, and if so, how did you feel and what did you do?

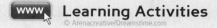 **Learning Activities**
© Arenacreative/Dreamstime.com

1. Develop a teaching scenario for a unit that illustrates EBP at the point of care.
2. Meet with an interprofessional team to identify an evidence-based intervention for your unit.
    a. Appraise the evidence for the identified problem.
    b. Meet with leadership to discuss the potential practice change.
    c. Integrate the evidence, team's expertise, and patient preferences into the practice change.
    d. Evaluate the integration and sustainability of this evidence-based practice at the point of care.

References

Adams, S., & Titler, M. G. (2009). Implementing evidence-based practice. In M. A. Mateo & K. T. Kirchoff (Eds.), *Research for advance practice nurses: From evidence to practice.* (pp. 329–360). New York, NY: Springer Publishing Company.

Benner, P. E., Hughes, R. G., & Sutphen, M. (2008). Clinical reasoning, decision making, and action: Thinking critically and clinically. In R. G. Hughes (Ed.) *Patient safety and quality— An evidence-based handbook for nurses.* Rockville, MD: Agency for Healthcare Research and Quality AHRQ Publication No. 08-0043. Retrieved from http://www.ahrq.gov/qual /nurseshdbk/

Benner, P. E., & Leonard, V. W. (2011). Patient concerns, choices, and clinical judgment in evidence-based practice. In B. M. Melnyk & E. Fineout-Overholt. (Eds.). *Evidence-based practice in nursing and healthcare: A guide to best practice* (2nd ed.). Philadelphia, PA: Wolters Kluwer, Lippincott Williams & Wilkins.

Centers for Medicare and Medicaid Services. (2003). Health care quality improvement program. In *Quality improvement organization manual.* Retrieved from https://www.cms.gov/manuals /downloads/qio110c16.pdf

Cullen, L., & Adams, S. L. (2012). Planning for implementation of evidence-based practices. *Journal of Nursing Administration, 42,* 222–230. doi: 10.1097?NNA.0b013e31824cc0a

Dearholt, S. L., & Dang, D. (Eds.). (2012). *Johns Hopkins Nursing evidence-based practice: Models and guidelines* (2nd ed.). Indianapolis, IN: Sigma Theta Tau, International.

DiCenso, A., Ciliska, D., & Guyatt, G. (2005). Introduction to evidence-based nursing. In A. DiCenso, G. Guyatt, & D. Ciliska (Eds.), *Evidence-based nursing: A guide to clinical practice*. St. Louis, MO: Elsevier Mosby.

EBBP. (n.d.). Steps for evidence-based behavioral practice. Retrieved from http://ebbp.org/steps .html

Fineout-Overholt, E., Melnyk, B. M., Stillwell, S. B., & Williamson, K. M. (2010a). Evidence-based practice, step by step. Critical appraisal of the evidence: Part II: Digging deeper— Examining the "keeper" studies. *American Journal of Nursing, 110*(9), 41–48. doi: 10.1097/01NAJ.0000388264.49427.f9

Fineout-Overholt, E., Melnyk, B. M., Stillwell, S. B., & Williamson, K. M. (2010b). Evidence-based practice, step by step: Critical appraisal of the evidence: Part III. *American Nursing, 110*(11), 43–51. doi: 10.1097/01.NAJ.0000390523.99066.b5

Hagg, H. W., Workman-Germann, J., Flanagan, M., Suskovich, D., Schachitti, S., Corum, C., & Doebbeling, B. N. (n.d.). *Implementation of systems redesign: Approaches to spread and sustain adoption* (white paper). Washington, DC: Association for Healthcare Research and Quality. Retrieved from http://www.ahrq.gov/downloads/pub/advances2/vol2/advances-hagg_80.pdf

Houser, J., & Oman, K. S. (2010). *Evidence-based practice: An implementation guide for healthcare organizations*. Sudbury, MA: Jones and Bartlett.

Institute of Medicine. (2001). *Crossing the quality chasm: A new health system for the 21st century*. Washington, DC: National Academy Press.

Institute of Medicine. (2003). *Priority areas for national action: Transforming health care quality*. Washington, DC: National Academy Press.

Institute of Medicine. (2011). *The future of nursing: Leading change, advancing health*. Washington, DC: National Academy Press.

Kroke, A., Boeing, H., Rossnagel, K., & Willich, S. N. (2003). History of the concept of "levels of evidence" and their current status in relation to primary prevention through lifestyle interventions. *Public Health Nutrition, 7*, 279–284. Retrieved from http://www.ncbi.nlm.nih .gov/pubmed/15003135

Melnyk, B. M., & Fineout-Overholt, E. (2011). *Evidence-based practice in nursing and healthcare: A guide to best practice* (2nd ed.). Philadelphia, PA: Wolters Kluwer/Lippincott Williams & Wilkins.

Melnyk, B. M., Fineout-Overholt, E., Stillwell, S. B., & Williamson, K. M. (2010). Evidence-based practice: Step by step. The seven steps of evidence-based practice: Following this progressive, sequential approach will lead to improved healthcare and patient outcomes. *American Journal of Nursing, 110*(1), 51–53.

Moseley, M. J. (2012). The role of the advanced practice registered nurse in ensuring evidence-based practice. *Nursing Clinics of North America, 47*, 269–281.

Nilsen, P., Roback, K., Brostrom, A., & Ellstrom, P. (2012). Creatures of habit: Accounting for the role of habit in implementation research on clinical behavior change. *Implementation Science, 7*, 53. doi: 10.1186/1748-5908-7-53

O'Connor, A. M., Stacey, D., Tuzwell, P., & Guyatt, G. (2005). Incorporating patient values. In A. DiCenso, G. Guyatt, & D.Giliska (Eds.), Evidence-based nursing: A guide to clinical practice. Toronto, Canada: Mosby.

Oxman, A. D., Sackett, D. L., & Guyatt, G. H. (1993). Users' guides to the medical literature: 1. How to get started. *Journal of the American Medical Association, 270,* 2093–2095.

Pincock, T., Bernstein, P., Warthman, S., & Holst, E. (2012). Bundling hand hygiene interventions and measurement to decrease health care associated infections. *American Journal of Infection Control, 40,* S18–S27. doi:10.1016/j.ajic.2012.02.008

Posa, P. J., Harrison, D., & Vollman, K. M. (2006). Elimination of central line-associated bloodstream infections: Applications of the evidence. *AACN Advanced Clinical Care, 17,* 446–454.

Rosswurm, M. A., & Larrabee, J. H. (1999). A model for change to evidence-based practice. *Image Journal of Nursing Scholarship, 31*(4), 317–322.

Sackett, D. L., Rosenberg, W. M. C., Gray, J. A. M., Haynes, R. B., & Richardson, W. S. (1996). Evidence based medicine: What it is and what it isn't. *British Medical Journal, 312*(7023), 71–72.

Sigma Theta Tau, International, 2005–2007 Research and Scholarship Advisory Committee. (2008). Sigma Theta Tau internal position statement on evidence-based practice, February 2007, Summary. *Worldviews on Evidence-Based Nursing, 5,* 57–59.

Straus, S. E., Richardson, W. S., Glasziou, P., & Haynes, R. B. (2005). *Evidence-based medicine: How to practice and teach EBM* (3rd ed.). Edinburgh, UK: Elsevier Churchill Livingstone.

Sullivan, C., Gleason, K. M., Rooney, D., Groszek, J. M., & Bernard, C. (2005). Medication reconciliation is the acute care setting: Opportunity and challenge for nursing. *Journal of Nursing Care Quality, 20*(2), 95–98.

Titler, M. G. (2010). The evidence for evidence-based practice implementation. In R. G. Hughes (Ed). *Patient safety and quality: An evidence-based handbook for nurses.* Rockville, MD: Agency for Healthcare Research and Quality AHRQ Publication No. 08-0043. Retrieved from http://www.ahrq.gov/qual/nurseshdbk/

U.S. Department of Health and Human Services. (2005). Code of Federal Regulations, Title 45 Public Welfare Part 46, Protection of Human Subjects. Retrieved from http://www.hhs.gov /ohrp/policy/ohrpregulations.pdf

The Effectiveness of a Central Line Care and Maintenance Bundle in Promoting Compliance and Consistency in Central Line Care: A CNL's Vision for an Evidence-Based Central Line Care Model That Bridges Current Gaps in Nursing Practice to Achieve Superior Outcomes

Sona H. Mahal

This quasiexperimental capstone study was completed in two acute care inpatient populations, a medical unit and a surgical unit, to improve central line (CL) care consistency and compliance with timely nursing care.

The Rosswurm and Larrabbee (1999) conceptual model of translating evidence into practice was chosen for this study because it clearly links nursing care and its outcomes to theoretical concepts. For example, educating nurses about the basic mechanism of biofilm formation on CLs prior to educating them on evidence-based practices creates a core knowledge base that helps guide practice. This model also supports the implementation of an evidenced-based project from start to finish. Finally, it includes a framework for evaluation.

A thorough review of the related literature revealed that a bundle approach is effective in achieving sustainable compliance that contributes to improved patient care outcomes. The CL care and maintenance bundle consisted of seven preexisting evidence-based practices that are proven to prevent central line blood stream infections (CLBSIs). This bundle prevents CLBSIs by intercepting the formation of intraluminal and extraluminal biofilm on the central catheter, at the insertion site, and where infusion devices and solution bag(s) are attached.

The bundle was implemented only on the medical unit, in conjunction with ongoing nursing education and reinforcement of the importance of timeliness and consistency in providing CL care. The quantitative and qualitative data were collected on both the medical and surgical units before, during, and after the bundle implementation on the medical unit. After reviewing 60 CLs over 5 months for compliance with bundle components, the findings strongly suggested that a bundle approach to evidence-based practices on the medical unit, in conjunction with ongoing education, improved nurses' compliance with timely and consistent CL care.

The CNL roles of risk anticipator, lateral integrator, systems analyzer, outcomes manager, patient advocate, and educator were utilized throughout the study. In addition to these roles, the CNL competencies on critical thinking, effective communication, and resource management were the key factors in successful completion of the study. In conclusion, this capstone study exemplified how proper utilization of the CNL role in a healthcare organization can result in sustainable improvement in delivering quality care to its customers while bridging the gap between process and outcome at the microsystems level.

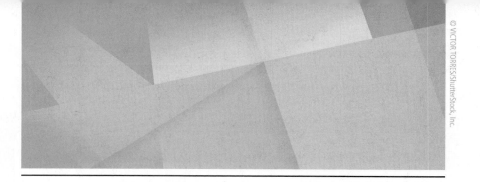

SIXTEEN

From Change to Transformation: Evidence-Based Practice in Action

■ Beverly A. Priefer, Melissa V. Taylor, and Anna C. Alt-White

© VICTOR TORRES/ShutterStock, Inc.

www. **Learning Objectives**

© Arenacreative/Dreamstime.com

- Discuss the merits of a clinical nurse leader–nurse manager dyad and requisite steps for advancing evidence-based practice
- Provide examples of how clinical nurse leaders and nurse managers can form an evidence-based practice question and the criteria for identifying evidence-based practice projects
- Identify how clinical nurse leader–nurse manager partnerships can facilitate evidence-based practice teams that translate evidence into practice to create meaningful and sustainable change

> Transformation doesn't describe our future by referencing the past; it births a future that is entirely new.
>
> Chris McGoff

Key Terms

Evidence-based practice
Evidence-based practice projects
Meaningful and sustainable change

Dyad
Partnership

CNL Roles

Communicator
Risk anticipator/averter

Team member
Life-long learner

Project manager
Partner

CNL Professional Values

Diversity Dignity Accountability Integrity

CNL Core Competencies

Information and healthcare technologies
Nursing technology and resource management

Critical thinking
Communication

Introduction

Provision of evidence-based practice (EBP; American Association of Colleges of Nursing [AACN], 2007) is one of the fundamental roles of the clinical nurse leader (CNL). Although the AACN's white paper on the CNL, as well as several recent articles (Lammon, Stanley, & Blakney, 2010; Ott et al., 2009; Porter-O'Grady, Clark, & Higgins, 2010; Reid & Dennison, 2011; Stanton, Barnett Lammon, & Williams, 2011; Thompson & Lulham, 2007) describe EBP as one aspect of the CNL's many roles, there is little guidance on how the CNL is to promote and role model EBP at the microsystem level.

Promoting and role modeling EBP at the point of care depends on a microsystem culture that values EBP and demonstrates this value through a vision and supportive infrastructure. This chapter focuses on how the CNL and nurse manager collaborate to create and support a culture of EBP.

Culture and Transformation

Stetler (2003) defines culture as "'how things are done' in an organization based on actual norms, beliefs, and values" (p. 101). McGoff (2012) views culture as a line separating those behaviors that are tolerated from those that are not and suggests that values and guiding principles are the building blocks of culture. Both of these definitions suggest that culture is reflected in behavior, and this behavior is a manifestation of underlying values, beliefs, and norms. Observing the behaviors of leadership and staff will provide insight into the microsystem culture and the underlying values, beliefs, and norms driving that culture.

Scott-Findley and Golden-Biddle (2005) suggest that many healthcare organizations value "doing work." When doing work is valued, "being busy" and working at a fast past are likely to be valued as well. When an organization or microsystem values doing work and being busy, nurses may rely on their practical knowledge or the knowledge of coworkers for answers to clinical questions, as opposed to taking time to search the evidence, especially if peers view the time spent searching or reflecting as nonproductive. Furthermore, when doing work and being busy are valued, leaders may expect nurses to search for evidence and engage in scholarly activities on their own time (Scott-Findlay & Golden-Biddle, 2005). Although many nurse leaders espouse commitment to EBP, incongruence between the "talk" and the "walk" becomes apparent when the behaviors of the staff are incompatible with an evidence-based practice.

According to McGoff (2012), "culture always exists" and is built by default or with intention. The first step in building an intentional EBP culture requires the CNL and nurse manager to critically examine and identify if the behaviors of the members of the microsystem reflect a practice where evidence-based interventions, clinical expertise, and patient preferences are integrated at the point of care. If not, the next action for the CNL and the nurse manager is to create a vision that establishes EBP as "a way of practicing" and to make that vision explicit by writing a vision statement.

"Creating a vision is about designing the future and inventing ways to bring it into reality" (McGoff, 2012). It is a transformation of practice.

To begin creating a vision for the microsystem, the nurse manager and the CNL identify the key elements of the vision and create in writing an overall framework for the vision statement. This statement is presented to staff with the explanation that it is an incomplete vision and that staff input is necessary to make it whole (McGoff,

2012). Including all staff in the development of the microsystem vision ensures shared ownership and responsibility to make the vision a reality. An example of a vision statement is:

> We recognize that patients on our unit trust us to communicate openly and to provide safe, high quality care. We honor that trust by engaging in a point-of-care practice that integrates evidence-based interventions, our clinical expertise, and the preferences of the patients we serve.

This vision statement makes explicit that the microsystem values EBP. From this statement flow the behavioral expectations required to make this vision a reality. These behavioral expectations also can be made explicit in a document that is provided to all new employees.

An example of an EBP behavioral expectation is:

> When implementing a nursing intervention, all nurses will communicate to the patient the intent of the intervention and be prepared to discuss the evidence supporting the intervention.

Creating Infrastructure

Organizational infrastructure is foundational for the support and delivery of patient care (Flodgren, Rojas-Reyes, & Foxcroft, 2012). A commitment to an EBP culture requires providing the necessary resources to educate, role model, and support staff to acquire and sustain these behaviors. A variety of resources comprise an EBP infrastructure, and human and material resources must be combined to support staff as they engage in an evidence-based practice (Newhouse, 2005). Many of the key points about organizational infrastructure can be adapted at the microsystem level. **Figure 16-1** depicts both the human and material resources that, when combined, form the infrastructure strategies that support EBP behaviors.

Human Resources

Leadership

Evidence suggests that role modeling and support are two nurse manager characteristics that contribute to the implementation of EBP (Sandström, Borglin, Nilsson, & Willman, 2011). Serving as a role model means that the unit nurse manager leads by example (Sandström et al., 2011) and understands the difference between evidence-based practice, evidence-based practices, and the evidence-based practice process.

Figure 16-1   EBP culture.

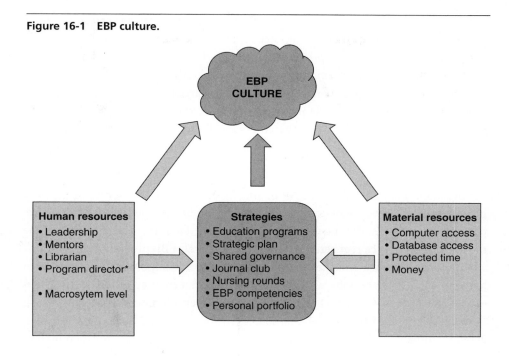

Because EBP content was not included in the undergraduate or graduate curriculum of many nurse managers, lack of knowledge about EBP not only may cause the nurse manager to underestimate the complexity of EBP but also may contribute to the gap between EBP rhetoric and practice (Wilkinson, Nutley, & Davies, 2011). One way for nurse managers to increase their knowledge of and support for EBP is to participate, along with the CNL, in an EBP workshop for the purpose of understanding EBP concepts and process. A federal healthcare system tested such a workshop attended by nurse manager–CNL dyads. The goal for the CNL was to develop the EBP skills necessary to serve as the microsystem EBP expert and mentor. The goal for the nurse manager was to develop an understanding and appreciation of the complexity of the EBP process and to identify the infrastructure needed to develop and sustain an EBP culture.

One nurse manager–CNL dyad that attended this workshop identified that those patients on their unit undergoing total hip and total knee replacement did not receive consistent preoperative education about postoperative pain management. The dyad, using the steps of the EBP process, asked whether there was evidence to guide the development of a preoperative pain management education program for veterans undergoing total hip or knee replacement. From their evidence review, they developed an education program and taught the ambulatory care nurse how to implement this program during the patients' preoperative visit.

When both the nurse manager and the CNL participate jointly in EBP education, it is more likely the nurse manager will understand that EBP is not the sole responsibility of the CNL. It is a shared responsibility of both the nurse manager and the CNL.

Mentors

Melnyk (2007) suggests that an EBP mentor is that person who serves as the "key mechanism" to implement and sustain EBP despite competing priorities. The person who assumes the mentor role varies among facilities. The mentor may be the advanced practice registered nurse who has overall EBP programmatic responsibility for the facility. Another mentor option is to educate several staff nurses to become process champions who understand and can mentor others in the steps of the EBP process (Aitken et al., 2011; Fineout-Overholt, Levin, & Melnyk, 2004; Fineout-Overholt, Melnyk, & Schultz, 2005; Newhouse, 2007a; Newhouse & Johnson, 2009; Schulman, 2008). Melnyk (2012) suggests that "when clinicians are mentored in EBP, their cognitive beliefs about the value of EBP and their ability to implement it are strengthened, which results in greater implementation of EBP" (p. 312).

Although the literature addresses supporting EBP as one aspect of the CNL role, there is little discussion about the CNL serving as the EBP mentor at the microsystem level. The EBP mentor is a critical CNL role if the unit strives for an EBP culture. As the EBP mentor, the CNL not only encourages nurses to question practice but also facilitates answering these questions by guiding nurses through the EBP process.

Not all CNLs acknowledge skill as EBP process mentors, but for those who would like to gain additional expertise, there are several national workshops and conferences that teach such skills. It is important to remember that acquiring process skills to identify and implement evidence-based interventions does not guarantee integration of these interventions with patient preferences and clinical expertise at the point of care. CNL mentoring skills extend beyond process facilitation; CNLs ensure, through role modeling and nursing rounds, that nurses understand and implement these interventions at the point of care.

Librarian

A librarian is a valuable resource to assist with refining key terms when searching for evidence to answer clinical questions (Aitken et al., 2011; Beck & Staffileno, 2012; Newhouse, 2007a; Newhouse, 2007b; Schulman, 2008). Traditionally, the place to find a librarian was the facility library. Today, however, many librarians are out and about and may attend nursing practice council meetings or accompany nurses and other health professionals on walk rounds. The librarian's presence on the unit provides quick access to evidence that facilitates answering clinical questions. The CNL can establish a working relationship with the facility librarian and schedule times for the librarian to attend unit council meetings, deliver presentations on basic search strategies, and participate in nursing rounds. If a facility does not have a librarian, an option for the CNL is to establish a relationship with a librarian at a local college or university with a nursing program.

Material Resources

Computer Access to Evidence-Based Practice Resources

Internet computer access is the gateway to numerous and varied online EBP resources including searchable databases, university and healthcare facility sponsored tool kits and tutorials, PowerPoint presentations, YouTube videos, and peer-reviewed articles. With the widespread conversion to electronic medical records, nurses have access to computers, but this does not necessarily translate into access to EBP Internet resources. CNLs, in collaboration with the facility librarian and unit managers, can make recommendations to organizational leadership about those resources most likely to provide evidence to answer clinical questions. Key database sources include Medline (through OVID or PubMed), the Cumulative Index for Nursing and Allied Health Literature (CINAHL), the Cochrane Library, the Agency for Healthcare Research and Quality (AHRQ), and Guidelines.gov.

Protected Time

CNLs may encounter some incongruity between the nurse manager's verbal commitment to EBP and the lack of protected time provided to nurses for EBP education, for nursing walk rounds, for participation in EBP work groups aimed at recommending EBP practice changes and writing evidence-based policies, and for participation in various council meetings where practice changes are discussed and vetted. Nurse managers may schedule protected time for staff but cancel this time when staffing is low because patient care must come first. Although patient care always is a priority, the nurse manager must determine what type of patient care is valued as a priority—is it care that is rooted in tradition and "the way we always do it," or is it care that incorporates evidence-based interventions, clinical expertise, and patient preferences at the point of care? If tradition and "staying the same" is what is valued, then cancelling protected time is not likely to matter, as changes to improve care are likely to be met with resistance. If, however, developing and sustaining an EBP culture is valued, except in emergencies, the nurse manager will not cancel this protected time because it is during this time that transformational work is accomplished. Kerfoot (2006), writing about protected time in the organization, states, "Think time provides the soil in which creativity and professional practice can grow and should be an important concept in an organizational culture" (p. 169).

The issue of protected time for scholarship and reflection cannot be separated from vision. If the microsystem's vision for practice is that nurses will engage in EBP, the only way rhetoric and practice can be compatible is if nursing leadership builds protected time into staffing schedules.

Strategies

Strategies to support an EBP culture result from the coming together of human and material resources and are those activities that promote behaviors consistent with an evidence-based practice.

Education

The EBP vision must be in place prior to identifying EBP educational needs so that staff who are invigorated with new ideas and skills are supported in their efforts to transform practice. Achieving the vision of evidence-based practice requires all nurses to understand the difference between evidence-based practice, evidence-based practices, and the evidence-based practice process and to acquire the skills necessary to engage in evidence-based practice at the point-of-care. Depending on the organization, this education may be provided by members of the education department, the EBP program director, or the CNL. The CNL can identify gaps in EBP knowledge of staff and help to design education tailored to the needs of the unit staff.

Regardless who educates, EBP education should focus on three questions:

1. *What is an evidence-based practice—what does it look and feel like?* One way to facilitate answering this question is to use nurse–patient scenarios to examine point-of-care behaviors and to identify and analyze whether these behaviors incorporate evidence, clinical expertise, and patient preferences. The goal for this strategy is for staff to experience "ah-ha" moments as they realize what it means to engage in EBP.

2. *What are evidence-based practices?* This education focuses on the importance of asking these questions: "What is the evidence that supports the interventions carried out at the point of care?" and "Should we be doing something different?" Staff are taught a process for critically examining and/or writing policies that include statements about the supporting evidence.

3. *What is the EBP process?* All staff need to understand the EBP process used to determine whether there is sufficient evidence to implement a practice change based on a clinical question. There are several models for educating those staff who desire to become proficient in the EBP process and serve as process mentors for other staff (Cullen, Titler, & Rempel, 2011; Newhouse 2007b; Selig & Lewanowicz, 2008; Wallen et al., 2010; Weeks, Moore, & Allender, 2011).

The nurse manager and CNL select a number of direct care nurses to become EBP mentors in both EBP at the point of care and the EBP process. These mentors will be the project leaders for EBP projects. There is consensus that EBP mentors are important (Aitken et al., 2011; Cullen, Greiner, Greiner, Bombei, & Comried, 2005; Fineout-Overholt et al., 2005; Melnyk, 2007; Rycroft-Malone, 2008), and given the emphasis on EBP in the AACN CNL curriculum, the CNL is the logical unit-based EBP mentor. As such, the CNL understands the difference between an evidence-based practice, evidence-based practices, and the evidence-based practice process (EBP process), and collaborates with the facility educators to develop an education program targeted to the needs of the unit staff.

Strategic Plan

The strategic plan is the document that establishes the goals for realizing the vision created by members of the microsystem. This plan establishes the expectation that EBP is a "way of practicing" and outlines the actions that will support the EBP vision such as education, protected time for scholarly work, shared governance, nursing rounds, and nursing competencies (Newhouse, 2007b). Like the microsystem vision, the framework for the strategic plan can be developed by the nurse manager and CNL and refined and finalized with input from the direct care nurses.

Shared Governance

EBP is a practice that encourages direct care nurses to continuously question practice. Shared governance provides the functional structure within which direct care nurses ask questions, make practice decisions, and assume accountability for practice. When nurses do ask questions about practice, they need both a mechanism by which to answer and apply those answers to their practice (the EBP process) and a mechanism for vetting, communicating, and sharing practice changes (shared governance). Without some type of organizing structure that provides a framework for discussing and vetting clinical questions, first at the microsystem and then the macrosystem level, there is the possibility that more than one EBP workgroup will attempt to answer the same or similar clinical questions (Newman, 2011).

Journal Club

Before initiating a journal club at the microsystem level, the CNL, along with the nurse manager, should identify the purpose of the journal club. Traditionally, the format for a journal club is to choose an article of interest, identify the various components of the article, discuss the article strengths and weaknesses, and discuss how the reported findings might be used in clinical practice. In the context of an EBP culture, the focus of the journal club may broaden to include critiques of systematic reviews, evidence-based guidelines, and nonresearch publications (case reports, opinion pieces) using one of the several critical appraisal formats (Dearholt & Dang, 2012; Fineout-Overholt, Melynk, Stillwell, & Williamson, 2010; Melnyk & Fineout-Overholt, 2011). Participation in the journal club may be greater if the materials chosen for discussion are those that provide evidence to answer questions relevant to the microsystem. Writing a charter or purpose statement will help focus the facilitator and journal club members during journal club discussions.

There are several different formats for journal clubs, and the best format is the one chosen by the staff, as participation in this decision will likely increase commitment and attendance. Formats include an online journal club, where articles are posted online and comments are shared through an electronic format such as SharePoint. This online format is readily available to all shifts because staff can log into the journal club site any time of the day or night. Some facilities may prefer the more robust discussions that occur during face-to-face journal clubs, and, if so, it may be necessary to vary the journal club schedule so that different shifts can attend these discussions. A third option is to embed the journal club into an existing meeting schedule. For example, if the nursing practice council meets the first and third Wednesday of the month for 2 hours, journal club could be held during the second hour of one of the meetings.

Offering continuing education units (CEUs) for journal club participation provides an additional incentive for attendance. The nursing education staff generally can complete the necessary paperwork for obtaining CEUs.

Nursing Rounds

Using a format borrowed from physician teaching rounds, nursing rounds, led by the CNL, are a skillful way for the CNL to educate and role model EBP (Aitken et al., 2011; Fineout-Overholt et al., 2005; Schulman, 2008). Nursing rounds take place at the patient's bedside and are attended by the CNL, the nurse assigned to the patient, and support staff. The staff nurse explains the reason for the patient's admission and discusses the patient's nursing care needs. The CNL observes the way in which the nurse communicates and assesses how this nurse–patient interaction reflects the integration of evidence-based interventions, clinical expertise, and patient preferences at the point of care. The CNL questions the nurse about the supporting evidence for the nursing interventions that comprise the plan of care. When the underlying evidence for a particular intervention is unclear, the CNL encourages the staff nurses to discuss this question at the unit-based practice council or the service-level practice council to determine if this question needs to be answered using the steps of the EBP process. If so, the CNL offers to mentor the staff nurse(s) who originally asked questions during nursing rounds and encourages the nurse(s) to charter EBP project work groups to answer clinical questions.

Nursing rounds also provide an opportunity for the CNL to role model how to communicate to patients the evidence that supports nursing interventions, how to elicit the patients' preferences about their care, and how to draw on clinical expertise to individualize care based on those identified preferences.

EBP Competencies

Expectations for staff behavior flow from the vision and culture statements. Once behavioral expectations are explicit, the nurse manager and CNL can develop the competencies necessary to demonstrate these behaviors. For the novice nurse, EBP competencies might focus on the ability to explain to patients the evidence base for nursing interventions and to elicit from patients their understanding of and willingness to accept these interventions. As nurses become more experienced, competencies focus on how nurses integrate clinical expertise into their EBP at the point of care and how they use that expertise to modify approaches to care when patient preferences trump evidence-based interventions. Competencies for expert nurses focus on the acquisition of EBP process skills necessary to lead an EBP workgroup.

Microsystem and Macrosystem Interaction

The microsystem has been identified as "key" to delivering safe, high-quality patient-focused care (Mohr, Batalden, & Barach, 2004); and although efforts to embed EBP at the microsystem level underlie high-quality patient outcomes, it is important for the CNL to understand the integral link between the microsystem and the macrosystem. Nelson and colleagues (2002) identified macro-level organizational support as one of the nine common characteristic of high-performing clinical microsystems. They define organizational support as facilitating the work of the microsystem through the provision of "recognition, information, and resources to enhance and legitimize the work of the microsystem" (p. 485).

The support of the organization at a broader level is essential as the CNL and nurse manager build a business case for the infrastructure resources required to support an EBP culture at the microsystem level. Additionally, organizational level support will likely be critical for the success of implementing new evidence-based practices at the microsystem level. For example, implementing a hand-off communication system requires collaboration and resources across microsystems (Nelson et al., 2002). The CNL, concentrating on building and sustaining a vision-based culture of EBP at the microsystem level, also needs to consider the complex interconnections between the various organizational microsystems and the overall culture and context of the macrosystem.

Summary

- Provision of EBP is one of the fundamental roles of the CNL.
- Development of a vision statement makes explicit that the microsystem values EBP.
- A commitment to an EBP culture requires providing the necessary resources to educate, role model, and support staff to acquire and sustain these behaviors.

 Reflection Questions

© Arenacreative/Dreamstime.com

Think about the daily interaction between you and the nurse manager on your unit:

1. What activities can you both engage in to strengthen your partnership?
2. How do you regularly identify practice issues?

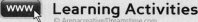 **Learning Activities**

© Arenacreative/Dreamstime.com

1. Identify the behaviors that reflect a microsystem's culture.
2. Write an EBP vision statement for a nursing unit.
3. Identify the infrastructure components on a unit that support EBP.

References

Aitken, L. M., Hackwood, B., Crouch, S., West, N., Carney, D., & Jack, L. (2011). Creating an environment to implement and sustain evidence based practice: A development process. *Australian Critical Care, 24*(4), 244–254. doi:10.1016/j.aucc.2011.01.004

American Association of Colleges of Nursing. (2007). AACN white paper on the role of the clinical nurse leader. Retrieved from http://www.aacn.nche.edu/publications/white-papers/cnl

Beck, M. S., & Staffileno, B. A. (2012). Implementing evidence-based practice during an economic downturn. *Journal of Nursing Administration, 42*, 350–352.

Cullen, L., Greiner, J., Greiner, J., Bombei, C., & Comried, L. (2005). Excellence in evidence-based practice: Organizational and unit exemplars. *Critical Care Nursing Clinics of North America, 17*, 127–142.

Cullen, L., Titler, M. G., & Rempel, G. (2011). An advanced educational program promoting evidence-based practice. *Western Journal of Nursing Research, 33*(3), 345–364.

Dearholt, S. L., & Dang, D. (Eds.). (2012). *Johns Hopkins nursing evidence-based practice: Models and guidelines* (2nd ed.). Indianapolis, IN: Sigma Theta Tau, International.

Fineout-Overholt, E., Levin, R., & Melnyk, B. (2004). Strategies for advancing evidence-based practice in clinical settings. *Journal of the New York State Nurses' Association, 35*(2), 28–32.

Fineout-Overholt, E., Melnyk, B. M., & Schultz, A. (2005). Transforming healthcare from the inside out: Advancing evidence-based practice in the 21st century. *Journal of Professional Nursing, 21*(6), 335–344.

Fineout-Overholt, E., Melnyk, B. M., Stillwell, S. B., & Williamson, K. M. (2010). Evidence-based practice step by step. Critical appraisal of the evidence: Part I: An introduction to gathering, evaluating, and recording the evidence. *American Journal of Nursing, 110*(7), 47–52.

Flodgren, G., Rojas-Reyes, M. X., & Foxcroft, D. R. (2012). Effectiveness of organizational infrastructures to promote evidence-based nursing practice. *Cochrane Database of Systematic Reviews, 2*, CD002212. doi:10.1002/14651858

Kerfoot, K. (2006). Reliability between nurse managers: The key to the high-reliability organization. *Nursing Economic$, 24*(5), 274–275.

Lammon, C. A., Stanton, M. P., & Blakney, J. L. (2010). Innovative partnerships: The clinical nurse leader role in diverse clinical settings. *Journal of Professional Nursing, 26*(5), 258–263. doi:10.1016/j.profnurs.2010.06.004

McGoff, C. (2012). *The primes: How any group can solve any problem*. Hoboken, NJ: John Wiley & Sons, Inc.

Melnyk, B. M. (2007). The evidence-based practice mentor: A promising strategy for implementing and sustaining EBP in healthcare systems. *WorldViews on Evidence-Based Nursing, 4*(3), 123–125.

Melnyk, B. M. (2012). Achieving a high-reliability organization through implementation of the ARCC model for systemwide sustainability of evidence-based practice. *Nursing: Administration Quarterly, 36*(2), 127–135.

Melnyk, B. M., & Fineout-Overholt, E. (2011). *Evidence-based practice in nursing and healthcare: A guide to best practice* (2nd ed.). Philadelphia, PA: Wolters Kluwer/Lippincott Williams & Wilkins.

Mohr, J. J., Batalden, P., & Barach, P. (2004). Integrating patient safety into the clinical microsystem. *Quality & Safety in Healthcare, 13*(Suppl. II), ii34–ii38.

Nelson, E. C., Batalden, P. B., Huber, T. P., Mohr, J. J., Godfrey, M. M., Headrick, L. A., & Wasson, J. H. (2002). Microsystems in healthcare: Part 1. Learning from high-performing front-line clinical units. *Joint Commission Journal on Quality Improvement, 28*(9), 472–493.

Newhouse, R. P. (2005). Evidence-based infrastructure (letter). *Hospitals and Health Networks, 79*(11), 10.

Newhouse, R. P. (2007a). Creating infrastructure supportive of evidence-based nursing practice: Leadership strategies. *WorldViews on Evidence-Based Nursing, 4*(1), 21–29.

Newhouse, R. P. (2007b). Organizational change strategies for evidence-based practice. *Journal of Nursing Administration, 37*, 552–557.

Newhouse, R. P., & Johnson, K. (2009). A case study in evaluating infrastructure for EBP and selecting a model. *Journal of Nursing Administration, 39,* 409–411.

Newman, P. (2011). Transforming organization culture through nursing shared governance. *Nursing Clinics of North America, 46*(1), 45–58.

Ott, K. M., Haddock, K. S., Fox, S. E., Shinn, J. K., Walters, S. E., Hadin, J. W., ... Harris, J. L. (2009). The clinical nurse leader: Impact on practice outcomes in the Veterans Health Administration. *Nursing Economic$, 27*(6), 363–370, 383.

Porter-O'Grady, T., Clark, J. S., & Higgins, M. S. (2010). The case for the clinical nurse leader: Guiding nursing practice into the 21st century. *Nurse Leader, 8*(1), 37–41.

Reid, K. B., & Dennison, P. (2011, September 30). The clinical nurse leader (CNL)™: Point of care safety clinician. *The Online Journal of Issues in Nursing, 16*(3), 4.

Rycroft-Malone, J. (2008). Evidence-informed practice: From individual to context. *Journal of Nursing Management, 16,* 404–408.

Sandström, B., Borglin, G., Nilsson, R., & Willman, A. (2011). Promoting the implementation of evidence-based practice: A literature review focusing on the role of nursing leadership. *WorldViews on Evidence-Based Nursing, 8*(4), 212–223. doi:10.1111/j.1741-6787.2011.00216.x

Schulman, C. S. (2008). Strategies for starting a successful evidence-based practice program. *AACN Advanced Critical Care, 19*(3), 301–311. doi:10.1097/01.AACN. 0000330381.41766.2a

Scott-Findlay, S., & Golden-Biddle, K. (2005). Understanding how organizational culture shapes research use. *Journal of Nursing Administration, 35,* 359–365.

Selig P. M., & Lewanowicz, W. (2008). Translation to practice: Developing an evidence-based practice nurse internship program. *AACN Advanced Critical Care, 19*(3), 325–332. doi: 10/1097/01.AACN.0000330381.64637.14

Stanton, M. P., Barnett Lammon, C. A., & Williams, E. S. (2011). The clinical nurse leader: A comparative study of the American Association of Colleges of Nursing. *Journal of Professional Nursing, 27,* 78–83. doi:10.1016/j.profnurs.2010.09.014

Stetler, C. (2003). Role of the organization in translating research into evidence-based practice. *Outcomes Management, 7*(3), 97–105.

Thompson, P., & Lulham, K. (2007). Clinical nurse leaders and clinical nurse specialists role delineation in the acute care setting. *Journal of Nursing Administration, 37,* 429–431.

Wallen, G. R., Mitchell, S. A., Melnyk, B. M., Fineout-Overholt, E. Miller-Davis, C., Yates, J. & Hastings, C. (2010). Implementing evidence-based practice: Effectiveness of a structure multifaceted mentorship programme. *Journal of Advanced Nursing, 66*(12), 2761–2771.

Weeks, S. M., Moore, P., & Allender, M. (2011). A regional evidence-based practice fellowship. *Journal of Nursing Administration, 41,* 10–14.

Wilkinson, J. E., Nutley, S. M., & Davies, H. T. O. (2011). An exploration of the roles of nurse managers in evidence-based practice implementation. *WorldViews on Evidence-Based Nursing, 8*(4), 236–246. doi:10/1111/j.1741-6787.2011.00225.x

WellStar Health System Partners with University of West Georgia

Donna Whitehead

WellStar Health System (WHS) recognized the need for the implementation of the CNL role as part of their vision to provide world-class health care in their community. The system's strategic goals include providing excellence in the patient's experience as well as coordination of care, resulting in a streamlined and efficient inpatient processes. To meet these goals there is a nursing focus on strengthening the nursing workforce through the additional support of CNLs on every inpatient unit. Senior nursing leaders recognize that demands on the bedside nurse have increased due to the higher acuity of patients coupled with the multitude of regulatory requirements. Future reimbursement for performance on nursing-sensitive indicators and the need for evidence-based practice at the point of care are additional indicators for the implementation of CNLs. WHS practices Lean principles that support process improvement initiatives. Through microsystem assessments, CNLs will drive best practices, utilizing Lean principles to improve system processes so that safe, efficient quality care is delivered to every inpatient.

WHS partnered with the University of West Georgia to bring their master's of science in nursing CNL program to the WHS campus. WHS has fully funded 40 full-time registered nurses to participate in the model A program of study. Through a robust selection process, 17 nurses were chosen for the first cohort to graduate April 2013, and 23 nurses are in the second cohort. WHS is paying students their salary during the 300-hour clinical immersion so that their focus will be on learning and implementing new skills. WHS hopes the vision of having CNLs on every inpatient unit will improve the care delivered to over 600,000 patients annually.

Hourly Rounding and Increased Patient Satisfaction Scores

Marie San Pedro

On one medical–surgical unit, patient satisfaction scores were well below the state and national averages, based on Hospital Consumer Assessment of Healthcare Providers and System (HCAHPS) scores. The CNL's goal was to improve these scores over a period of six months. Applying evidence-based practice, hourly rounding was implemented to meet patient needs more quickly and consistently. By acting as a change agent, the CNL was able to educate the staff, teaching them to observe the 4 Ps (pain, potty, positioning, and placement of belongings) when doing their rounds. A script was also implemented as a guide for staff on what to say to their patients while rounding. Within a four-month period the call bell was used less and patient satisfaction scores increased by almost 20%.

© VICTOR TORRES/ShutterStock, Inc.

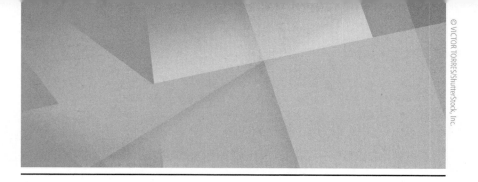

SEVENTEEN

Improvement Science and Team Science: Links to Innovation, Effectiveness, and Safety*

Kathleen R. Stevens

Learning Objectives

© Arenacreative/Dreamstime.com

- Define improvement science and its role in ensuring safe and efficient care delivery
- Describe the goals of improvement science in promoting evidence-based practice for clinical nurse leaders

Introduction

Heightened interest in evidence-based quality and safety of health care has created a sense of urgency around developing a focused program of improvement science that can guide the transformation of health care. Clinical nurse leaders (CNLs), in their roles as clinician, advocate, information manager,

*Acknowledgments: Portions of this work are supported by a federal grant from the National Institute for Nursing Research (NIH 1RC2 NR011946-01).

Key Terms

Improvement science efficiency   Effectiveness   Quality

Evidence-based practice   Safety   Innovation

CNL Roles

Clinician   Advocate   Information manager

Life-long learner   Member of a profession   Outcomes manager

Educator

CNL Professional Values

Accountability   Outcome measurement   Quality improvement

Integrity   Social justice

Microsystems management   Evidence-based practice

Interprofessional teams   Quality patient care and safety

CNL Core Competencies

Critical thinking   Ethical decision making   Member of a profession

Team leader   Communication   Assessment

Healthcare systems and policy

Design/management/coordination of care

Assessment environment of care manager

and outcomes manager, use the highest level of evidence to support patient-centered care. Improvement science has raised the bar in translating research evidence at the bedside and at the point of care. The National Institutes of Health (NIH)-funded Improvement Science Research Network (ISRN) has systematically developed consensus priorities for improvement research in order to ensure that research resources are first applied to the nation's most urgent knowledge gaps in improvement science. This chapter explores this new field, describes the approach used to establish the nation's first research agenda in improvement science, and presents the research agenda. The role of improvement science for the CNL will be discussed in relationship to evidence-based practice and communication of results in a collaborative manner.

> **Without continual growth and progress, such words as improvement, achievement, and success have no meaning.**
>
> Benjamin Franklin

Background

Healthcare quality problems are widespread and often glaring, but the underlying causes of these problems remain unclear (McGlynn et al., 2003). Attempts to achieve optimal care have been expressed via a wide array of approaches, including translational research targets, evidence-based care, accreditation and external accountability for quality and safety, risk management, error prevention, organizational development, leadership and frontline enhancement, and complex adaptive systems frameworks (Grol, Baker, & Moss, 2004). Nevertheless, effective methods of achieving improvement have not been confirmed by the simple tests pursued in the context of these approaches; more complex, well-designed interventions and testing strategies are required. The CNL's understanding of improvement underscores his or her role in evidence-based care and innovation. Skills such as use of measurement tools as the foundation for assessment and clinical decisions and applying clinical judgment and decision-making skills in designing, coordinating, implementing, and evaluating client-focused care are the cornerstones to improvement science for the CNL (King, 2013).

The Importance of Improvement Science

Quality improvement and patient safety are imperative clinical targets supported by policy, patient advocacy, and healthcare professional groups, yet research to determine which improvement strategies are effective has been insufficient at best. Despite the critical need for improvement research evidence, corresponding infrastructure and capacity among health scientists to conduct rigorous, well-designed and action-oriented studies are lacking.

This gap is caused in part by the lack of rigorous research approaches in the field of improvement science. Shojania and Grimshaw (2005) questioned, "Why would we exempt research in quality improvement from scientific standards that we routinely

> The improvement of understanding is for two ends; first, our own increase of knowledge; secondly, to enable us to deliver that knowledge to others.
>
> John Locke

apply to the leading causes of morbidity and mortality" (p. 74)? Some research approaches remain to be invented. In addition, the theories, methods, and designs for achieving rigorous research in the field are newly arising, and many healthcare scientists are not yet skilled in applying these new research methods. Training programs are only beginning to include these topics in the education of future healthcare scientists (Rubio et al., 2010).

CNLs understand that there are critical barriers to progress in improvement research and seek to develop their knowledge base of implementation and translational science. Barriers recently underscored by an expert panel of the Institute of Medicine (IOM) include the following (IOM, 2007):

1. Improvement initiatives are conducted for different purposes than scientific research, instead emphasizing experiential learning and compromising the understanding of generalizable truths.
2. Specific contexts of improvement initiatives limit generalizability.
3. Improvement science does not have a scientific home and requires interdisciplinary research.
4. There is a mismatch between training and practice—those conducting improvement projects have little research training.
5. Ethical oversight principles are not clear-cut.
6. Improvement studies are not subject to rigor, and causality is difficult to establish.
7. In the rare instance when improvement studies are published, they are often poorly conducted and not generalizable.
8. Lack of a common vocabulary and taxonomy for improvement research terms hinders progress.

Improvement research has the potential to help transform health care, and these barriers can be overcome. Exploration of terminology and establishing research priorities will help clarify collective thinking about the most fruitful first steps. These are important steps in the CNL's informed evidence-based practice and the sustained improvement of innovative strategies that CNLs tackle in their role.

Terminology in the Field

A flurry of terms has emerged and, in at least some regard, this language is related to increasing the understanding of what is effective in making changes that are intended to improve care and outcomes. In this discussion, the umbrella term "improvement science" is used to refer to the collection of terms. Terms in the field are often inter-related and overlapping (e.g., complexity science, science of change, implementation science, systems research and, of course, improvement science). None are adequately defined by experts in the field yet, hence the IOM's reference to Barrier #8.

The paradigm shift to emphasizing the science underlying healthcare quality improvement is a recent one. Research directions began to change in the last decade and were heavily influenced by the IOM's quality initiative reports (IOM, 1999, 2001, 2008a, 2008c). The escalating movement has spawned a number of terms and approaches, adding to the initial scatter of the effort. Among the terms used are improvement science (preferred in this discussion and offered as a term meant to include others), translational science, science of change, and implementation sci-ence. Evolution and final determination of terminology in the field is beyond the scope of this discussion, but the term "improvement science" will be discussed in juxtaposition to the other terms, such as translational science.

Added to the traditional research on clinical efficacy of interventions, the interest in "what works in improvement strategies" and "how it works" has rap-idly grown. This major shift was catapulted forward with the issuance of the NIH Roadmap, which set new directions and coined new terms; in fact, the term "trans-lational science" was used in this 2005 report (Zerhouni, 2005). The concepts were outlined and further dubbed "Translation 1" (T1—from bench to clinical trials) and "Translation 2" (T2—from trials to widespread clinical adoption). These terms were further cemented with the establishment of the NIH's Clinical Translational Research Awards (CTSA), intended to firmly link bench research to bedside care by setting requirements (e.g., translational science and community outreach) that are intended to transform the clinical research enterprise.

This chapter's definition of improvement science includes T2 as originally defined, as well as expanding to include translational science, or T3. T3 research seeks to discover the "how" of effective and safe care delivery so that "evidence-based treatment, prevention, and other interventions are delivered reliably to all patients in all settings of care and improve the health of individuals and populations" (Dough-erty & Conway, 2008, p. 2320). The CNL focuses on the "why" and "how," thus supporting evidence-based care in collaborative teams. The CNL provides clinical leadership for changing practice based on evidence-based research and improvement science methods. Through assessment, critiquing, and analysis of information sources, the CNL becomes an informed consumer, thus enhancing synthesis of knowledge to evaluate and achieve optimal client outcomes.

In this schema, translational science engages multidisciplinary collaboration to accelerate application of the discoveries across all stages and moves toward improved healthcare quality and value and population health (Dougherty & Conway, 2008). The CNL is truly primed for this application. Extended from T1 and T2, T3 represents the practice-oriented stage; T3 relies on dissemination and answers questions about whether the effective practices are now being used in the world at large. Questions in T3 research are: What is the best method to reach clinicians and patients with a policy concerning a given treatment so that they will (1) understand the new treatment and (2) start to use it? Also in T3, new widespread practices are standardized as scientific and new evidence-based policies are formulized. Additional questions focus on effective ways to make systems changes and create organizational cultures of quality. It takes all three stages to move what is discovered in a lab into the common care of the general population. The CNL understands microsystem change, action-oriented research supported by implementation science.

Each of these stages brings to light important research, and the attendant research methods and frameworks of each of these stages will differ. T1 and T2 research methods in basic science and clinical trials are well defined and executed through a long history of methodological and theoretical evolution. The rigorous methods of basic "bench" research follow well-established standards for scientific discovery in a controlled laboratory. Many of the standards are also used in clinical research trials, where the randomized control trial (RCT) is the "gold standard" for testing.

This is not the case with T3—research methods in this stage of translational science are embryonic. The methods more closely follow the broad field of health services research. Two paradigmatic shifts will be necessary to hasten the evolution of improvement science methods in the T3 stage. The first shift is from quality improvement strategies to the science of improvement that tests the improvement strategies. The second shift is from classic experimental research with highly controlled variables to research about complex and dynamic phenomena. Relatively highly controlled designs, such as RCTs, are ill fitted to provide explanations for phenomena within complex adaptive systems (such as change within clinical care units); designs that include triangulation of qualitative and quantitative data within such frameworks are more useful. The CNL is expected to critically appraise research evidence, while focusing on a microsystem's change during his or her immersion experience. Knowing the "metrics that matter" will further help him or her determine the best qualitative and quantitative data to collect. Evaluation of the process goes hand in glove with the quality improvement initiatives. Add to this the collaborative nature of the work, which further provides the translation of local improvement.

Recently, innovation has been added to the emphasis on healthcare improvement, and the seeds of improvement science can be traced in the methods employed. The Agency for Healthcare Research & Quality (AHRQ) Innovations Exchange, launched in 2008, profiles improvement innovations and includes information about how the innovations were evaluated to answer the question, "Did it work?" Included in this resource are innovations of national import that have been evaluated and have yielded significant improvement in care processes and patient outcomes— most often within a local context. The 500-plus innovations profiled in this online resource reflect the nationwide interest in improvement science (AHRQ, 2008).

Following a recent IOM report, *Knowing What Works in Health Care*, scientists have begun to explore further the scientific approaches to systematic reviews and development of evidence-based clinical practice guidelines (IOM, 2008b). Methodological questions were raised about rigor in systematic reviews of the credibility of clinical guidelines. These, too, are important research designs in improvement science, and it is recommended that national scientific standards be established for these methods (IOM, 2008b).

Experts have asserted that unique research designs are required to capture cause and effect from improvement interventions (Pawson & Tilley, 1997). A series of articles highlighted the specific aspects necessary to adequately study improvement. Indeed some suggest that new academic posts, "translationally oriented," are urgently needed to raise awareness and accomplish reorganization of academic teams to address translational research (Kermaris, Kanadaris, Tziopis, Kontakis, & Giannoudis, 2008). The CNL as a lateral integrator is important to this end. The CNL identifies relevant outcomes and measurement strategies that will improve patient outcomes and promote cost-effective care.

Indeed, the recently funded ISRN is further proof of the nation's interest in this field (Stevens, 2009). This NIH-funded project (NIH 1RC2 NR011946-01) created a research network to increase the quantity and quality of improvement research in acute care settings. As part of the network, national healthcare leaders have joined together in a project advisory steering council ; they are keen to advance improvement science through multiple interprofessional venues, including this proposed scholarly work.

This report draws from the work done by the steering council and coordinating center team of the ISRN. ISRN research priorities were introduced on July 7, 2010, at a news conference, the Improvement Science Summit, which was one of the nation's few gathering points for improvement scientists.

Research Priorities in Improvement Science

The overriding goal of improvement science is to ensure that quality improvement efforts are based as much on evidence as the best practices they seek to implement (Shojania & Grimshaw, 2005). Simply put, strategies for implementing evidence-based quality improvement need an evidence base of their own. CNLs recognize the importance of this work and are front and center to these efforts to improve patient-centered care in a collaborative way.

With a heightened interest in the quality of health care comes a burgeoning concern about the science underlying practices and delivery of care. However, insufficient progress has been made in improvement science.

In characterizing the current status of improvement research, the following shortcomings were noted: Studies are performed in single organizations and do not yield generalizability information; imprecise measurement and insufficient description of the improvement intervention are apparent; studies do not produce information about sustainability of changes; contexts affecting implementation are not considered; cost or value are not estimated; and such research tends to be opportunistic rather than systematically planned (IOM, 2008a).

Experts point to the increasing challenge of translating and disseminating improvement evaluation results in a way that makes them useful in decision-making processes that strive to improve health and health care. Indeed, research is considered a driving force for change in healthcare improvement and is at the core of the business case for quality improvement. Among the recommendations to advance improvement research is an improved infrastructure involving multiple institutions from a variety of regions and practices. The ideal infrastructure would enable cross-institutional studies, multidisciplinary studies, researcher training, and funding, all of which are necessary to improve the improvement research infrastructure. Along with these new directions, experts emphasize that a priority agenda for quality improvement research would stimulate and validate such research efforts (IOM, 2008a).

The revolutionary direction outlined in the NIH's Roadmap brought with it the impetus to redesign the very foundation of the health research enterprise—the Clinical and Translational Science Awards (Zerhouni, 2005). The goal of these awards was to create research infrastructure that would translate basic research through clinical trials into widespread use in patient care, thus impacting patient outcomes. Included in the redesign was the requirement to effectively involve the public and clinicians in clinical and translational research priority setting and participation through community engagement groups (NIH, 2007).

Taken together, these recommendations and funding directions have launched improvement science and pointed to the need for a research agenda for the field. The nascent field has many challenges in moving forward. One of the most urgent is to set a course toward highly relevant improvement research studies. This discussion presents the first major action of the ISRN—to establish consensus for priorities in improvement research (Stevens, 2009).

The Need for Priorities for Improvement Research

The great need for improvement science carries with it the opportunity for myriad priorities to be defined. Consensus priorities can highlight the most important and urgent gaps in improvement knowledge as identified by clinical and academic scholars, leaders, and change agents in acute healthcare settings. The need for improvement research is great, yet today's resources are limited, and advancements in the field are hampered by the lack of a national research agenda with clearly defined priorities to systematically build knowledge.

There is a limited cadre of improvement scientists, a situation that may not be remedied in the near future because current training is inadequate and often unrelated to improvement research (IOM, 2008c). In addition, research dollars in the field are constrained. Federal and foundation spending for T2 and quality improvement research is estimated to be only 1.5% of total biomedical research funding (Moses, Dorsey, Mattheson, & Thier, 2005).

The call for quality improvement research to be relevant, useful, and practical to decision makers anchors the development of improvement science priorities. This situation accentuates the need for a well-targeted agenda for improvement science. Clear priorities will pave the way for today's limited brain trust and fiscal capacity to be focused on the most urgent improvement topics, enabling research to become a driving force in quality improvement. CNLs sitting at the table are important to this ongoing discussion, as they are translational in their role.

Developing Consensus on Improvement Research Priorities

As part of the strategic plan to build an infrastructure for improvement science, an early target of the ISRN was to establish consensus on high-priority research, development, and evaluation needs to guide the scientific field. Because the ISRN aims to promote a national program of research to advance what is known about improvement strategies, it was urgent to outline an agenda of priority research studies and topic areas as a place to begin. Such an agenda serves as a common rallying point to focus resources and attract improvement scientists and scholars into a collaborative around these common research goals.

The ISRN research priorities are intended to define the most urgent research studies needed to determine effective strategies in quality improvement and patient safety at this point in time. By networking to conduct improvement studies on these first targets, the ISRN will be able to intensify research efforts and produce seminal research-based knowledge quickly.

The ISRN's priority-setting process was informed by a number of sources. These included environmental scans of major concerns in health care, reviews of professional and scientific literature, research priorities for quality and patient safety established by other entities (e.g., the World Health Organization), a targeted interprofessional stakeholder survey, and a RAND Delphi process with the ISRN steering council , the council itself being representative of a wide array of stakeholders with interprofessional perspectives. Multiple points of information and multiple iterations of consensus building were used to ensure that the research agenda merits a high level of attention.

Development was accomplished through four major phases (1) multiple iterations of survey development, (2) administration of online survey to stakeholders, (3) the RAND Delphi technique with steering council members, and (4) refinement through steering council discussion.

Stakeholder opinions were sought through an online structured survey. The survey was developed, tested with various groups of stakeholders, and revised over an 8-month period (June 2009 to February 2010) and went through three revisions. The final survey included 33 improvement topics organized into 9 dimensions of quality and safety. The online survey was preceded with an advance email invitation, followed by the invitation and survey link, and a reminder, each sent at 1-week intervals. During a 5-week period (February 2010 to March 2010), the survey was distributed to 2,777 stakeholders identified through a variety of methods, including identifying interprofessional groups and organized associations of health scientists, healthcare clinical leaders, and thought leaders in improvement and patient safety. Data were gathered from 560 respondents (a 20% response rate).

Responses were analyzed using descriptive statistics and presented to the ISRN steering council at its on-site meeting March 25, 2010. A RAND Delphi approach was used during facilitated consensus formation discussion at this meeting, which took place in Houston, Texas.

Results of the steering council's multiple iterations were captured by the ISRN coordinating team and vetted once again during the April 2010 steering council meeting. Through these processes, consensus on the ISRN research priorities was established and framed as the ISRN research agenda. The research priorities represented in **Table 17-1** were adopted by the ISRN as the best thinking to date about the direction that should be taken in improvement science.

The research agenda is organized into four broad priority categories or domains. Although it is acknowledged that, within each of these four areas, investigators could pose questions to investigate structure, process, outcome, and knowledge, the four clusters provide one way to emphasize various perspectives on quality and safety. To further circumscribe each research domain, priority topics and examples of improvement strategies were added. The order of topics does not reflect the order of priority.

This agenda for development of improvement science represents the first in the nation. The ISRN is creating collaborative research teams of academic and clinical partners in acute-care settings to conduct improvement studies aligned with these priorities (ISRN, 2010).

The directions established through this research agenda will advance knowledge translation, clinical decisions, and ultimately inform policy related to quality improvement, driving healthcare transformation. By making substantial progress in these areas over the next 3 to 5 years, the ISRN will contribute significantly to improvement science for patient outcomes in our nation.

Table 17-1 Research Priorities of the Improvement Science Research Network

---

A. COORDINATION AND TRANSITIONS OF CARE—this category emphasizes strategies for care improvement to care processes in specific clinical conditions. At this time, care coordination and transitions of care are the key clinical focus.

Priority Topics:
Evaluate strategies and methods to assure coordination and continuity of care across transitions in given clinical populations.
Test and refine methods of handoffs and other strategies to assure safe, effective, and efficient transitions in given clinical populations.

Examples of Improvement Strategies and Research Issues:
Team performance, medication reconciliation, discharge for prevention of early readmission, patient-centered care, measurement of targeted outcomes.

B. HIGH-PERFORMING CLINICAL SYSTEMS AND MICROSYSTEMS APPROACHES TO IMPROVEMENT—this category emphasizes structure and process in clinical care and healthcare as complex adaptive systems.

Priority Topics:
Determine effectiveness and efficiency of various methods and models for integrating and sustaining best practices in improving care processes and patient outcomes.

Investigate strategies to engage front-line providers in improving quality and patient safety.

Evaluate strategies for preventing targeted patient safety incidents.

Establish reliable quality indicators to measure impact of improvement and isolate nursing care impact on outcomes.

Examples of Improvement Strategies and Research Issues:
Front-line provider engagement, factors related to uptake, adoption, and implementation, sustaining improvements and improvement processes.

C. EVIDENCE-BASED QUALITY IMPROVEMENT AND BEST PRACTICE—this category emphasizes closing the gap between knowledge and practice through translating knowledge and designating and implementing best practices.

Priority Topics:
Evaluate strategies and impact of employing evidence-based practice in clinical care for process and outcomes improvement.

Determine gaps and bridge gaps between knowledge and practice.

Transform evidence for practice through conducting systematic reviews, developing practice guidelines, and integrating into clinical decision making.

Develop new research methods in evidence-based quality improvement, including comparative effectiveness research and practice-based evidence.

Examples of Improvement Strategies and Research Issues:
Develop and critically appraise clinical practice guidelines, adoption and spread of best practices, customization of best practices, institutional elements in adoption, defining best practice in absence of evidence, consumers in EBP, technology-based integration.

Table 17-1   Research Priorities of the Improvement Science Research Network (continued)

D. LEARNING ORGANIZATIONS AND CULTURE OF QUALITY AND SAFETY—this category emphasizes human factors and other aspects of a system related to organizational culture and commitment to quality and safety.

Priority Topics:

Investigate strategies for creating organizational environments, processes that support cultures fully linked to maintaining quality, patient safety to maximizing patient outcomes.

Determine effective approaches to develop organizational climates for change, innovation, and organizational learning.

Examples of Improvement Strategies and Research Issues:

Unit-based nursing quality teams, protecting strategy from culture, engendering values and beliefs for culture of patient safety.

Source: Improvement Science Research Network (ISRN). (2010). Research priorities. Retrieved from http://www.isrn.net/research. Reproduced with permission.

Summary

- CNLs can use their understanding of improvement science to advance their roles as lateral integrators, advocates, information managers, life-long learners, educators, and outcomes managers.
- Knowing the intersection of critical appraisal of the research and profiles of improvement innovations, the CNL uses this information about how an innovation was evaluated to answer the question, "Did it work?"
- Understanding resources of innovations of national import can yield significant improvement in care processes and patient outcomes—most often within the local context of the innovation.
- CNLs as clinical leaders in microsystem change are optimally positioned to bring teams together to sustain improvement.

WWW Reflection Questions
© Arenacreative/Dreamstime.com

1. Consider the research priorities of the ISRN (refer to Table 17-1). What microsystem change projects that you are currently engaged in fit into a

particular priority area? Does an understanding of improvement science inform your project? How so?

2. Using the example of your change project from Question 1, what improvement strategies best describe your approach to sustaining your innovation? Is there a fit for one of the ISRN's priority areas (refer to Table 17-1)?

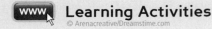

Learning Activities

1. What critical barriers to progress in improvement research, discussed in this chapter, have you noted as you embark on your microsystem improvement change? Describe how you could overcome these barriers.
2. When critically appraising evidence to support your microsystem's change, what have you noted regarding T1, T2, and T3? What lessons did you learn when critically appraising a variety of research evidence documents, such as systematic reviews?

References

Agency for Healthcare Research & Quality. (2008). Health care innovations exchange, Retrieved from http://innovations.ahrq.gov/

Dougherty D., & Conway, P. H. (2008). The "3T's" road map to transform US health care: The "how" of high quality care. *Journal of the American Medical Association, 299*(19), 2319–2321.

Grol, R., Baker, R., & Moss, F. (2004). *Quality improvement research: Understanding the science of change in health care.* London, England: BMJ Books.

Improvement Science Research Network (ISRN). (2010). Research priorities. Retrieved from http://www.improvementscienceresearch.net/research

Institute of Medicine. (1999). *To err is human: Building a safer health system.* L. T. Kohn, J. M. Corrigan, & M.S. Donaldson (Eds.). Washington, DC: National Academies Press. Retrieved from http://www.iom.edu/Reports/1999/To-Err-is-Human-Building-A-Safer-Health-System.aspx

Institute of Medicine. (2001). *Crossing the quality chasm: A new health system for the 21st century.* Washington, DC: National Academies Press. Retrieved from http://www.iom.edu/Reports/2001/Crossing-the-Quality-Chasm-A-New-Health-System-for-the-21st-Century.aspx

Institute of Medicine. (2007). *The state of quality improvement and implementation research: Expert views. Workshop summary.* Washington, DC: National Academies Press. Retrieved from http://www.iom.edu/Reports/2007/The-State-of-Quality-Improvement-and-Implementation-Research-Expert-Views-Workshop-Summary.aspx

Institute of Medicine. (2008a). *Creating a business case for quality improvement research: Expert views. Workshop summary.* Washington, DC: National Academies Press. Retrieved from http://www.nap.edu/catalog.php?record_id=12137

Institute of Medicine. (2008b). *Knowing what works in health care: A roadmap for the nation.* J. Eden, B. Wheatley, B. McNeil, & H. Sox (Eds.). Washington, DC: National Academies Press. Retrieved from http://www.iom.edu/Reports/2008/Knowing-What-Works-in-Health -Care-A-Roadmap-for-the-Nation.aspx

Institute of Medicine. (2008c). *Training the workforce in quality improvement and quality improvement research.* IOM Forum Workshop. Washington, DC.

Kermaris N. C., Kanadaris N. K., Tziopis G., Kontakis, G., & Giannoudis, P. V. (2008). Translational research: From bench to bedside. *Injury, 39*(6), 643–650.

King, C. R. (2013). Evidence-based practice. In C. R. King & G. S. O'Toole (Eds.), *Clinical nurse leader certification review.* New York, NY: Springer Publishing Company.

McGlynn, E. A., Asch, S. M., Adams, J., Keesey, J., Hicks, J., DeCristofaro, A., & Kerr, E. A. (2003). The quality of health care delivered to adults in the United States. *New England Journal of Medicine, 348*(26), 2635–2645.

Moses, H., 3rd, Dorsey, E. R., Mattheson, D. H., & Thier, S. O. (2005). Financial anatomy of biomedical research. *Journal of the American Medical Association, 294*(11), 1333–1342.

National Institutes of Health. (2007). Part II—Full text of announcement. Section I. Funding opportunity description. 1. Research objectives. IN: Institutional Clinical and Translational Science Award (U54). RFARM-07-007. Retrieved from http://grants.nih.gov grants/guide /rfa-files/rfa-rm-07-007.html#PartII

Pawson, R., & Tilley, N. (1997). *Realistic evaluation.* London, England: Sage.

Rubio, D. M., Schoenbaum, E. E., Lee, L. S., Schteingart, D. E., Marantz, P. R., Anderson, K. E.,... Esposito, K. (2010). Defining translational research: Implications for training. *Academic Medicine, 85*(3), 470–475.

Shojania, K. G., & Grimshaw, J. M. (2005). Evidence-based quality improvement: The state of the science. *Health Affairs (Millwood), 24*(1), 138–150.

Stevens, K. R. (2009). *A research network for improvement science: The Improvement Science Research Network.* NIH 1 RC2 NR011946-01.

Zerhouni, E. A. (2005). Translational and clinical science—time for a new vision. *New England Journal of Medicine, 353*(15), 1621–1623.

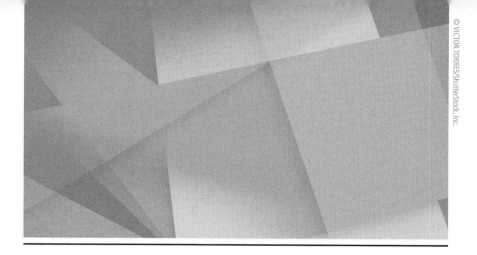

UNIT 4
Health Promotion and Disease Prevention: Essentials for the CNL

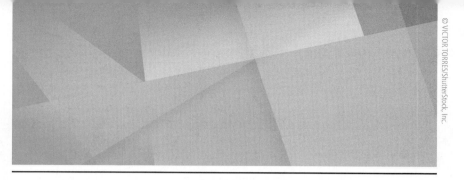

EIGHTEEN

Community Resource Awareness and Networking Through Advocacy

Linda Roussel, Alice J. Godfrey, and Lonnie Williams

www Learning Objectives

- Describe the clinical nurse leader's roles as patient advocate and community leader
- Evaluate tools and models used in discharge planning and assurance of continuity of care
- Outline creative tools for team building and collaboration
- Identify community outreach and networking opportunities for the clinical nurse leader

> **Teamwork divides the task and multiplies the success.**
>
> **Author Unknown**

Key Terms

Discharge planning   Community outreach   Social justice

CNL Roles

Outcomes manager   Client advocate
Educator   Information manager
Systems analyst and risk anticipator   Team manager

CNL Professional Values

Accountability   Human dignity
Social justice

CNL Core Competencies

Communication   Assessment
Nursing technology   Health promotion
Resource management   Risk reduction
Disease prevention   Information and healthcare technologies
Ethics   Human care systems and policy
Complexity and community networking
Design/management/coordination of care

Introduction

The clinical nurse leader (CNL), as the designer, manager, and coordinator of care, provides and assembles comprehensive care for clients—individuals, families, groups, and communities—in multiple and varied settings. According to the American Association of Colleges of Nursing (AACN, 2007), the CNL guides the patient through the health system using skills essential to this role. Such skills include communication, collaboration, negotiation, delegation, coordination, and evaluation of interdisciplinary work, and the application, design, and evaluation of outcome-based practice models (pp. 25–26).

Preparation of the CNL

Preparing the CNL for community resource management and networking includes course work in leadership, interdisciplinary team building, organizational skills, information management, delegation, and cost–benefit analysis. The CNL considers the environment's readiness for change and the processes that are important to that end. Understanding organization and community culture and how decisions are made in translating best practices, as well as identifying key stakeholders, gives the CNL skill sets to accomplish these goals. The CNL does not work alone. Creating a vision for the stakeholders with those at the point of care (patients, family, staff, multidisciplinary teams, and community members) helps to spread and sustain quality and safe care. Patients' involvement in their care, working to facilitate decision making and self-management, is strengthened when interdisciplinary teams and community networks are involved.

> Never doubt that a small group of thoughtful committed citizens can change the world, indeed it's the only thing that ever has.
>
> Margaret Mead

Leadership and Interdisciplinary Team Building

As a horizontal leader, the CNL is pivotal to the healthcare team, serving as a critical navigator through the microsystem. The CNL knows the roles of the various team members and the value they add to the transition of the patient into the community. The CNL understands concepts of team building and the skills necessary to build quality teams. Such skills include visioning, group dynamics, accountability, and the basics of how to conduct a meeting. Complexity science advances concepts for the larger view of social systems and community networking, important knowledge for the CNL to possess.

Complexity and Community Networking

Complexity theory provides new insights into the behavior and emergent properties of social systems. Complexity theory purports that the experience of community is both an outcome and the context of informal networking. A well-connected community is achieved when people feel part of a web of diverse and interlocking relationships. These networks sustain and shape an integrated and dynamic social and organizational environment. They support the familiar patterns of interaction and collective organization that characterize the voluntary and community sectors. Community development involves creating and managing opportunities for connection and communication across social identity and geographical boundaries. Termed "meta-networking," it is a core function of the professional role. The community can be envisioned as part of the microsystem when the population of patients at the microsystem level is cared for within this system. Failing to take into consideration where patients are going (and coming from) and the neighborhood and community support available creates a fissure in the system. This failure underscores the silos that health care continues to reinforce, which are often related to reimbursement methods.

The professional values of the CNL support active involvement with the community. When assuming responsibility for the comprehensive care of individuals, families, and population groups, the CNL participates in the care of the communities where their clients live, work, and play. The CNL advocates for the worth and value of all persons and individualizes a plan for continuity of care that reflects a commitment to the principle of social justice. Social justice is tied to the CNL's responsibility for fair, equitable care. Competency in providing health care to diverse populations and working with diversity is also integrated into social justice.

Tools and Models for the CNL's Roles in Advocacy and Networking

Discharge Planning

Discharge planning is a process that has long been recognized as essential in the delivery of quality health care. The process rose to the forefront in healthcare management with the passage of legislation that mandated it as an essential service. Today, discharge planning is a critical process that requires interprofessional teamwork. The identification of cost-effective healthcare resources, as well as evaluation of these resources, is essential to the implementation of the CNL's role.

The key features of the discharge planning process are as follows:

- Planned and coordinated events in any patient care setting
- Contribution to the continuity of patient care services
- Promotion of health maintenance and safety of patients as they access and consume healthcare services
- Contribution to the cost effectiveness of healthcare services
- An interprofessional process

Discharge planning begins with the first encounter with the patient. The individual patient assessment tools include information about the patient's diagnosis as well as living arrangements, family, and significant others. Each microsystem has standard tools for patient assessments. Information obtained in the patient's initial assessment serves to direct the CNL to tools that will assist with the identification of discharge needs, as well as diagnosing community needs.

Transition Care Model

The Care Transitions Program developed by Coleman (2007) refines the process of coordinated care and discharge planning by identifying specific goals for the process of moving patients between healthcare providers and healthcare settings. According to Coleman, the goals of transition care are to support patients and families; increase skills among healthcare providers; enhance the ability of health information technology to promote health information exchange across care settings; implement system level interventions to improve quality and safety; develop performance measures and public reporting mechanisms; and influence health policy at the national level.

Networking and Interprofessional Team Building

The CNL will identify the persons in the clinical microsystem who contribute to the process. These individuals form the interprofessional team that becomes the patient and the community's source for direct care, primary prevention, and continued care and rehabilitation. The interprofessional team today reflects the expertise of providers from many disciplines: medicine, allied health, nursing, social services, clinical laboratory providers, and long-term care providers. In addition to these professionals, the family members and lay providers must be identified. These individuals provide essential support and validation for the patient.

The Epidemiological Triad

Disease in humans is typically explained in terms of the epidemiological triad, which is a tool that is central to community diagnosis. The epidemiological triad describes the complex interaction of the human host with a disease-causing agent and the environment in which the interaction occurs. Host characteristics can be such factors as age, sex, race, religion, customs, occupation, previous disease, and immune status. Types of disease-causing agents may include biological, bacterial, viral, chemical, and nutritional. Temperature, humidity, altitude, crowding, food, water, air pollution, and noise are identified environmental factors that can cause an increased risk of human disease. It is the interaction of these factors (host, agent, and environment) that contributes to disease. Analysis of the host characteristics, possible agents, and environmental factors enable the CNL to identify risks that can contribute to the onset of disease and disability. According to Gordis (2009), disease can be caused by biological, physical, chemical factors. Psychosocial factors also contribute to disease occurrence but may not fit into the usual categorization of factors.

The Natural History of Disease Model

The natural history of disease model is a classic tool developed by Leavell and Clark (1965). The model describes the progression of disease. There are two disease periods in this model: the prepathogenesis period and the pathogenesis period. The prepathogenesis period begins with the interaction of the host, agent, and environmental factors. As disease develops in a person, the model includes the phases of pathogenesis that the person experiences. The levels of prevention are correlated to the periods of prepathogenesis and pathogenesis (primary, secondary, and tertiary). Primary prevention focuses on the prepathogenesis period, whereas secondary and tertiary prevention focus on the pathogenesis period. Primary prevention considers health promotion and may include such interventions as health education; provision of adequate housing, recreation, and working conditions; and periodic selective examinations. Primary prevention can be related to specific protection against occupational hazards, accidents, and carcinogens; use of specific nutrients; and avoidance of allergens. Secondary prevention related to early diagnosis, prompt treatment, and disability limitation includes such interventions as case-finding measures, screening surveys, and adequate treatment to arrest the disease process and prevent further complications and contraindications. Tertiary prevention is included in the period of pathogenesis. Rehabilitation is central to tertiary prevention. Provision of hospital and community facilities for retraining and education for maximum use of remaining capacities describe important interventions in rehabilitation (tertiary prevention). Additional rehabilitation interventions may include education of the public and industry to employ the rehabilitated, selective work placement, and work therapy in hospitals. This model offers a blueprint for health promotion as well as disease management in individuals and at the community level. For example, the CNL who documents an increase in young males who are injured in motorcycle accidents will investigate primary prevention strategies for preventing accidents at the community level. A community diagnosis emerges when the absence of a needed service or the presence of an agent that contributes to disease is identified at the community level.

Mind Maps

Mind maps provide an excellent tool for leading teams through innovation. According to Buzan (2004), mind maps give depth and breadth of scope that a list of ideas cannot. (See **Figure 18-1** for an example of a mind map.) "By working from the centre outwards, mind map encourages your thoughts to behave in the same way (Buzan, 2004, p. 8)." The framework provides an illustrative view of ideas and their expansion and alternatives, radiating creative thinking. By using letters and numbers, colors and images, mind maps engage the left and the right sides of the brain. Starting from the center, working outwardly with ideas, symbols, colors, numbers, and other symbols, mind maps engage thinking power that increases synergistically. "Each side of the brain simultaneously feeds off and strengthens the other in a manner which provides limitless creative potential (Buzan, 2004, p. 9)." Mind maps are useful for short- and long-term planning. Working with teams can be more efficient when employing mind maps. They can help a team focus on the way ahead and bring together a shared, creative, and imaginative vision. Techniques include incorporating equal time to listen and speak; showing interest in people and ideas; and having a clear idea of where the CNL, the team, and the organization are all headed.

For example, using mind maps, the CNL can focus the team on the core of his or her innovation; then, using brainstorm sessions, the team can work out specific strategies and ideas. Mind maps can be revisited as ideas are advanced or carried out, with new options surfacing with the changes. The mind map can serve as an agenda, a business plan, and the basis for developing project plans. Considering this nonlinear (complexity) way of thinking, mind maps offer a natural way to innovate.

Figure 18-1 Process evaluation TX mind map.

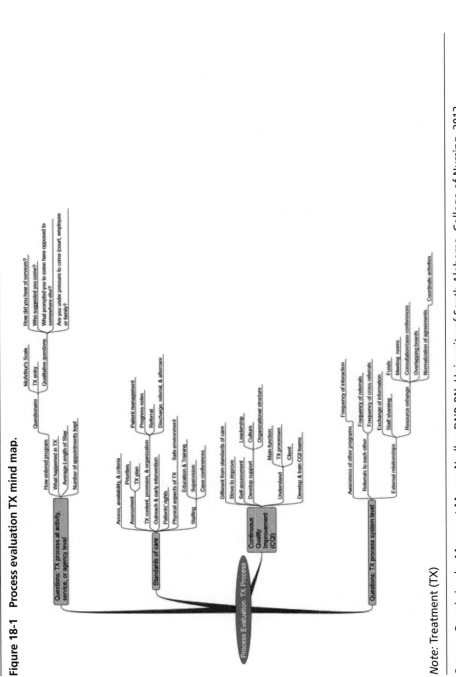

Note: Treatment (TX)

Source: Permission by Margaret Moore-Nadler, DNP, RN, University of South Alabama, College of Nursing, 2013.

Buzan also offers the TEFCAS model (trial, event, feedback, check, adjust, and success) as a successful mechanism for working with mind maps. Each aspect of TEFCAS identifies tools, a checklist, and strategies for applying a different way of thinking. TEFCAS helps to monitor and react to the outcome of project plans, focusing on goals and outcomes. This model reinforces project planning, adding new insights to ongoing processes.

The Use of Story: Messages to Innovate Team Collaboration

Loehr (2007) described the power of story as a means of changing one's destiny in business and in life. Loehr shared the following:

> By "story," then, I mean those tales we create and tell ourselves and others, and which form the only reality we will ever know in this life. Our stories may or may not conform to the real world. They may or may not inspire us to take hope-filled action to better our lives. They may or may not take us where we ultimately want to go. But since our destiny follows our stories, it's imperative that we do everything in our power to get our stories right. (p. 5)

Bringing about ways to understand the CNL's story and that of the CNL's organization can be critical to understanding the mission and goals to be carried out. Knowing the CNL's own story (about success, challenges, and use of opportunities and challenges) is a good place to start. Reflecting on values and beliefs, the "private voice" in the CNL's head is part of self-awareness and self-reflection, qualities that are necessary for helping others to understand their stories and to mutually create one story for the team. Loehr identifies three rules of storytelling: purpose, truth, and action. *Purpose* considers the motives and overall intention of the story. What is the team striving for? What principle? What end? What goal? What does the team want to see at the end of the day or the year? Is the story taking the team where it wants to go? What is nonnegotiable? These are questions that can guide clarity of purpose (Loehr, 2007, p. 138). A shared vision through story can engage head and heart.

Truth relates to the authenticity of the story. "Is it grounded in objective reality as fully as possible; that is, does it coincide with generally agreed-upon portrayal of the world? Or is it true only if I'm living in a dreamland" (Loehr, 2007, p. 138)? Being truthful gives credibility to leading innovation in patient care delivery. *Action* relates to the purpose and the truthfulness of the story being told. "Does the story move others to action?" Knowing how explicit actions (plan) will be played out for desired outcomes can provide a dynamic template for the team. This action plan involves the stakeholders, their engagement in the process and outcomes, and how the story plays out.

Stories engage the heart and the mind. The CNL can use a story to bring alive what may seem like static processes, policies, and procedures that may be considered mechanistic and carried out in robotic fashion.

Equipped with knowledge and skills in discharge planning, community outreach, and creative collaboration, the CNL furthers the business case for safe, quality continuity of care. Effective discharge planning through a greater understanding of community outreach, networking, and tools such as mind maps and story can improve financial, quality, safety, and satisfaction outcomes as teams come together.

Community Assessment

The CNL will demonstrate leadership, as well as creativity, in the provision of continuity of care. No skill better displays leadership qualities and the development of strategies for improving care for individuals, families, and communities than that of community assessment. Community assessment requires interprofessional communication and collaboration, along with the ability to prioritize. Community assessments identify resources and gaps in services in the community. Anderson and McFarlane (2000) identified eight elements of a comprehensive community assessment:

1. Physical environment
2. Recreation
3. Education
4. Economics
5. Communication
6. Health and social services
7. Politics and government
8. Safety and transportation

Box 18-1 provides an example of a community outreach assignment.

Any service or resource considered for a patient needs to be evaluated. The questions in **Box 18-2** can serve as a guide to evaluating community resources.

A case study in leadership and advocacy is also provided at the end of the chapter.

Box 18-1   Community Outreach Assignment

This assignment gives you the opportunity to evaluate community services, referrals, and other community resources that your patients/consumers access in your clinical microsystem. Consider patient discharge planning and how patients on your unit (in your microsystem) use community services (your major referral support services). In the same vein, where are patients being admitted from (in your community)? What patterns do you see regarding admissions and discharges? In other words, are patients coming from the same communities and settings (home, nursing homes, senior centers, etc.)? Are patients being discharged back to their same settings?

What have you learned from this assignment?

_____

_____

_____

Describe your microsystem's discharge plan considering referral and support sources. Do you observe any patterns? If so, what are the patterns?

_____

_____

_____

Outline primary sources and follow-up plans. Do you have contact with your patients after discharge? If so, describe the continuity of care and how this impacts the quality and safe delivery of services and patient satisfaction.

_____

_____

_____

Outline recommendations to improve community outreach and ongoing continuity of patient care in your microsystem.

_____

_____

_____

Assignment is in APA style, has a scholarly presentation, and uses reference citations liberally.

_____

_____

_____

Box 18-2   Evaluating Community Resources

- Is the agency an official or governmental agency?
- Is the agency a private or voluntary agency?
- What is the level of prevention addressed by the services of the agency?
- What are the eligibility requirements for the services?
- What are the costs of services, and what payment sources are accepted?
- How are referrals made?
- How are families and significant others included in the services provided?
- What is the preparation and expertise of the service provider?

Summary

- As reimbursement tightens and there are greater demands for efficient, effective care, discharge planning and community networking become more critical.
- The CNL—in the role of outcomes manager, client advocate, and team manager—provides an understanding of quality improvement data, using evidence-based practice methods to promote a smooth transition of care from setting to setting.
- As an educator, information manager, systems analyst, and risk anticipator, the CNL uses tools for discharge planning and community diagnosing, including the epidemiological triad and the natural history of disease model.
- Additional strategies include mind maps and story, which contribute to engaging staff and communicating and collaborating with teams.
- CNL core competencies—such as communication, assessment, nursing technology and resource management, health promotion, and risk reduction—are essential to CNL success in community outreach and participating in patient-centered care.
- Core competencies also include integrating disease prevention, information and healthcare technologies, ethics, and human care systems.

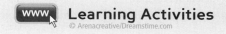

Reflection Questions
© Arenacreative/Dreamstime.com

1. As a CNL, how do you determine the best strategies for networking with community partners?
2. What are the best communication strategies for beginning a dialogue with community leaders and stakeholders?

Learning Activities
© Arenacreative/Dreamstime.com

As a CNL on a fast-paced surgical orthopedic unit, suppose you have noted that after most of your patients are discharged into their community, they return just weeks later. You note that many of the patients require after-hospital care, including home health services, support groups, long-term care, and assisted living services. Other services, such as Meals on Wheels, medication assistance programs, and assistance with durable medical equipment, are also important to your patients' discharge planning. You begin to see a pattern of inadequate resources within your community. You have also noted that your hospital has programs that may be useful to the community.

1. As an outcomes manager, what specific outcomes would be appropriate for you to address these issues?
2. What are the advocacy issues? As a client advocate, what are your responsibilities? How are these evaluated?
3. As an educator and information manager, how would you determine educational needs and how would you manage this information?
4. As a systems analyst/risk anticipator, how would complexity theory guide you in managing community resources?
5. Who would need to be at the "table" as you serve as a team manager?

Recommended Reading

Bourgeault, I. L., & Mulvale, G. (2006). Collaborative health care teams in Canada and the USA: Confronting the structural embeddedness of medical dominance. *Health Sociology Review, 15*(5), 481–494.

Hagenow, N. (2003). Why not person-centered care? The challenges of implementation. *Nursing Administration Quarterly, 27*(3), 203–207.

Summers, L., Marton, K., Barbaccia, J., & Randolph, J. (2000). Physician, nurse, and social work collaboration in primary care for chronically ill seniors. *Archives of Internal Medicine, 160*(12), 1825–1833.

Virginia Regional Medical Program. (1974). *Discharge planning.* Richmond, VA: Author.

References

American Association of Colleges of Nursing. (2007). *White paper on the education and role of the clinical nurse leader.* Washington, DC: Author. pp. 6–10. Retrieved from http://www.aacn .nche.edu/Publications/WhitePapers/ClinicalNurseLeader07.pdf

Anderson, E. T., & McFarlane, J. M. (2000). *Community as partner: Theory and practice in nursing* (3rd ed.). Philadelphia, PA: Lippincott.

Buzan, T. (2004). *Mind maps at work: How to be the best at your job and still have time to play.* New York, NY: Penguin Group.

Coleman, E. A. (2007). *Care transitions intervention.* Retrieved from http://www.caretransitions .org/definitions.asp

Gordis, L. (2009). *Epidemiology* (4th ed.). Philadelphia, PA: W. B. Saunders.

Leavell, H. F., & Clark, E. G. (1965). *Preventive medicine for the doctor in his community: An epidemiologic approach.* New York, NY: McGraw-Hill.

Loehr, J. (2007). *The power of story.* New York, NY: Simon and Schuster.

Tools of the Trade: Case Studies

Case Study 1: Individual Level

A 21-year-old pregnant woman who has a history of intravenous drug abuse is admitted through the emergency department. As the CNL on the labor and delivery unit, you admit the patient and begin the initial assessment and discharge planning. Consider the following questions as the discharge planning begins.

1. Who does the patient consider her family?
2. Where does the patient currently live, and where will she go when she leaves the hospital?
3. What personal, environmental, and safety concerns will the patient have when she leaves the hospital?
4. What health and medical follow-up care (including pre-/postnatal care) will be needed?
5. After considering Questions 1–4, use the natural history of disease model to identify primary, tertiary, and prevention interventions that might help the patient.

Case Study 2: Community Level

Examine the histories and assessment data of the patients on your unit or in your microsystem. Focus on the demographic profiles of the patients. Do the patients come from one community or neighborhood? Are the patients referred by primary providers or by another agency, such as a nursing home or home care agency, or are they admitted through the emergency department? Are patients being discharged back to the same setting, or are they referred to another level of care?

1. Describe your microsystem's discharge process, and consider the referral and support resources used. Do you observe any patterns? If so, what are they?
2. Describe your microsystem's follow-up plan for patients. If the follow-up plan includes contact with the patients after discharge, describe that process.
3. How does your microsystem evaluate the discharge process and its effect on the patient and community? Is there a method for documenting outcomes?

Case Study 3: Leadership and Advocacy in the Community

Assessment of patient data, as well as the discharge planning process in your microsystem, reveals the following information.

A significant number of patients with type II diabetes have been admitted over the last year. The patients reside in the zip code where a new retirement community that provides housing for low-income persons over age 65 has just been established. The patients have different primary care providers. The neighborhood is on the public bus route that transports residents to a chain grocery and shopping center.

1. Who are the stakeholders in this neighborhood?
2. How would you go about initiating a diabetic management clinic for the retirement community?
3. What are the resources that will assist with the patients' care, and what is the first step you would take with each client?

Population of Complex Care

Lauran Hardin

Friday afternoon at 3 pm the classic complex call came in over the pager. "There's a patient here with multiple admissions who has no insurance, needs a new heart valve, is schizophrenic, homeless, and is discharging in 2 hours—can you take care of this?" It would take a village to resolve this situation in 2 hours.

After reading the patient's chart and assessing the root cause of her readmissions, it was clear that there were cross-continuum issues that needed to be addressed. The patient needed a safe place to live and a primary care physician (PCP) to lead her team. She needed insurance to get access to the complex medical care she required. She needed help to stop smoking crack. She needed to learn how to take critical medicines to prevent her from being overcome by heart failure. She needed transportation, and so much more.

Engaging the CNL core competencies of healthcare systems coordinator of care and facilitator of interprofessional teams, the CNL called the hospitalist, the master's prepared social worker (MSW), the case manager, the new PCP, and the PCP's lead nurse. A collaborative complex care conference was organized in the patient's room within the hour. After hearing a summary by the CNL of key issues that needed to be solved, each discipline stepped up to the plate to offer its best. The hospitalist was linked with the new PCP to give direct patient reports, decreasing fragmentation in care. A Medicaid application was completed, housing obtained, and bus tickets provided by the MSW. The case manager obtained the medications gratis. The staff nurse set up the medication box and provided teaching. The CNL coordinated the team and set up a joint care conference with the patient, the PCP, and the lead nurse on the following Monday to transfer the plan of care and link the patient with her new physician. A focus on solutions, combined with the facilitation to make it happen, allowed the patient to leave in 2 hours, with everything she needed to start over again.

Community-Based Wound Care Integration

Ann Nguyen

Problem Statement

The current communication tools, patient education, and wound care network have not worked effectively within a healthcare system in San Francisco, CA. Sending copies of current medication lists from skilled nursing facilities (SNFs) to wound care centers (WCC) and faxing wound care orders from WCCs to SNFs do not provide nurses with adequate information about patients' conditions and comorbidities related to wound etiologies and treatment modalities. In addition, the lack of a networking system between the inpatient wound care team and the outpatient WCC delays the follow-up. Therefore, the number of wound care readmissions is high and the time of healing is prolonged.

Team Development

Key terms: collaboration, lateral integration, and patient centeredness

This project was developed by using Kotter's theory and Six Sigma methodology to achieve the positive goal of achieving effective and efficient wound-healing outcomes. This project had three parts:

1. Creating the SCAN (status/condition/any laboratory result/new wound) communication tool: collaboration between the wound care nurse and community-based setting nurse: SCAN tool included at the end of this exemplar
2. Patient teaching handouts: patient centeredness
3. Inpatient/outpatient wound care network: lateral integration

Implementation

1. Providing the tools, continuing education, and presentation of materials to the WCC staff, 5 SNFs, 5 Home Health Aides (HHAs), and case managers
2. Working with community-setting partners for individual patients and every wound care visit through the SCAN communication book
3. Collaborating with case managers and attending physicians on discharge plans for wound care patients

Financial Impact and Outcomes

1. The SCAN communication tool saved $280,560 in 4 months for all WCCs, SNFs, and home health agencies and positively impacted patient/customer satisfaction
2. The patient teaching handout saved $635, $130 in 4 months for the WCC by reducing the length of treatment
3. Wound care network implementation saved $ 567,00 in 4 months by reducing the readmission rate

Wound Care "SCAN" Communication

PATIENT NAME: **DATE:**

PREVISIT NURSE: **PHONE:**

STATUS	Last FSBS/ Treatment	Last Dressing Change	On Coumadin		Others
			□ YES *Dose:*	□ NO	

CONDITION	Fever (T⁰)		Loose Bowel Movement		Others
	□ YES	□ NO	□ YES *Treatment:*	□ NO	

ANY LAB WORK	Current Lab Result (Date)			Wound Culture		Others
	CBC	Hemoglobin / Hematocrit	Hb A1C	□ YES	□ NO	

NEW WOUND	Location	Date identified	Current treatment

POSTVISIT   **NURSE/DATE:**   **PHONE: (408) 272-6450**

STATUS	Please refer to Nursing Assessment Sheets		
CONDITION	Stable		Others
	□ YES	□ NO	
ANY LAB WORK	New Lab Order	Culture Result		Others
		□ YES	□ N/A	
NEW WOUND	Location	Diagnosis	Treatment
			Please refer to the Physician Order and Home Care Instruction

NINETEEN

Promoting Health and Preventing Illness

 Margaret Moore-Nadler

WWW Learning Objectives
© Arenacreative/Dreamstime.com

- Compare and contrast health promotion and illness prevention
- Discuss the *Healthy People 2020* indicators and how health promotion strategies contribute to the achievement of national healthcare goals
- Discuss the clinical nurse leader's role in promoting wellness and prevention efforts
- Describe the clinical nurse leader's role in patient engagement, including health literacy, motivational interviewing, and readiness for change

(continues)

> Mothers, the newborn and children represent the well-being of a society and its potential for the future. Their health needs cannot be left unmet without harming the whole of society.
>
> Lee Jong-wook, former director-general, World Health Organization, Make Every Mother and Child Count, Geneva, April 2005

Key Terms

Health promotion	Wellness	Illness prevention
Secondary prevention	Health literacy	Self-care
Self-management	Motivational interviewing	
Cultural sensitivity	Readiness for change	
Patient engagement		

CNL Roles

Clinician	Outcomes manager	Team manager
Educator	Client advocate	Life-long learner

CNL Professional Values

Altruism	Human dignity	Social justice
Accountability	Integrity	

CNL Core Competencies

Communication	Health promotion	Disease prevention
Illness and disease management		
Healthcare systems and policy		
Design/management/coordination of care		
Assessment	Risk reduction	Human diversity
Provide and manage care	Member of a profession	

Learning Objectives (continued)

- Outline strategies for secondary prevention and promotion
- Identify and describe tactics that promote wellness
- Discuss the impact of culture on promoting health and preventing disease

Health Promotion and Illness Prevention: Overview

Health promotion is not just a healthcare system or healthcare provider responsibility. Promoting health and preventing disease require collaboration with both governmental and nongovernmental agencies (Interprofessional Education Collaborative Expert Panel, 2011). Governments, businesses, and the healthcare system collaborating and developing partnerships can promote health effectively and efficiently by linking social and health determinates that endorse a health promotion infrastructure focused on the whole individual (Jia, Moriarty, & Kanarek, 2009; Kjellstrom et al., 2007). Political and business leaders (local, national, and international) must recognize that the social determinants of poverty, education, employment, and environment strongly impact physical and mental health (Jia et al., 2009; Kjellstrom, et al., 2007). Acknowledging and correcting the social determinants reduces morbidity and mortality rates for all humanity (Kjellstrom et al., 2007; World Health Organization, 2012b). Clinical nurse leaders (CNLs)—armed with an understanding and historical perspective of health promotion and illness prevention locally, nationally, internationally, and globally—are well equipped to intervene in positive ways.

> Our greatest concern must always rest with disadvantaged and vulnerable groups. These groups are often hidden, living in remote rural areas or shantytowns and having little political voice.
>
> Dr. Margaret Chan, director-general, World Health Organization, 2007

Historical Perspective: International Governments/ United Nations

Governmental involvement in health safety dates back to 1851, when international collaboration began with the first International Sanitary Conference in Paris, France. The focus of the convention was to decrease costly quarantine requirements while simultaneously maintaining health for European nations. The first three conferences focused on cholera. In 1897, the conference addressed preventing the spread of plague. In 1903, the European community established the International Sanitary Convention (World Health Organization, 2012a).

After World War II, the United Nations proposed the development of an international organization to engage in improving the global health and the welfare of all people. The World Health Organization (WHO) was born in 1948; it took on the responsibility of international sanitary conventions and international epidemiological reporting (WHO, 2012a).

For the past 60 years, WHO's involvement in global public health has included persuading nations, private sectors, and communities to examine the possibilities of improving health outcomes on a global scale. WHO's current agenda has a six-point plan to improve health, strategic planning, and collaboration designed to improve health outcomes: (1) promoting socioeconomic development; (2) limiting health epidemics; (3) supporting and strengthening health systems and professionals; (4) applying research, information, and evidence; (5) enhancing and supporting collaboration; and (6) improving competence and quality (WHO, 2012b).

Global Trends in Health

According to Toffler (1970), a futurist and author, the world started shifting to a new paradigm of a "super industrial" society over 40 years ago. He predicted that this new paradigm would have an overwhelming impact on society, causing stress and disorientation (Toffler, 1970). Are Toller's predictions about the 21st century correct?

The United Nations (2011a) predicts that by 2030 the majority of the world population will be living in urban areas. Interestingly, urban growth has increased over the past 50 years due to industry offering economic growth and stability to people living in rural areas (Frieden & Garfield, 2012; United Nations, 2011a). Urbanization has created both benefits and challenges for society. The benefit for many countries is economic growth that, in turn, provides opportunities to improve the health and well-being of residents. In contrast, the impact on urban planning, health, social, and economic development has been challenging, causing a new set of concerns (United Nations, 2011a). According to Gracey (2002), urbanization has created a "New World Syndrome," which is characterized by lifestyle diseases, or noncommunicable diseases (NCDs; Gracey, 2002).

Individuals and families are transitioning from rural to urban living in search of financial, physical, and emotional stability. Transitioning to urban living has brought an alarming rate of overweight, obesity, stress, alcohol, tobacco, and illicit drug use, as well as physical, emotional, and sexual abuse that increases health risk factors (Bloom et al., 2012; Organisation for Economic Co-operation and Development [OECD], 2011; WHO, 2011). These risk factors have taken center stage, threatening the health and welfare of the world (Bloom et al., 2012; United Nations, 2011b; WHO, 2011). These combined risk factors are what created the new world syndrome, with NCDs such as hypertension, diabetes, and cardiovascular disease developing from unhealthy lifestyles (Gracey, 2002).

The health status of the world—in particular NCDs—has become a major concern for global leaders (Bloom et al., 2012; OECD, 2011; WHO, 2011). The OECD has monitored the health of nations related to the delivery of healthcare services and finances using statistical and analytical data for the past 50 years. Participating countries monitoring the health of their nations have identified risk factors influencing the health status of their residents. Responding to global health concerns, the United Nations held a high-level meeting to promote health and prevent a human and economic crisis related to NCDs (see **Figure 19-1**; United Nations, 2011b, 2011c).

According to Ki-moon, secretary-general of the United Nations, private and public sectors developing partnerships can avoid a devastating global health crisis within the next 20 years if nations actively promote health (United Nations, 2012). Global health and economic growth are reliant on protecting and improving the health of humanity through education, clean and safe environments, social supports, and health care (Chao, Carpio, De Geyndt, Shaabdullaeva, & Shi, 2011). In 2011, the OECD reported three trends in global health: a significant increase in life expectancy, a change of health risk factors, and an increase in health expenditures (OECD, 2011).

Health Implications Related to Life Expectancy

According to the OECD (2011), the past 50 years have demonstrated an increase in life expectancy due to education and improvements in environmental regulations and medical technology and treatments. This increase in longevity was observed across the life span for all OECD countries. Countries with a higher national income and larger expenditures in health care have a corresponding positive correlation in life expectancy. Infant mortality rates in these countries have sharply dropped, and people are living up to 80 years of age. Mortality rates due to cardiovascular disease have declined significantly. Men are now living up to 76.7 years and women up to 82.2 years of age (see **Figure 19-2**).

Figure 19-1   A vicious circle: poverty contributes to noncommunicable disease and noncommunicable diseases contribute to poverty.

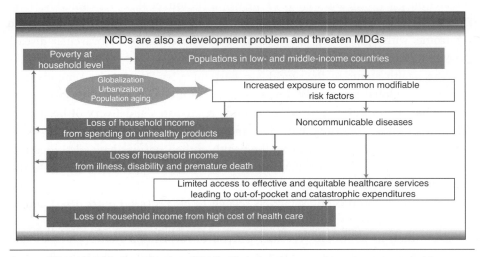

Source: World Health Organization. (2011). *Global status report on noncommunicable diseases 2010.* Geneva, Switzerland: World Health Organization.

The health status of the Japanese has improved the most, with a 15.2-year gain in life expectancy, from birth to 83.0 years of age, since 1960 (OECD, 2011). The United States leads the world in healthcare expenditures, which have increased faster and have become more costly than all other high-income countries since 1970 (Institute of Medicine [IOM], 2002; Majette, 2011; OECD, 2011). However, life expectancy at birth in the United States is 78.2 years, an increase of 8.3 years in longevity; the United States ranks 27 out of the 40 countries participating in the OECD health status report (see **Figure 19-3**).

According to Pham (2012), calculating life expectancy in the United States is more challenging than some other countries due to residents emigrating from a variety of countries with diverse environmental and living conditions. Pham's (2012) 60-year study, from 1946 to 2005, found a difference in life expectancy for both sexes at 84 (male 81.9 years, female, 84.6 years) in contrast to the findings of the Centers for Disease Control and Prevention (CDC), which found a life expectancy for both sexes of 77.8 years (males 77.8 years, female 80.4 years; Pham, 2012). Whatever

Figure 19-2   Total deaths by broad cause group, by WHO region, World Bank income group and by sex, 2008.

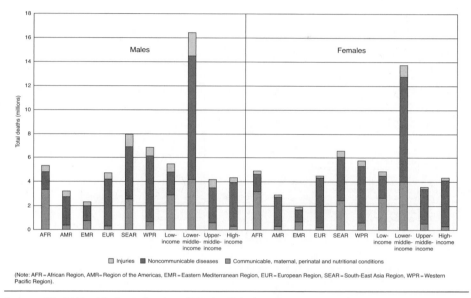

(Note: AFR = African Region, AMR = Region of the Americas, EMR = Eastern Mediterranean Region, EUR = European Region, SEAR = South-East Asia Region, WPR = Western Pacific Region).

Source: World Health Organization. (2011). *Global status report on noncommunicable diseases 2010.* Geneva, Switzerland: World Health Organization.

the case may be in the United States, longevity creates another issue for healthcare services—addressing the needs of an aging population (OECD, 2011). However, the trends of longevity are about to change.

Increase in Health Risks

Looming in the near future is a recognized epidemic of noninfectious diseases or NCDs that includes diabetes, cancer, cardiovascular diseases, respiratory disorders, and mental health issues (Bloom et al., 2012; Marrero, Bloom, & Asashi, 2012). Global longevity may decline by 2030 if risk factors are not addressed. The death toll from NCDs is estimated to increase to five times the death toll of communicable disease, influencing quality of life and creating a global economic crisis (Bloom et al., 2012; Marrero et al., 2012).

Figure 19-3   Life expectancy at birth, 2009 (or nearest year available), and years gained since 1960.

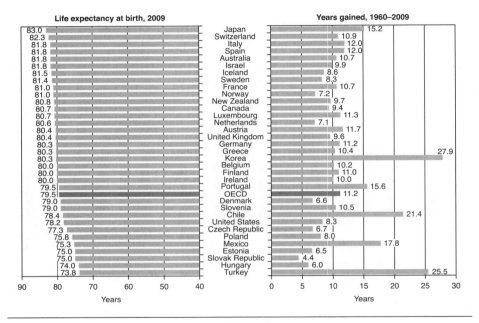

Source: OECD, Health at a Glance 2011: OECD Indicators.

Increase in Health Expenditures

In 2010, NCDs accounted for a 75% loss in global gross domestic product (GDP), equal to 63 trillion U.S. dollars. NCDs are still in the budding stage, yet they have the potential to decrease the supply of labor and capital growth globally (Bloom et al., 2012). An economist conference held in Geneva, Switzerland reported the banking crisis will seem insignificant in comparison to the global cost of NCDs (Tan, 2012). Developing countries will be the most significantly debilitated by the lack a healthy workforce (Bloom et al., 2012). It is predicted that the cost of NCDs and mental health issues will create a macroeconomic output loss over the next two decades of nearly 47 trillion U.S. dollars (Bloom et al., 2012; Tan, 2012). Bloom and colleagues (2012) calculated the global economic burden of NCDs and mental health using three diverse economic methods: (1) cost of illness, (2) global economic impact, and

(3) the value of statistical life. However, investments in health promotion activities would cost less than 0.40 per day in U.S. dollars (Bloom et al., 2012).

Currently, the United States spends more on money on health care than any other nation (Kapustin, 2010; Majette, 2011). The cost of heart disease and stroke were $448 billion and cancer $89 billion, respectively, in 2008, and management of chronic diseases uses 75% of the $2 trillion spent on annual medical expenditures (Kapustin, 2010). However, if the United States begins to make healthy lifestyle changes, $1.6 trillion could be saved. Presently, the United States spends only 5% of allocated healthcare costs for health promotion; 95% is spent on chronic diseases (Kapustin, 2010).

Another increase related to healthcare costs is employer-sponsored health insurance. Premiums have varied over the years, with a progressive increase in cost for employers and employees. The variation is due to the number of employees, geographical location, benefits, and sharing of costs with single or married employees. From 2002 to 2012, employers paid a 97% increase in healthcare premiums ($15,745 compared to $8,003 in 2002). Employee contributions increased 102% ($4,316, in contrast to $2,137 in 2002) (Claxton, Rae, Panchal, Damico, & Lundy, 2012). Over 50 years, the United States' healthcare costs increased from 5.2% of the GDP to 17.9% in 2010. The increasing costs of insurance and health care in the United States can be attributed to healthcare technology, an older population, changes in health status and chronic diseases, and wasteful spending that includes overtreating patients (Henry J. Kaiser Family Foundation, 2012).

Understanding the Larger Perspective

For the past 30 years, the *Healthy People* initiative, managed by the U.S. Department of Health and Human Services and the Office of Disease Prevention and Health Promotion, has encouraged a national agenda to improve the health status of U.S. residents. *Healthy People* strives to improve the health of the nation, as well as to educate and support individuals in choosing healthy lifestyles. According to *Healthy People 2020*, applying the concepts of social and physical environments, health services, individual behaviors, and biology and genetics will improve national health outcomes (U.S. Department of Health and Human Services, 2012a).

Healthy People 2020 measures national health improvement by 12 leading health indicator topics:

1. Access to health services
2. Clinical preventive services
3. Environmental quality
4. Injury and violence
5. Maternal, infant, and child health
6. Mental health
7. Nutrition, physical activity, and obesity
8. Oral health
9. Reproductive and sexual health
10. Social determinants
11. Substance abuse
12. Tobacco

Each topic has one or more measureable outcomes. Moreover, *Healthy People 2020* provides individuals and communities with evidence-based strategies for implementing health promotion and prevention (U.S. Department of Health and Human Services, 2012a).

Protecting the health of U.S. citizens began in the formative years of the country's independence. In 1798, the federal government enacted a bill to provide health care to sick and disabled sailors. A marine hospital network was established, and over the next hundred years it evolved into the Public Health Department. In 1887, the federal government began researching disease, which resulted in the National Institutes of Health. In 1902, the United States established the International Sanitary Bureau in Washington, D.C. (World Health Organization, 2012a).

Throughout the 20th century, the federal government has implemented a variety of agencies designed to protect and provide services for all residents regardless of race, creed, age, or gender in the United States (U.S. Department of Health & Human Services, 2012b). The health of the nation has improved because epidemiologists stepped into unknown paths to find the causes of infectious diseases and discovered methods to prevent reoccurrences of disabling and deadly infections (Frieden & Garfield, 2012). Health has improved significantly in the United States during the 20th century (Altman, 2012). New and improved treatments and therapies have reduced mortality and disability and improved the quality of life for people suffering from cancer or heart disease (DeVol & Bedroussian, 2007).

The lead agency for public health in the United States is the CDC in Atlanta, Georgia. The CDC's role is to provide leadership in public health that protects the health of a diverse population and to educate healthcare professionals to promote healthy lifestyles (Communicable Disease Center, 2012). Public health in the United States has made great strides over the past 100 years with reducing preventable injuries, illness, and premature deaths and increasing life expectancy throughout the country (IOM, 2002; OECD, 2011).

In recent years, the U.S. healthcare system has come under great scrutiny, with the high cost of health care and patients being harmed by the system that is designed to help and protect them (Altman, 2012; IOM, 1999). Current reports on the public health system indicate that it lacks adequate funding, and there is inadequate collaboration within communities to support public health (Majette, 2011). Recommendations to improve public health have been presented to Congress, including redesigning local public health departments so that they become proactive and lead their communities in promoting and protecting health, as well as develop collaborations within the community to promote healthy lifestyles (IOM, 2002).

Public health experts testified to Congress about the significant impact of creating a framework based on health promotion, prevention, and wellness in the U.S. healthcare system and improving public health. The national debate resulted in Congress supporting the recommendations for a healthcare act that became the Patient Protection and Affordable Care Act (PPACA). President Obama signed this legislation into law on March 23, 2011 (Majette, 2011). Now the national agenda in health care requires a focus on health promotion and wellness, as opposed to a system focused on sick care or cure. Implementing a new healthcare agenda will require partnerships with public and private sectors working together to overhaul the healthcare system (National Prevention Council, 2011).

The CDC will lead health promotion, prevention, and preparedness efforts in the United States. The public health system has developed a new framework to strengthen public health infrastructure, develop partnerships, improve communication, use evidence to support actions, develop accountability systems, and address multiple determinants of health for communities (IOM, 2002). To become effective and efficient, the CDC has identified five strategic areas for improvement:

1. Supporting state and local health departments
2. Improving global health
3. Implementing measures to decrease leading causes of death
4. Strengthening surveillance and epidemiology
5. Reforming health policies (Communicable Disease Center, 2012).

The Business of Health Care

In the early 1900s, employers began contributing to the health of their employees with employer-sponsored insurance for employees and their families (Heinen & Darling, 2009). Offering health insurance to job seekers made employers more inclined to hire and maintain a workforce that was loyal to the company. Several historical events contributed to this relationship with employers, the new healthcare system, and employees (McCarter, Daly, & Cooper, 2010). Knowing the historical perspective of wellness and prevention better positions the CNL to play a significant role in making the United States a healthier nation.

The Great Depression limited people seeking health care, which caused a near collapse of the still growing and developing healthcare system. In addition, World War II created a demand for a new and healthy workforce, with many young men out of the country. Employers were not able to offer increased wages; however, they could offer free healthcare insurance to employees as an incentive to work in their business or industry, and this increased the workforce (McCarter et al., 2010). Business and industry became the security blanket for an infant healthcare system (Heinen & Darling, 2009; Ricci & Chee, 2005).

Business and industry have a stake in keeping employees healthy. Without a healthy workforce, the country's economic base would falter. In 1970, the federal government implemented the Occupational Safety and Health Administration (OSHA) to assist employers and employees with education, training, and guidance to maintain a safe work environment. Employers and employees have rights and responsibilities to identify risks or hazards to prevent being harmed at work. OHSA's standards guide employers to promote a safe workplace, provide training to employees to keep them safe from harm, and provide an avenue to report safety concerns while upholding the confidentiality of individuals filing reports (U.S. Department of Labor, 2011).

The business sector, in recent years, has become more concerned with employee absenteeism as it relates to lower productively (Pelletier, 2011). A healthy workforce increases the GDP and decreases the use of disease management programs. As a result, many employers are incorporating worksite healthcare clinics. Pelletier's (2011) analysis reports that the business sector would be well advised to develop worksite clinics that focus on health promotion and disease management. A worksite clinic designed to meet the needs of employees' health concerns decreases absenteeism, improves the health of employees, and is cost effective (Goetzel, Roemer, Liss-Levinson, & Samoly, 2008; Pelletier, 2011). Depending on the health promotion programming, employers are reporting a positive return on their investments, dollar for dollar, from \$1.40 to \$4.70 during a 3-year time frame (Goetzel et al., 2008). CNLs can play a leading role through health coaching, assisting with transitional care strategies to improve the nation's health.

The CNL's Role in the Evolving Healthcare System

Health care has evolved since the 1900s, when it was a cash or barter system for services provided by physicians, to the current system, which is supported by employer insurance packages, federally funded programs for older and chronically disabled Americans, or private insurance (McCarter et al., 2010). Today, the healthcare system is complex, with many services provided, plus internal and external oversight, communication, safety and environmental concerns, and behavioral choices of professionals and patients. Professional boundaries are challenged, mental models held by providers may not be shared, and systems within systems can create misunderstandings that build tension and can result in a lack of predictability (Plsek & Greenhalgh, 2001).

A major challenge to CNLs' leadership in health care is contending with the complexity of healthcare organizations while attempting to improve the quality of health care. Improving the healthcare system requires a multidimensional, interprofessional, interagency approach with the goal of eliminating gaps or silos in health care by leaders at the macro-, meso-, and microsystems levels (Dartmouth Institute for Health Policy & Clinical Practice, 2010). CNLs are educated and socialized to address these gaps and silos, bringing teams together through lateral integration.

The significance of CNL collaboration is the exchange of information and knowledge while building partnerships to reduce redundancies of services and developing or refining programs to avoid gaps or barriers to healthcare services (Harris, Provan, Johnson, & Leischow, 2012). With the CNL's exchange of information and knowledge, services provided to patients will be centered on their needs in a timely, effective, efficient, and safe approach (Institute for Healthcare Improvement, 2000; IOM, 2001).

Meeting the IOM's aims is not enough to improve the health of a nation, however. Healthcare leaders must analyze and link social and health determinants to reduce preventable diseases such as obesity, diabetes, and heart disease (DeVol & Bedroussian, 2007; Majette, 2011). According to Plesk and Greenhalgh (2001), the zone of simplicity is using reductionist thinking—discover the problem and fix it. Alternatively, the edge of chaos is a lack of leadership, where agreement or action is not clear. On the other hand, the zone of complexity allows multiple options to be explored that help with problem solving. The zone of complexity is deep thinking, challenging ideas, asking difficult questions, searching for solutions, and coming to a group consensus for a solution that requires continuous performance improvement (Plsek & Greenhalgh, 2001). CNLs as advanced generalists have a keen understanding of microsystem complexity and change, and they can lead efforts to reduce disparities.

Globally health care has reduced premature mortality, with an increase in life expectancy over the past 50 years (OECD, 2011; WHO, 2009). Despite this, the IOM's (1999) report card on health care in the United States indicates that as many as 98,000 people die yearly due to medical errors in health care. Medical errors are costing hospitals $17 to $29 billion annually (IOM, 2001). The high cost of health care in the United States is preventable; leaders need to clearly define roles and responsibilities and collaborate and communicate at the micro-, meso-, and macrosystem levels (Campbell, 2009; Martin, Lloyd, & Nolan, 2007). The delivery of health care across all settings must focus on developing leadership, implementing evidenced-based research in clinical practice, patient safety, and establishing national and agency performance indicators with measurable outcomes (IOM, 2001). CNLs are pivotal to these efforts.

The CNL's Role in Increasing Patient Engagement and Partnerships

Nurse–patient partnerships share leadership, with each member taking responsibility for his or her role (Cribb & Entwistle, 2011). First, the CNL's role is to hear the patient's perspective and share the health-related concerns, risks, and treatment options for the patient (Bensing et al., 2011; Cribb & Entwistle, 2011; Rollnick, Miller, & Butler, 2008). The CNL who listens to the patient develops a therapeutic relationship with a person who is a member of a family that lives and interacts in a community and who is a part of society (Cribb & Entwistle, 2011).

CNLs play a key and critical role on the healthcare team. In the delivery of health care, nurses spend more time with patients than other health team members. Quality patient care can be provided when CNLs collaborate, educate, and apply theory and evidenced-based research in clinical practice (IOM, 2003). However, communication and education are currently insufficient, with issues related to patient safety, hospital readmission rates, and medication education reported by regulatory agencies such as The Joint Commission and the Centers for Medicare and Medicaid Services (Seidl, 2011). The standards of professional nursing performance view CNLs as educators who collaborate and advocate for quality and ethical care based upon research while using resources appropriately (American Nurses Association, 2004).

Jallinoja and colleagues (2007) reported that nurses and physicians think patients should accept responsibility for health behaviors. The nurses in this study reported that their primary duies were to educate, motivate, and support patients in changing health behaviors. However, 50% of the nurses reported that other nursing responsibilities did not allow them to intervene with patients living risky lifestyles. Interestingly, nurses with less experience were more likely to provide education about healthy living (Jallinoja et al., 2007).

The CNL's Role in Shared Responsibility and Accountability

CNLs, comprehending the complexity of health care, need to collaborate to link the healthcare system with governmental and nongovernmental agencies that will focus on promoting and preventing disease (CDC, 2009; DeVol & Bedroussian, 2007; Martin et al., 2007; Suhrcke, Nugent, Stuckler, & Rocco, 2006; United Nations, 2011b; WHO, 2008, 2011). A healthy community shares responsibility for making behavioral changes that will be sustainable for future generations. Public and private entities working collaboratively must interconnect activities promoting healthy living in school systems, business, advertising, the community, and public and private healthcare systems, and engage civic leaders in planning a supportive environment. Community and individual involvement can help prevent physical and emotional suffering throughout the life span for low- or high-income communities (CDC, 2009; Gostin, 2012; United Nations, 2011c; WHO, 2008).

The CNL's Role in Changing Health Risk Factors

Demographic changes from rural to urban living have increased from 14% to greater than 50% since the 1900s (Allender, Foster, Hutchinson, & Arambepola, 2008). According to Gracey (2002), two-thirds of the world's population will live in metropolitan areas by 2030. Urbanization demonstrates profound effects on lifestyles and diseases (Allender et al., 2008). Because of the demographic shift to urbanization, morbidity and mortality are increasing (Allender et al., 2008; Gracey, 2002). Governments and the healthcare system are not adequately planning for the changing demographics of communities (Gracey, 2002). Understanding changes in health risk factors provides the CNL with information to better inform and improve healthcare outcomes.

People transitioning to metropolitan living experience dietary changes, poor nutrition, limited exercise, overcrowding, and stress, and they often lack a social support network. The new city dwellers' lifestyle changes result in overweight, obesity, social isolation, and depression. Moreover, many of the new residents lack coping skills to contend with diversity or contrary social or environmental systems. Lacking coping skills to live in the new social environment can result in behavioral changes, such as abuse (physical, sexual, and emotional) or using tobacco, alcohol, or street drugs to cope or fit in with the new culture (DeVol & Bedroussian, 2007; Gracey, 2002; OECD, 2011; WHO, 2011).

In 2008, 36 million people died from NCDs (OECD, 2011; WHO, 2011). Countries not promoting health and wellness can expect that an estimated 7.5 million will die by 2020 just from tobacco use, with 71% of the smokers' deaths related to lung cancer, 42% to chronic respiratory disease, and 10% to cardiovascular disease. In 2030, an estimated 82% incidence of cancer will occur; moreover, the increase in obesity creates new risk factors for NCDs such as cardiovascular disease, cancer, diabetes, and chronic lung disease, which are now the leading causes of global death (Clarke, 2010).

The leading cause of death and disability in the United States is chronic diseases. Understanding that chronic diseases affect 1 in 10 American activities of daily living, the CNL is armed to better plan and intervene to prevent further deterioration. Between 2007 and 2008, over 33.8% of Americans were obese, 23.6 million had diabetes, 26 million had chronic kidney disease, 53.7% of men and 55.8% of women between 55 and 64 years of age had hypertension, and in 2009, 292,540 men and 269,800 women died from cancer (Clarke, 2010). In 2006, deaths from heart disease and stroke numbered 768,755, cancer 559,888, chronic lower respiratory diseases 124,583, and diabetes 72,449 (Kapustin, 2010). In 2029, the youngest of the baby boomers will be 65 years of age. If the current trend with chronic disease continues, the U.S. healthcare system will not be not be able to meet demands (Kapustin, 2010; Tan, 2012).

Moreover, a U.S. national survey of 153,000 people discovered that only 3% of the U.S. population maintains a healthy lifestyle, using four key characteristics such eating fruits, eating vegetables, health, weight, exercising, and not smoking. On the other hand, 20% of adolescents and 43 million U.S. adults smoke tobacco (Clarke, 2010). The morbidity and mortality rates due to NCDs can be significantly reduced with health education and promotion and counseling in primary care (OECD, 2011). CNLs, through health education and counseling, focus on behavioral risk factors by increasing physical activity, decreasing use of alcohol and tobacco, and stressing eating a healthy diet to help reduce the morbidity and mortality rates due to NCDs.

The CNL's Role in Health Promotion/ Primary Prevention

Global, national, and local leaders in government, the business sector, and health care must collaborate at the macro-, meso-, and microsystem levels to reduce NCD risk factors (CDC, 2009; United Nations, 2011b; WHO, 2011). Organizational leaders must change mental models to a culture that operates within a conceptual framework of performance improvement linked to a strategic plan that integrates health promotion policies across the spectrum (CDC, 2009; Martin et al., 2007; Smith, 2001; United Nations, 2011b).

Health promotion, or primary prevention, is an upstream activity intended to prevent people from putting themselves or others at risk of harm or injury (Cypress, 2004; Institute for Work & Health, 2006). Promoting health and wellness requires a multidimensional approach and shared responsibility, with government and nongovernment sectors supporting mental and physical health (WHO, 2009). Social determinants must be equalized among communities to include healthy food, safe housing, education, employment, safe and healthy environments, and social justice that protects everyone (Perdue, Richards, Acree, & Stroup, 2005).

The global epidemic of NCDs, the new world syndrome, is preventable; however, leaders must understand that globalization and urbanization are contributing to premature death due to processed foods that are high in saturated and trans fats, salt, and refined sugars (Bloom et al., 2012; CDC, 2009; United Nations, 2011b). Governmental and nongovernmental agencies need to develop policies promoting healthier foods. For example, limiting sugars in foods and beverages can help reduce obesity. Incentives could be offered to supermarkets to locate in underserved areas, food chains could be encouraged to offer healthier foods and drinks in underserved areas, local farmers could be encouraged to sell their products in farmers' markets, and strategies could be provided for preparing and serving healthy portion-controlled meals (CDC, 2009). CNLs have the skill set to impact healthier outcomes.

CNLs as community leaders can help create policies that provide a safe environment and increase outdoor activities, such as suggesting bike lanes or paved sidewalks for children to walk or bicycle to and from school. They can advocate that schools increase physical education and extracurricular physical activities to reduce obesity, and that families have increased access to public recreation and transportation, strategically located in neighborhoods to promote physical activities (CDC, 2009).

CNLs working with public health departments can address responsibilities by providing immunizations for infectious disease and educating people to seek regular health exams and screenings for illnesses. CNLs can address education needs that are comprehensive and provided by schools, businesses, governmental agencies, and within the healthcare system. CNLs work with individuals and communities that need to understand and apply the basics of nutrition and exercise; the risks of alcohol, drugs, tobacco, and firearms; plus home, highway, and workplace safety and dangers. Funding research and education regarding healthy lifestyles is cost effective, as compared to the cost of morbidity or mortality (Pelletier, 2011). CNLs can engage in community planning or redesign, for example adding sidewalks to encourage walking, with bus stops located within neighborhoods for easy access. Parks can be located within walking distance of neighborhoods, offering activities that encourage physical activity and socialization (CDC, 2009).

The CNL's Role in Disease/Secondary Prevention

Individuals or communities that have fallen into the river are identified with risk traits or diagnosed with a disease or disorder. The CNL has the goal of providing early interventions for patients that have the possibility of limiting or preventing long-term suffering and disability (Institute for Work & Health, 2006). With the new world syndrome threatening global health, health care will be overwhelmed attempting to rescue people suffering from preventable diseases (CDC, 2009; Clarke, 2010; DeVol & Bedroussian, 2007; United Nations, 2011b). For example, people who are overweight or obese are at risk for heart disease or diabetes. Dietary changes, exercise, and scheduling regular exams and health screenings could prevent a decline in health status.

The CNL's Role in Rehabilitation/Tertiary Prevention

CNLs understand that downstream rescuing is more complicated to manage and prevent further mental and physical deterioration. Rehabilitation is more costly with human suffering. The cost of health care, loss of healthy workforce, and GDP creates a loss for the United States and the global economy (Bloom et al., 2012). Interventions for NCDs or chronic disease must be specialized to prevent further physical or mental deterioration (Institute for Work & Health, 2006).

The CNL's Role in Promoting Health

The role of the CNL is providing direct patient care in a microsystem that may be located in any setting within the continuum of care. The CNL role was developed to lead, guide, and direct other nursing staff to provide patient-centered care based upon best practice guidelines, providing care that has measurable outcomes while reducing healthcare disparities and improving health literacy (American Association of Colleges of Nursing [AACN], 2007). The CNL's praxis must include emotional intelligence, attitude, and good communication skills to develop the CNL role within a microsystem (Bradberry & Greaves, 2009).

The praxis of the CNL role is underpinned by a conceptual and theoretical framework (Cody, 2013). Patient-centered care is a vital component as an underpinning in nursing praxis (Frampton et al., 2008; IOM, 2003). Nurses and other healthcare professionals, valuing the diversity of humanity, develop collaborative relationships with patients that honor and respect individuals as the experts on their body (Cribb & Entwistle, 2011). CNLs and other nurses promoting health, preventing disease, or rehabilitating patients must understand the patient's perspective of health, the process of behavioral change, and motivational approaches to empower patients to change risky health behaviors.

Patient-Centered Care

In health care, a patient is an individual, a family, a community, a nation, or the world. Keeping the patient at the center of all care activities, including health promotion activities, is key to successful behavioral change (Frampton et al., 2008). Providers must have a fundamental knowledge and understand the world of diversity (ethnic, cultural, and spiritual background) patients come from and the environments they live in (Leininger & McFarland, 2006). All patients seeking health care bring a lived experience, hopes, and desires (Collins & Selina, 2010). Healthcare professionals hearing the patient's perspective build professional relationships. The respect, trust, and confidence between the healthcare professional and the patient develop a team, allowing the patient expert and the healthcare expert to share in decision making (Cribb & Entwistle, 2011).

Assessing the patient's needs using a patient-centered approach provides insight into readiness, willingness, and motivation to change health behaviors (DiClemente, 2007; Frampton et al., 2008; Rubak, Sanboek, Lauritzen, & Christensen, 2005). Healthcare teams listening and understanding the perceptions of the patient and collaborating to identify the patient's concerns, goals, and desired outcomes empowers patients to make behavioral changes (Frampton et al., 2008). Promoting health or preventing disease risks fails when the patient is not considered the expert on his or her body and lifestyle (Seear, 2009). Self-care and adherence to treatment or therapy are more likely when the patient expert and provider expert develop a collaborative partnership (Kaye et al., 2010; Seear, 2009).

Professional relationships can become conflicted between the nurse and the patient when the paternalistic approach, the "notably scientific expert" (Seear, 2009), attempts to correct noncompliance. The scientific expert attempts to correct the patient in a logical and objective manner, expecting the patient to respond positively to the directive (Cribb & Entwistle, 2011). However, the patient may view the interaction as demeaning and a barrier to health care. As a result, many nurses and healthcare providers will identify the avoidant patient behaviors as noncompliance with medical treatment (Seear, 2009).

Motivational Interviewing

A trusting nurse–patient relationship begins with the nurse listening to the patient's health concerns (Cribb & Entwistle, 2011; Rollnick et al., 2008). CNLs engage in communication and patient engagement to best meet patients' needs. Motivational interviewing (MI) is a nonconfrontational communication approach that is patient-centered care. MI is a well-established, evidence-based communication approach designed to help providers understand the patient's perspective and empower the patient to move toward a healthier lifestyle (Rubak et al., 2005).

Three communication styles are used with patients depending on the situation: (1) directing, (2) guiding, or (3) following the patient. Using the guidance style of communication means always taking more time to ask, listen, and inform patients. MI has basic guidelines that are easy to follow. The primary "RULE" is to *r*esist giving advice, *u*nderstand the patient's perspective, *l*isten for the DARN (*d*esire, *a*bility, *r*eason, or *n*eed) words and *e*licit feedback (Rollnick et al., 2008). Providers facilitate a supportive environment in order to help patients ponder the risks and benefits of behavioral change. Creating this milieu can happen only after you have asked permission from the patient to share your concern regarding his or her health (Rollnick et al., 2008; Rubak et al., 2005). Depending on the circumstances, acknowledgement of pain, discomfort, or coping with the issue is addressed, followed by the concerns for health and safety. Hearing the DARN words is an indicator for the patient's readiness to change.

The Transtheoretical Model of Change

Behavioral change is a complex process of thinking about the importance, willingness, and confidence to change (Nidecker, DiClemente, Bennett, & Bellack, 2008). The transtheoretical model of change guides providers to identify the stages of change as precontemplation, contemplation, action, and maintenance (DiClemente, 2007; Prochaska, 2008). Changing risky health behaviors is a challenge for patients, as well as for the providers attempting to provide healthcare services (Chase, Osann, Sepina, Wenzel, & Tewari, 2012; Seear, 2009).

Patients need time and words of encouragement to take steps toward changing behaviors (Rollnick et al., 2008). For example, a patient in the precontemplation stage is unaware of a need to change. The best intervention at this stage is for the nurse to share his or her health concerns and information about risk factors, and allow the patient time to think about this. Applying the correct intervention for the stage of change based on the patient's needs is more likely to help him or her move to successful behavioral change. Even with a relapse in behavior change, patients make progressive improvements with longer lasting maintenance stages.

Readiness to Change Ruler

A "readiness to change ruler" is a valid and reliable patient-centered approach to help healthcare providers understand patients' thinking about behavioral change (Center on Alcoholism Substance Abuse and Addictions [CASAA], 1995). The readiness ruler identifies the willingness, importance, and confidence to change

Case Study

Nurse-Managed Clinic

Our Neighborhood Healthcare Clinic (ONHC) operates under the umbrella of the University of South Alabama's College of Nursing. The primary clinic is located in the USA Medical Center in Mobile, Alabama. ONHC, located at 15 Place, is one of three outreach centers and is located within a day shelter for homeless people.

The purpose of opening the doors for ONHC at 15 Place was to promote health and wellness for homeless people. Health education, guidance, and counseling are followed with referrals to agencies that provide care for the homeless population. Developing relationships and linking community stakeholders is intended to improve the health status of the community's most vulnerable population and is vital to reduce gaps and barriers to health care.

Theoretical Underpinnings

The transtheoretical model was used to identify the individuals' readiness to change. Nurses used the strategy of motivational interviewing, a powerful communication approach that is patient centered, respectful, and encourages the individual to think about making decisions to exchange poor health habits with healthier habits.

Collaboration

The clinical team included a doctor of nursing practice (DNP), a biomedical librarian, and a premedical student. A CNL student was also involved, completing his CNL immersion experience at the center. In addition to collaborating with the homeless people and 15 Place, OHNC has developed collaborative relationships with community agencies and within the USA system that includes the Department of Social Work and Allied Health. The faculty at USA is placing physician's assistants, social workers, and emergency medical technician students in the clinic to learn the value of providing care to a vulnerable and disenfranchised population.

Health Promotion Clinic

Patients were screened for the premetabolic syndrome. Individuals identified with the metabolic syndrome, heart disease, or diabetes were encouraged to

Case Study (continued)

seek health care from a clinic providing services for the homeless. Education was linked in with health screening. The goal was to empower individuals to learn to manage self-care. Patients were encouraged to return to the clinic for guidance and support to self-manage their health care.

Conclusion

Healthy individuals and communities are a result of upstream efforts by governmental and nongovernmental sectors linking social and health determinants to benefit all residents. Healthy communities are working together to keep the environment clean and safe for everyone to enjoy outdoor physical activities. Employers and employees in healthy communities have a sound financial foundation due to a healthy workforce. When individuals or families are at risk, communities offer support and guidance to help them regain the ability to self-manage daily living. Social and health determinants are addressed simultaneously because communities understand health promotion is the right thing to do; furthermore, it is cost effective compared to attempting to cure a problem.

health behaviors. Assessments help the nurse understand the patient's perspective and guide the provider to empower the patient, as well as to apply the correct intervention with the stage of change.

Promoting healthy behaviors with some patients may result in avoidance issues due to sociodemographic factors, personal or provider issues, and administrative barriers (Byrne, 2008). Providers who focus on the patient's needs and concerns are more likely to influence behavioral change. Interventions for the patient must be designed based on the patient's stage of thinking about change. Implementing an intervention prematurely (before the patient is in the appropriate stage) can abort the change process or cause a delay in behavioral improvements (Armitage, 2009; DiClemente, 2007; Miller & Rose, 2009; Prochaska, 2008; Rubak et al., 2005).

Providers sharing concerns, risks, or treatment options must communicate in terms that the patient is able to obtain, process, and understand. The Joint Commission's national patient safety goals require health information be presented verbally and in writing at a level that is understandable to the patient (Stonecypher,

2009). Jointly the team explores options that may challenge each other. Challenging dialogue regarding options or negotiating should happen only when the patient is comfortable with that approach (Cribb & Entwistle, 2011). The overarching goal for healthcare teams is empowering the patient to self-manage his or her health care based on the level of readiness to change and to choose the best option for a healthy outcome (Barrie, 2011; Prochaska, 2008).

Summary

- Promoting health and preventing disease require collaboration with governmental and nongovernmental agencies.
- WHO's current agenda has established a six-point plan to improve health, strategic planning, and collaboration designed to improve health outcomes: (1) promoting socioeconomic development; (2) limiting health epidemics; (3) supporting and strengthening health systems and professionals; (4) applying research, information, and evidence; (5) enhancing and supporting collaboration; and (6) improving competence and quality.
- The increased cost of insurance and health care in the United States can be attributed to healthcare technology, an older population, changes in health status and chronic diseases, and wasteful spending that includes overtreating patients.
- CNLs can engage in community planning or redesign and advocate improvements such as the inclusion of sidewalks to encourage walking and parks located within walking distance of neighborhoods that offer activities that encourage physical activity and socialization.
- The CNL's praxis must include emotional intelligence, attitude, and good communication skills to develop the CNL role within a microsystem.
- Behavioral change is a complex process of thinking about the importance, willingness, and confidence to change.
- Promoting healthy behaviors with some patients may result in avoidance issues due to sociodemographic factors, personal or provider issues, and administrative barriers.
- The overarching goal for healthcare teams is empowering the patient to self-manage his or her health care based on the level of readiness to change and to choose the best option for a healthy outcome.

www **Reflection Questions**
© Arenacreative/Dreamstime.com

1. According to Gracy (2002), urbanization has created the new world syndrome characterized by lifestyle diseases or NCDs. What lifestyle diseases impact your clinical microsystem?
2. The increased cost of insurance and health care in the United States can be attributed to healthcare technology, an older population, changes in health status and chronic diseases, and wasteful spending that includes overtreating patients (Henry J. Kaiser Family Foundation, 2012). What are the implications for your clinical microsystem?

www **Learning Activities**
© Arenacreative/Dreamstime.com

1. Consider motivational interviewing and readiness for change. Using tools from these theoretical underpinnings, describe improvement strategies.
2. Promoting healthy behaviors with some patients may result in avoidance issues due to sociodemographic factors, personal or provider issues, and administrative barriers (Byrne, 2008). Give examples from your clinical microsystem.

References

Allender, S., Foster, C., Hutchinson, L., & Arambepola, C. (2008). Quantification of urbanization in relation to chronic disease in developing countries: A systematic review. *Journal of Urban Health: Bulletin of the New York Academy of Medicine, 85*(6). doi: 10.1007/s11524-008-9325-4

Altman, D. (2012). Pulling it together: Reflections on this year's four percent premium increase. *The Henry Kaiser Family Foundation.* Retrieved from http://www.kff.org/pullingittogether/altman_premium_increase.cfm

American Association of Colleges of Nursing. (2007). *White paper on the education and role of the clinical nurse leader.* Washington, DC: Author, pp. 6–10. Retrieved from http://www.aacn.nche.edu/Publications/WhitePapers/ClinicalNurseLeader07.pdf

American Nurses Association (Ed.). (2004). *Nursing: Scope and standards of practice.* Silver Spring, MD: nursesbooks.org.

Armitage, C. J. (2009). Is there utility in the transtheoretical model? *British Journal of Health Psychology, 14*(Pt 2), 195–210.

Barrie, J. (2011). Patient empowerment and choice in chronic pain management. *Nursing Standard, 25*(31), 38–41.

Bensing, J. M., Deveugele, M., Moretti, F., Fletcher, I., van Vliet, L., Van Bogaert, M., & Rimondini, M. (2011). How to make the medical consultation more successful from a patient's perspective? Tips for doctors and patients from lay people in the United Kingdom, Italy, Belgium and the Netherlands. *Patient Education & Counseling, 84*(3), 287–293. doi: 10.1016/j.pec.2011.06.008

Bloom, D. E., Cafiero, E. T., Jane-Llopis, E., Abrahams-Gessel, S., Bloom, L. R., Fathima, S., ... Weinstein, C. (2012). *The global economic burden of noncommunicable diseases. Working paper series*. Geneva, Switzerland: World Economic Forum and Harvard School of Public Health.

Bradberry, T., & Greaves, J. (2009). *Emotional Intelligenace 2.0*. San Diego, CA: TalentSmart.

Byrne, S. K. (2008). Healthcare avoidance: A critical review. *Holistic Nursing Practice, 22*(5), 280–292.

Campbell, R. J. (2009). Creating a winning organizational culture. *Health Care Manager, 28*(4), 328–343.

Center on Alcoholism Substance Abuse and Addictions, University of New Mexico. (1995). Readiness ruler. Retrieved from http://casaa.unm.edu/inst/Readiness%20Ruler.pdf

Centers for Disease Control and Prevention. (2009). *CDC's recommended community strategies and measurements to prevent obesity in the United States*. Atlanta, GA: Author. Available at http://www.cdc.gov/nccdphp/dnpao/publications/index.html

Chao, S., Carpio, C., De Geyndt, W., Shaabdullaeva, Z., & Shi, Y. (2011). *The growing burden of non-comunicable disease in the eastern Caribbean: Human development unit Latin American and the Caribbean region*. Washington DC: The World Bank.

Chase, D. M., Osann, K., Sepina, N., Wenzel, L., & Tewari, K. S. (2012). The challenge of follow-up in a low-income colposcopy clinic: Characteristics associated with noncompliance in high-risk populations. *Journal of Lower Genital Tract Disease, 16*(4), 345–351. doi: 10.1097/LGT.0b013e318249640f

Clarke, J. L. (2010). Preventive medicine: A ready solution for a health care system in crisis. *Population Health Management, 13*(2). doi: 10.1089/pop.2010.1382

Claxton, G., Rae, M., Panchal, N., Damico, A., & Lundy, J. (2012). *Employer health benefits 2012 annual survey*. Chicago, IL: Henry J. Kaiser Family Foundation, Health Research & Education Trust, NORC at the University of Chicago. Retrieved from http://ehbs.kff.org/pdf/2012/8345.pdf

Cody, W. K. (Ed.). (2013). *Philosophical and theoretical perspectives for advanced nursing practice* (5th ed.). Burlington, MA: Jones & Bartlett Learning.

Collins, J., & Selina, H. (Eds.). (2010). *Introducing Heidegger: A graphic guide*. London, UK: Tatem Books, Ltd.

Communicable Disease Center. (2012). About CDC: Our story. Retreived from http://www.cdc.gov/about/history/ourstory.htm

Cribb, A., & Entwistle, V. A. (2011). Shared decision making: Trade-offs between narrower and broader conceptions. *Health Expectations, 14*(2), 210–219. doi: 10.1111/j.1369-7625.2011.00694.x

Cypress, M. (2004). Looking upstream. *Diabetes Spectrum, 17*(4), 249–253. doi: 10.2337/diaspect.17.4.249

Dartmouth Institute for Health Policy & Clinical Practice. (2010). Microsystems at a glance. In M. M. Godfrey (Ed.), *Developed by microsystem members for microsystem members.* Retrieved from www.clinicalmicrosystem.org

DeVol, R., & Bedroussian, A. (2007). *An unhealthy America: The economic burden of chronic disease—Charting a new course to save lives and increase productivity and economic growth.* Santa Monica, CA: Milken Institute.

DiClemente, C. C. (2007). The transtheoretical model of intentional behavior change. *Drugs & Alcohol Today, 7*(1), 29–33.

Frampton, S., Guastello, S., Brady, C., Hale, M., Horowitz, S., & Smith, S. B. S. (2008). *Patient-centered care improvement guide.* Derbee, CT: Planetree, Inc. and Picker Institute, Inc.

Frieden, T. R., & Garfield, R. M. (2012). The cover. *Journal American Medical Association, 307*(19), 2005–2006.

Goetzel, R. Z., Roemer, E. C., Liss-Levinson, R. C., & Samoly, D. K. (2008). *Workplace health promotion: Policy recommendations that encourage employers to support health improvement programs for their workers.* Washington, DC: Partnership for Prevention.

Gostin, L. O. (2012). A framework convention on global health: Health for all, justice for all. *Journal of American Medical Association, 307*(19), 2087–2092.

Gracey, M. (2002). Child health in an urbanizing world. *Acta Paediatrica, 91*(1), 1–8. doi: 10.1080/080352502753457842

Harris, J. K., Provan, K. G., Johnson, K. J., & Leischow, S. J. (2012). Drawbacks and benefits associated with inter-organizational collaboration along the discovery-development-delivery continuum: A cancer research network case study. *Implementation Science,* 7–69.

Heinen, L., & Darling, H. (2009). Addressing obesity in the workplace: The role of employers. *Milbank Quarterly, 87*(1), 101–122. doi: 10.1111/j.1468-0009.2009.00549.x

Henry J. Kaiser Family Foundation. (2012). *Health care costs: A primer.* Menlo Park, CA: Author.

Institute for Healthcare Improvement. (2000). Improvement methods. *How to improve.* Retrieved from http://www.ihi.org/IHI/Topics/Improvement/ImprovementMethods/HowToImprove/

Institute for Work & Health. (2006). Primary, secondary and tertiary prevention. *At work,* (43). Retrieved from http://www.iwh.on.ca/wrmb/primary-secondary-and-tertiary-prevention

Institute of Medicine. (1999). *To err is human: Building a safer health system.* Washington, DC: National Academies Press. Retrieved from http://www.iom.edu/~/media/Files/Report%20 Files/1999/To-Err-is-Human/To%20Err%20is%20Human%201999%20%20report%20 brief.ashx

Institute of Medicine. (2001). Crossing the quality chasm: A new health system for the 21st century. Washington, DC: National Academies Press. Retrieved from http://www.iom.edu/Reports /2001/Crossing-the-Quality-Chasm-A-New-Health-System-for-the-21st-Century.aspx

Institute of Medicine. (2002). *The future of the public's health in the 21st century.* Washington, DC: National Academies Press. Retrieved from http://www.iom.edu/~/media/Files/Report%20 Files/2002/The-Future-of-the-Publics-Health-in-the-21st-Century/Future%20of%20 Publics%20Health%202002%20Report%20Brief.pdf

Institute of Medicine. (2003). *Keeping patients safe: Transforming the work environment of nurses.* Washington, DC: National Academies Press. Retrieved from http://www.iom.edu/Reports/2003/Keeping-Patients-Safe-Transforming-the-Work-Environment-of-Nurses.aspx

Interprofessional Education Collaborative Expert Panel. (2011). *Core competencies for interprofessional collaborative practice: Report of an expert panel.* Washington, DC: Interprofessional Education Collaborative.

Jallinoja, P., Absetz, P., Kuronen, R., Nissinen, A., Talja, M., Uutela, A., & Patja, K. (2007). The dilemma of patient responsibility for lifestyle change: Perceptions among primary care physicians and nurses. *Scandinavian Journal of Primary Health Care, 25*(4), 244–249.

Jia, H., Moriarty, D. G., & Kanarek, N. (2009). County-level social environment determinants of health-related qulity of life among US adults: A multilevel analysis. *Journal of Community Health, 34,* 430–439.

Kapustin, J. (2010). Chronic disease prevention across the lifespan. *Journal for Nurse Practitioners, 6*(1), 16–24. doi: 10.1016/j.nurpra.2009.09.015

Kaye, J. D., Richstone, L., Cho, J. S., Tai, J. Y., Arrand, J., & Kavoussi, L. R. (2010). Patient noncompliance before surgery. *BJU International, 105*(2), 230–233. doi: 10.1111/j.1464-410X.2009.08760.x

Kjellstrom, T., Friel, S., Dixon, J., Corvalan, C., Rehfuess, E., Campbell-Lendrum, D., ...Bartram, J. (2007). Urban environmental health hazards and health equity. *Journal of Urban Health: Bulletin of the New York Academy of Medicine, 84*(1).

Leininger, M. M., & McFarland, M. R. (Eds.). (2006). *Culture care diversity and universality: A worldwide nursing theory.* Sudbury, MA: Jones and Bartlett.

Majette, G. R. (2011). PPACA and public health: Creating a framework to focus on prevention and wellness and improve the public's health. *Journal of Law, Medicine & Ethics, 39*(3), 366–379. doi: 10.1111/j.1748-720X.2011.00606.x

Marrero, S. L., Bloom, D. E., & Asashi, E. Y. (2012). Noncommunicable diseases: A global health crisis in a new world order. *Journal of American Medical Association, 307*(19), 2037–2038.

Martin, L. A., Lloyd, E. D., & Nolan, T. W. (2007). *Whole system measures. IHI innovation series white paper.* Cambridge, MA: Institute for Healthcare Improvement.

McCarter, T., Daly, F. N., & Cooper, K. (2010). The 5 eras of healthcare finance: Wellness as a clinical model. *American Health & Drug Benefits, 3*(2), S83–S88.

Miller, W. R., & Rose, G. S. (2009). Toward a theory of motivational interviewing. *American Psychologist, 64*(6), 527–537. Retrieved from http://libproxy2.usouthal.edu/login?url=http://search.ebscohost.com/login.aspx?direct=true&db=aph&AN=44468321&loginpage=login.asp&site=ehost-live&scope=site doi:10.1037/a0016830

National Prevention Council. (2011). *National prevention strategy.* Washington, DC: U.S. Department of Health and Human Services, Office of the Surgeon General.

Nidecker, M., DiClemente, C. C., Bennett, M. E., & Bellack, A. S. (2008). Application of the transtheoretical model of change: Psychometric properties of leading measures in patients with co-occurring drug abuse and severe mental illness. *Addictive Behaviors, 33*(8), 1021–1030.

Organisation for Economic Co-operation and Development. (2011). *Health at a glance: OECD Indicators*. Paris, France: Author.

Pelletier, K. R. (2011). A review and analysis of the clinical and cost-effectiveness studies of comprehensive health promotion and disease management programs at the worksite: Update VIII 2008 to 2010. *Journal of Occupational and Environmental Medicine/American College Of Occupational And Environmental Medicine, 53*(11), 1310–1331.

Perdue, W. C., Richards, E. P., Acree, K. H., & Stroup, D. F. (2005). Legal frameworks for preventing chronic disease. *Jounal of Law, Medicine and Ethics 33*. Retrieved from http://heinonline.org/HOL/LandingPage?collection=journals&handle=hein.journals/medeth33&div=122&id=&page=

Pham, H. (2012). Loving life longer. *Industrial Engineer: IE, 44*(4), 45.

Plsek, P. E., & Greenhalgh, T. (2001). Complex science: The challenge of complexity in health care. *British Medical Association, 323*, 625–628.

Prochaska, J. O. (2008). Decision making in the transtheoretical model of behavior change. *Medical Decision Making, 28*(6), 845–849.

Ricci, J. A., & Chee, E. (2005). Lost productive time associated with excess weight in the U.S. workforce. *Journal of Occupational & Environmental Medicine, 47*(12), 1227–1234. doi: 10.1097/01.jom.0000184871.20901.c3

Rollnick, S., Miller, W. R., & Butler, C. C. (Eds.). (2008). *Motivational interviewing in health care: Helping patients change behavior*. New York, NY: The Guilford Press.

Rubak, S., Sanboek, A., Lauritzen, T., & Christensen, B. (2005). Motivational interviewing: A systematic review and meta-analysis. *British Journal of General Practice, 55*(513), 305–312.

Seear, K. (2009). "Nobody really knows what it is or how to treat it": Why women with endometriosis do not comply with healthcare advice. *Health, Risk & Society, 11*(4), 367–385. doi: 10.1080/13698570903013649

Seidl, K. L. (2011). Patient education: Responsibility amidst mandates. *Bariatric Nursing and Surgical Patient Care, 6*(4), 165–166. doi: 10.1089/bar.2011.9941

Smith, M. K. (2001). Peter Senge and the learning organization. *The Encyclopedia of Informal Education*. Retrieved from www.infed.org/thinkers/senge.htm

Stonecypher, K. (2009). Creating a patient education tool. *Journal of Continuing Education in Nursing, 40*(10), 462–467.

Suhrcke, M., Nugent, R. A., Stuckler, D., & Rocco, L. (2006). *Chronic disease: An economic perspective*. London, England: Oxford Health Alliance.

Tan, B. (2012). Economist conferences: Cost of non-communicable disease to weigh on society more than the global financial crisis. *PRWeb Online Visibility from Vocus*. Retrieved from http://www.prweb.com/pdfdownload/10072655.pdf

Toffler, A. (1970). *Future shock*. New York, NY: Random House.

United Nations. (2011a). *Population distribution, urbanization, internal migration and development: An international perspective*. New York, NY: United Nations Department of Economic and Social Affairs.

United Nations. (2011b). *Prevention and control of non-communicable diseases: Report to the secretary-general: Follow-up to the outcome of the Millennium Summit.* New York, NY: Author.

United Nations. (2011c). *Scope, modalities format and organization of the high-level meeting of the General Assembly on the prevention and control of non-communicable diseases.* General Assembly, Sixty-fifth session.

United Nations. (2012). Millennium development Goal 8. *The global partnership for development: Making rhetoric a reality, MDG Gap task force report 2012.* New York, NY: Author.

U.S. Department of Health and Human Services. (2012a). Healthy People 2020: Leading health indicators, 2012. Retrieved from http://www.healthypeople.gov/2020/LHI/default.aspx

U.S. Department of Health & Human Services. (2012b). Historical highlights. Retrieved from http://www.hhs.gov/about/hhshist.html

U.S. Department of Labor. (2011). About OSHA. Retrieved from http://www.osha.gov/about.html

World Health Organization. (2008). *2008-2013 Action plan for the global strategy for the prevention and control of noncommunicable diseases.* Geneva, Switzerland: Author.

World Health Organization. (2009). *Milestones in health promotion: Statement from global conferences.* Geneva, Switzerland: Author.

World Health Organization. (2011). *Global status report on noncommunicable diseases 2010.* Geneva, Switzerland: Author.

World Health Organization. (2012a). Origin and development of health cooperation. Retrieved from http://www.who.int/global_health_histories/background/en/index.html

World Health Organization. (2012b). The WHO agenda. Retrieved from http://www.who.int/about/agenda/en/index.html

Health Promotion in an Acute Care Setting: A Quality and Process Improvement Initiative

Laurie Sayer and Kristin Mast

Influenza and pneumonia are major causes of hospitalization and death in the United States. As a clinician, the CNL promotes better health for populations by creating awareness, knowledge, and system changes to increase the adult inpatient immunization rate. This ensures improved compliance with the Centers for Medicare and Medicaid Services (CMS) quality-of-care measures and accountable care and will have a financial impact related to pay-for-performance standards. A higher immunization rate also aligns with the *Healthy People 2020* goal of increasing immunization levels and reducing preventable infectious diseases.

Our organization was not consistently meeting established benchmarks for pneumonia's quality core measures. In addition, a baseline audit undertaken October to December 2010 indicated that only 51% of patients actually received their ordered Pneumovax 23 (pneumococcal polysaccharides [PPSV]) vaccine and 41.7% their ordered influenza vaccine prior to discharge.

A CNL-led interdisciplinary task force was formed to look at current practice, analyze data, identify barriers, and develop a process improvement plan using Lean principles. At a system-wide and microsystem level, CNLs support immunization processes through both formal and informal education, mentoring, system changes, data awareness, and accountability.

A root cause analysis was performed with essential input from staff nurses to identify issues affecting immunization compliance. The team recognized several problems related to the immunization process and sought input from staff nurses to identify barriers to vaccine administration. Based on feedback from staff on all inpatient units, the team identified three main focus areas: education, accountability, and continual awareness of vaccine compliance.

CNLs were champions of the quality initiative. As outcome managers, unit CNLs received daily and monthly reports to monitor compliance and trends, and to evaluate gaps for unit specific improvement opportunities. Inpatient CNLs have been instrumental in obtaining accurate patient immunization history. This has created an increased awareness of up-to-date immunizations. The CNLs provided education at unit staff meetings and mentoring on the units and obtained feedback from the nurses about barriers and gaps in the process, which was then taken back to the team to address. CNLs were also instrumental in eliminating duplicate vaccinations by researching patients' vaccine histories and updating immunization histories. The CNLs also received daily reports for active vaccine orders to ensure just-in-time education and compliance. Each unit's PPSV and influenza vaccine monthly data reports are posted on their quality boards for awareness and transparency.

With the CNL initiative, PPSV and influenza vaccines ordered and given increased from a baseline of less than 52% to 89.3%. Several initiatives at our organization have failed to improve and sustain pneumococcal and influenza rates for the adult inpatient populations, thus affecting the quality of care and safety of our patients. A CNL-led interdisciplinary initiative using process improvement methods and supported by an accountability model has played an instrumental role in improving and sustaining the overall vaccination rate for the organization. Ongoing efforts are directed toward accurately assessing and providing immunizations to every patient every time (100% of the time).

Improving Geriatric Patient Safety by Restricting Sleep Aids

Leslie Phillips

CNL observations of increased incidence of hospitalization-induced delirium in a geriatric population led to chart audits that reflected similarities between patients of advanced age, a history of dementia, and the use of a sleep aids. The acute mental status changes displayed by these patients led to increased length of stay and diagnostic expenses. Complications also included emotional distress in patients and family members. Patient safety became compromised as patients often displayed the symptoms of hyperactive delirium. These behaviors demanded increased vigilance by the nursing staff to prevent injury. A review of the pharmacological evidence revealed the manufacturer's advice of restricted use in older adults, as the drug could induce increased confusion and motor dysfunction. When queried, the hospital pharmacist advised restricted use in geriatric patients. The unit medical director echoed this advice. Collaboration between the unit nursing manager, medical director, CNL, and pharmacy led to the adoption of a new unit guideline restricting the use of sleep aids in patients 65 years of age and older. On the advice of the unit medical director, "new starts" of sleep aids were to be avoided as well. The CNL was responsible for educating the nursing staff, performing medication audits on newly admitted patients, and advocating for change with attending physicians. Nursing was challenged to promote sleep with alternative medications such as mild analgesics, sedating antidepressants and antipsychotics, warm drinks, and soothing music. With diligence, education, and patient advocacy, the incidence of medication-induced delirium decreased, thereby improving patient safety.

Patient Satisfaction with Pain Management

Maureen Tait

In an effort to increase patient satisfaction in the pain management arena, a few CNLs decided to host a competition. We had been working within our units on a daily basis, educating staff about establishing a pain goal with their patients and developing a plan to meet it. The metrics that were used were the Press Ganey survey results, along with monthly unit audits. These measurements showed that further work was needed.

Working within a microsystem at times can give you tunnel vision. We individually knew that organizational goals were set at a high level and we strived to achieve them. But we were still falling short. What could we do to improve them? What were other units doing?

The CNLs who joined together on this project all work on surgical floors where pain management is a strong component of quality patient care. We decided that for a period of 1 week each of us would audit our units for pain goal documentation. Setting a pain goal with patients establishes a sense of trust and safety. It shows a concentrated effort to include patients in their plan of care. The results were posted on each unit's huddle board. The anticipation and interest in these numbers was beyond our expectations. Staff would clap and cheer when their numbers were greater than the others. On the other hand, staff would challenge each other to improve if they were not number one. At the end of the week a blue ribbon was presented to the winning unit. It is proudly displayed on its huddle board. Since then, when we have been challenged in a quality improvement project, the suggestion for a competition comes up frequently!

Improving Fall Outcomes: A CNL's Patient Safety Collaborative Initiative

Patricia Baker

The literature confirms that the population of elderly persons (age 65 and older) is growing rapidly, and this growth corresponds with an increased risk of injury from falling. The number of elderly persons is expected to increase from 31 million in 1990 to 68.1 million by 2040. This 45-bed medical telemetry unit averages 72% "high fall risk" patients, as shown by an evidence-based practice (EBP) fall assessment tool. The facility and unit-based leadership's top priority is to improve fall outcomes, as illustrated by National Database of Nursing Quality Indicators' (NDNQI) first and second quarter fiscal year (FY) 2010 data, with 7.18 and 6.74 falls per 1,000 patient days respectively, and 0.94 and 1.18 falls with injury per 1,000 patient days. This negatively impacts patient safety outcomes and detracts from the clinical excellence of the institution. Falls are considered a potential hazard of hospitalization for the frail, elderly individual. Annually, elderly persons fall at a rate that is three times higher in nursing homes and hospitals.

The microsystem's interdisciplinary team's specific aim was to decrease the number of total falls by 50% by the end of the third quarter of FY2010, which would meet NDNQI's 50th percentile. A strengths, weaknesses, opportunities, and threats (SWOT) analysis showed an insufficient supply of bed alarms. The team submitted a business proposal that suggested 100% of "high fall risk" patients be guaranteed a bed alarm in addition to the facility's other EBP fall precaution interventions, including patient/family-centered education. Utilizing the continuous quality improvement of plan, do, study, act (PDSA) monitoring, third quarter data revealed a marked improvement; there was a 2.98 fall rate and 0.32 falls with injury rate, exceeding NDNQI's 50th percentile. The return on investment was a benefit of $251,152.

Improving Glycemic Control

Ann Eubanks

Problem Statement

Surgical site infections, and particularly sternal and mediastinal infections, have implications for significantly increasing both morbidity and mortality, as well as their associated costs in both man hours and dollars spent. Postoperative hyperglycemia is associated with the development of surgical site infections among cardiac surgery patients. Adequate glycemic control has been shown to decrease the incidence of deep sternal wound infection. According to Furnary and colleagues (2003), continuous insulin infusion protocols should be the standard care for glycometabolic control in all patients undergoing cardiac surgical procedures. Furthermore, the Centers for Medicare and Medicaid Services (CMS) publicly reports on postoperative glycemic control as part of the Surgical Care Improvement Project (SCIP). The goal of this project is to increase the percentage of cardiac surgery patients to at least 90% meeting SCIP criteria for adequate glycemic control, with serum glucose levels less than 200 mg/dL on the first and second postoperative days.

Multidisciplinary Team

A multidisciplinary team was formed to address the design and implementation of updated glycemic control strategies to conform to current evidence-based practices. The team consisted of the nurse manager, staff nurses, diabetic educators, a clinical pharmacist, information systems analysts, and a cardiovascular surgeon. These individuals were chosen based on expertise in their respective disciplines. A retroactive chart review was performed to obtain baseline data; it revealed that glucose targets were only met in 40% of heart surgery patients.

Project Processes and Evaluation Methods

A microsystem assessment was performed in the cardiac recovery unit to determine knowledge levels regarding glycemic control and current methods of glucose management. Brainstorming and cause and effect analysis methods were used to determine possible causes of poor glycemic control. A literature review of best practices for postoperative glycemic control was undertaken by the team, and numerous

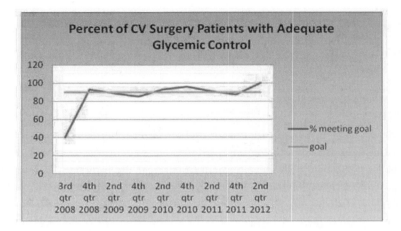

evidence-based protocols were evaluated. A mutually agreed upon continuous insulin infusion (CII) protocol was identified. Information systems analysts converted the protocol into an electronic form, which enabled bedside nurses to accurately titrate insulin infusion rates. The CII protocol was presented to the medical executive committee for approval as standing orders. The plan-do-study-act (PDSA) cycle was used to conduct tests of change using the agreed upon protocol. Bedside nurses received comprehensive education on glycemic control and utilization of the new protocol prior to implementation.

Outcomes

Upon implementation of the new CII protocol, close supervision and clinical support was provided for all shifts. Data was monitored daily to ensure safety and to quickly identify problems. After the first quarter using the CII protocol, adequate glycemic control was achieved in 93% of patients. Through ongoing surveillance, periodic decreases were analyzed and attributed to staffing changes. Additional education and training for staff resulted in measurable improvements.

Reference

Furnary A. P., Gao, G., Grunkemeier, G. L., YingXing, W., Zerr, K. J., Bookin, S. O., . . . & Starr, A. (2003). Continuous insulin infusion reduces mortality in patients with diabetes undergoing coronary artery bypass grafting. *Journal of Thoracic Cardiovascular Surgery, 125*, 1007–1021.

Innovation at the Bedside Improves Efficiency in Nursing Care and Nursing/Patient Satisfaction

Beth VanDam

Key terms: advocate, clinician, efficiency, nurse/patient satisfaction

The nurse on the oncology unit cares for many complex surgical patients. Patients who have had an operative Whipple procedure for pancreatic cancer need to be monitored for many changing medical needs, including electrolyte and fluid balance changes. I am the CNL with advanced clinical expertise, and these patients are prioritized for my involvement.

This past spring, Mrs. J. had a Whipple procedure to treat her pancreatic cancer. She had a long and rocky postoperative course, including continual high outputs from the gastrostomy tube. The physician had ordered all gastrostomy tube outputs to be refed every 4 hours into the jejunostomy tube (j-tube) in an effort to maintain electrolyte balance. I noted that the gastrostomy tube was putting out 500–800 cc every 4 hours. The nurse said that the refeeding took 45 minutes manually. The patient was reporting that she was exhausted from the frequent interruptions from the staff and the nurse voiced frustration with the nursing time required to complete this element of care.

I discussed other options to providing the refeeding with the nurse, such as getting another tube feeding pump, as well as an empty tube-feeding bag in which to pour the gastrostomy outputs. We also set up a Y connector so that both gastrostomy outputs and tube feedings could be run at the same time.

I discussed this option with the physician as well, who lacked a clear understanding regarding the amount of time it was taking for nursing to manually refeed. After further discussion and clarifying total hourly j-tube intake, between tube feedings and gastrostomy refeeds, the physician orders were modified to meet patient/nursing needs while ensuring the patient was receiving necessary nutrition and refeedings. The success of this set-up resulted in improved efficiency in nursing care and less interruption for the patient, leading to improved staff and patient satisfaction.

Enhancing Palliative and End-of-Life Care

Vidette Todaro-Franceschi

The End-of-Life Nursing Education Consortium (ELNEC) core training is incorporated into our CNL graduate program, which consists of eight modules (introduction, pain management, symptom management, ethical and legal aspects, cultural aspects, communication, grief/loss, and final hours). One of the clinical objectives and concurrent written assignments for the students is to complete an assessment of end-of-life/palliative care practices in their microcosm and then create an action plan to address any deficiencies that they have identified.

Our CNL program is in its infancy, with only 16 students thus far completing the assignment. However, the potential for change in this important area is notably tangible. Feedback from students who received ELNEC training has been positive, with the majority believing that end-of-life care pedagogy is a necessary component of CNL role development. Not only did the students realize that their own knowledge base and comfort level regarding dying and death had improved with ELNEC training, but many were then able to foster an increased awareness in staff as well.

One student who worked in an intensive care unit (ICU), upon having an open discussion with staff and identifying that many had difficulty facing death, offered educational sessions to assist them in becoming more comfortable communicating with patients who are dying and their loved ones. Another, noting that there were frequent anticipated deaths on his unit, had a private room dedicated for patients in transition so that there would be a quiet space for staff and loved ones to be with the patient. Yet another student spoke with her practice council in the emergency department about end-of-life care, and they then recognized a need to address staff and patient concerns related to unanticipated deaths. The outcome was the creation of a bereavement packet for the loved ones of patients who die suddenly.

The student clinical logs also indicated a change in awareness as the students shared instances where they intervened on behalf of patients who were nearing the end of life. For example, one noted that she had spoken with a family at length about end-of-life care choices for their 94-year-old loved one who had been in and out of the ICU four times. After discussing concerns, the family decided that their loved one did not need to be in an ICU and the patient was transitioned to comfort care. The student noted, "I would not have been able to have this discussion with the family had we not had classes on end-of-life care."

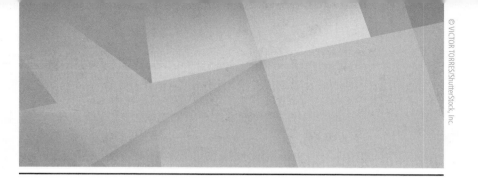

TWENTY

The Clinical Nurse Leader: Transforming Nursing Care in Acute Care, Ambulatory, and Long-Term Care Settings

■ Michelle A. Lucatorto, Evelyn Sommers, Larry Lemos, and Storm Morgan

 Learning Objectives

■ Describe the clinical nurse leader's role as a generalist and microsystem change agent in the acute care, ambulatory, and long-term healthcare settings
■ Discuss how advocacy and ethics manifest in the role of the clinical nurse leader
■ Describe how clinical nurse leaders contribute to transforming nursing care by implementing evidence in a microsystem using quality improvement redesign and lateral integration skills

> Most people spend more time and energy going around problems than in trying to solve them.
>
> Henry Ford

Key Terms

Transformation	Delivery models	Quality
Safety	Efficiency	Effectiveness
Financial stewardship	Advocacy	Ethics

CNL Roles

Clinician	Transformer	Coordinator of care
Team member	Risk anticipator	Outcomes manager
Advocate	Systems analyst	Ethical decision maker

CNL Professional Values

Advocacy	Accountability	Altruism	Integrity
Social justice	Human dignity		

CNL Core Competencies

Communication	Assessment	Health promotion
Risk reduction	Disease prevention	Ethics

Human care systems and policy
Information and healthcare technology
Nursing technology and resource management
Design/management/coordination of care

Introduction

The role of the clinical nurse leader (CNL) was developed in response to demands of increased technology, complex care coordination, and growth of clinical evidence experienced. The CNL role was designed as a generalist addressing safety and quality of care. The CNL's focus is the point of care and integration of care in a microsystem. The required basic skills for a CNL reflect the professional practice of nursing. The CNL role is distinguished from advanced practice nurses (APNs) by its focus on implementation of evidence in nursing-sensitive outcomes, system redesign expertise, and care coordination at the microsystem level. Understanding the role and using the CNL's abilities to translate evidence into practice and provide care coordination with expert understanding of the flow processes, system dynamics, and culture will result in measurable improvements in clinical outcomes, efficiency measures, care coordination, and staff and patient satisfaction (Rusch & Bakewell-Sachs, 2007).

The CNL role manifests core competencies of communication and coordination, assessment, health promotion, risk reduction, disease prevention, ethics, systems redesign, and health technology. A CNL is a master's prepared nurse who uses evidence-based practices to facilitate and coordinate care for a group of patients and to provide direct patient care in complex situations, engaging other nurses to collaborate in effecting positive patient outcomes. The CNL is well positioned by education and training to assess inpatient acute care (or intensive care), primary care, and long-term care microsystems.

The CNL is the first nursing role to focus on systems redesign or healthcare engineering principles. The CNL has been labeled a "point-of-care systems engineer" in health care by Reid and Dennison (2011). The redesign focus of the CNL role has origins in the Institute of Medicine's report, *Crossing the Quality Chasm: A New Health System for the 21st Century* (2001). This publication created a sense of urgency in the nursing profession to address quality and safety with redesign using informatics, to develop care coordination systems that promoted teamwork, to recognize the patient as the team lead, and to do this work at the microsystem level. Although the microsystem is small in relation to the overall organization, its reach is mighty, for no healthcare system can claim quality and safety outcomes as a whole if these positive outcomes are not occurring at the microsystem level (Nelson et al., 2003). The microsystem is the key area for evidence-based implementation and systems redesign to merge as the size and complexity of a microsystem is conducive to redesign and quality improvement processes. According to Kimball, Joynt, Cherner, and O'Neil (2007), innovation in healthcare systems is often driven by the development of new nursing roles and the expansion of existing roles.

Delays in the diffusion of clinical evidence into practice have historically been a barrier to improvements in quality and safety. A few of the most discussed examples that evidence a history of delays in implementation include the results of the Diabetes Prevention Program, use of beta blockers in myocardial disease, and interventions to prevent hospital-acquired infections. The success of implementation at the microsystem level requires the clinical insight of direct care staff, an understanding of the quality of the evidence supporting the recommendations, and the ability to engineer the evidence into the microsystem (Sherman, Clark, & Maloney, 2008). The CNL's advanced education in nursing and systems redesign, in addition to the CNL's direct care clinical role, is preparatory for implementation expertise. The identification of nursing outcomes that are amenable to improvement using clinical evidence is the work of the CNL. The interventions CNLs implement to achieve desired outcomes provide for the measurement of quality and safety outcomes of nursing care in a variety of settings. The development of interventions for nursing and the growth in the evidence to guide practice are tools that are actively used by CNLs.

The improvement in nursing-sensitive quality and safety indicators using both clinical evidence and a systems redesign approach is a major focus of the role of the CNL. The CNL can also influence the care provided to individual patients while providing direct care, mentoring staff in the provision of direct care, or collaborating with direct care and APNs in joint care planning. Although the mastery of health informatics and nursing technology and resources (staff and supplies) is often not thought of as a clinical competency, it is nonetheless a key element for the CNL's navigation of the microsystem (Stanton, 2006).

The CNL supports autonomy for the individual through competencies of ethics and advocacy. Assisting a patient in obtaining needed health care—which may include cost, language, and geographical barriers—is a common advocacy action. Formally and informally acknowledging a patient's rights and serving as a liaison between a patient and the healthcare system are other actions. In operationalizing the American Nurses Association's (ANA's) (2001) code of ethics, the CNL's primary commitment is to the individual patient and the collective patient group. An example of ethical judgment in the systems redesign work of the CNL is the inclusion of patient views in mapping work processes, the inclusion of patients as members of nursing committees, and the design of work processes that mandate informed patient choice.

The CNL role can be operationalized in a variety of nursing settings. This chapter focuses on the CNL's core roles and competencies in a variety of clinical microsystems. Content and case studies describe the use of evidence and systems redesign by CNLs in the acute, ambulatory, and long-term care settings. Readers are encouraged to apply the content presented through answering reflection questions and engaging in suggested learning activities.

Although the CNL may be based in the microsystem of a primary care team setting, knowledge of interacting microsystems and how to navigate through macrosystems is also required. The CNL can gain an understanding of the relationships between influencing systems by serving on system committees and engaging in interactions with nursing partners such as clinical nurse specialists, nurse educators, nurse informatics, and nurse administrators to develop a community. The staffing pattern of the CNL must allow for direct patient care, design of implementation of evidence, and coordination with interactions in other microsystems and with a macrosystem focus.

The CNL in the Acute Specialty Care Setting

The CNL in the acute care setting uses skills for the design of processes that lead to implementation of evidence, care coordination, and promotion of individual patient autonomy. An example of the CNL role in redesign to improve quality and safety related to nursing care is the prevention of central venous catheter (CVC) infections and ventilator-associated pneumonia (VAP). Nurses working in a variety of general or specialty care units provide care directed at the prevention of infection for those persons at risk.

The inpatient acute care setting provides the CNL with a unique role in the organizational microsystem. In the unit-based microsystem, the CNL influences nursing practice and clinical outcomes by incorporating clinical evidence, system redesign processes, and enhanced care related to nursing-sensitive indicators. Patients in the inpatient specialty care setting are often confronted with the burden of disease symptoms, a distress state, and risk for hospital-acquired events. The CNL implements interventions that are supported by clinical evidence to promote health, minimize risks of hospitalization, and reduce the effects of the disease state on the person. The CNL advocates for patients through development of a patient-centered culture that emphasizes quality and safety. Research examining the effect of the CNL on nursing-sensitive interventions and outcomes in the acute care setting is substantial and growing.

CNLs functioning in the acute care setting are rapidly demonstrating the usefulness of education, tools, and outreach combined with a systems redesign focus in producing meaningful improvements in inpatient care. DeBoer (2011) used the Iowa model of evidence-based practice, along with workflow analysis, to provide structure to improve the implementation of an intervention for the acute renal failure specialty care population.

The case study on the following page illustrates the ability of the CNL to role model and demonstrates a balance of clinical decision making, patient advocacy, and respect for human dignity in the delivery of care.

In addition to improvement of quality and safety at the microsystem level and improvement in direct patient care outcomes, the CNL can also contribute to the operational and fiscal improvements at the microsystem level. The ANA has developed several operational quality measures related to staffing that can be directly influenced by the CNL.

Unlike the APN, the CNL is a clinical and nursing microsystems engineer. The CNL uses nursing's scientific evidence combined with systems redesign principles to improve clinical outcomes by transforming care delivery at the microsystem level. Nursing has, like other components of the healthcare system, grown in complexity with advances in clinical evidence and technology. The CNL and the APN are complementary resources for such complex healthcare systems.

The CNL partners with the APN in the implementation and dissemination of evidence in the direct care setting. An example is the implementation plan for evidence-based skin care in an acute care system. The doctorally prepared APN works with the unit-based CNLs to develop a clinical question and provide evidence synthesis. The CNL group uses the understanding of the microsystem on units to tailor the evidence into an actionable plan. Because the CNL is a direct care component of the unit-based staffing, the CNL can additionally provide role modeling and expert end user feedback regarding the implementation plan. The APN works with information technology macrosystems engineers to develop data collection and reporting tools for the nursing staff.

The CNL in the Ambulatory Care Setting

Integration of the CNL role in the primary care ambulatory setting is relatively new, and less evidence is available to describe processes and outcomes. This is largely due to the historical trend of CNLs practicing mainly in inpatient acute care settings. Significant opportunities exist for expansion of the CNL role to drive change and promote quality and safety at the microsystem level in ambulatory care. Changes in healthcare reform currently focus on patient-centered medical homes, as described

Case Study

Sam is a 72-year-old Korean War veteran recently admitted to the cardiac care inpatient unit with worsening heart failure. Having recently become a widower, Sam lives alone with his small dog, Toby. Sam has been admitted to the cardiac care unit six times in the last year, and although he wishes desperately to stay home with Toby, he admits things usually seem to go downhill a few weeks after each discharge. The staff has a great relationship with Sam, and they are frustrated that they cannot seem to create a plan of care to help him. The staff members are hopeful that the new CNL who joined their unit a month ago can help with Sam's care plan.

The CNL uses systems-based knowledge and clinical evidence to help redesign Sam's system of managing heart failure. Sam and the CNL plot out the common path that follows each hospitalization. Together they discover that Sam has intense support in the first 10 days after discharge, including a visit by his son to shop and pick up medications, as well as a 2-day postdischarge call from his primary care nurse and a 7–10 day visit with his primary care provider. Sam says he feels confident and healthy during this time and is thankful for the help. When Sam and the CNL plot out the events that occur after day 10, Sam admits he feels lonely, and he forgets to take his medications and has more food "treats" than he should. Sam feels guilty because he knows what he should be doing. The CNL tells Sam that continued support is often needed, and that this is not a sign of weakness. The CNL also acknowledges that human interaction is as important a part of treatment as medications and diet. Sam is surprised, but because he now feels that planned follow-up is expected and not a sign of weakness, he is delighted to explore home health nursing, telehealth, and even day programs for adults.

In the end, Sam chooses telehealth, as he feels having a good conversation with someone once a week is the best supplement to the support he gets from his family, primary care team, and his dog, Toby. The nurses on the unit began to use the concept of plotting out the path of events that follow discharge with all patients as part of early discharge planning, rather than focusing on only the instruction portion.

by the American College of Physicians (ACP, n.d.). The medical home was developed primarily to provide for financial reimbursement for primary care physicians. Over time it is becoming clear that the medical home will transition to focus on patient activation and development of a community that supports health, combined with a team that uses evidence and data to design systems that support patients. A system that reimburses primary care is essential for the health of the population, and a successful model will be team based and patient led. The second-generation medical home that evolves will require the CNL role for success. The Dartmouth Institute for Clinical Microsystems has developed a microsystem academy that provides tool kits for the CNL in both specialty care and ambulatory care settings that include process and outcome tools (Dartmouth Institute, n.d.). CNLs in the ambulatory setting will use and build on these tool kits as they begin to publish evidence of improvement in outcomes for team processes, access, satisfaction, safety, and clinical quality.

In the primary care setting, there is a focus on chronic disease management, identification of high-risk patients through population health management, patient activation and engagement in health care, and prevention of unplanned urgent or emergency care. Much of the work builds on the chronic disease model's call for systems improvement and patient activation (Wagner et al., 2001). The chronic disease model moves ambulatory care away from the traditional medical model by recognizing that patient leadership in the clinical team and engaging the patient system and community resources will improve health and well-being (Coleman, Austin, Brach, & Wagner, 2009). The chronic disease model also requires a systematic implementation of evidence and the use of clinical informatics in care processes. Redesigning transition processes between episodes and healthcare teams can produce cost-effective, quality care and improve patient satisfaction. The case study on the next page demonstrates the implementation of evidence and the use of data in redesign processes to improve systems-based outcomes.

The CNL uses evidence-based practice to coach and mentor the clinical team. Implementing evidence adapted to the unique clinical setting, the CNL leads small changes in practice geared toward enhancement of patient centeredness, healing environments, patient flow, and staff movement and tasks and works with the primary care team members and patients to make improvements (Nelson et al., 2003). The CNL assists in moving successful interventions into the daily practice through clinical support software development, standardized tools and processes, education and training of team members, and negotiation and change management when resistance arises. The CNL also monitors the stabilization of changes in practice and

Case Study

An example of a CNL using redesign principles and clinical data systems to improve care processes comes from the primary care ambulatory setting in the Veterans Health Administration (VHA). The CNL led the clinical team to map the current "as is" process for a group of patients with high-risk diagnoses. The flow map included the inpatient stay, the discharge process, the procurement of medications for the home setting, the timing and decision flow for scheduling follow-up specialty and primary care, as well as use of home medical services such as home nursing and home telehealth. The CNL used published clinical evidence demonstrating reduction in readmission rates to redesign the discharge process. The actions included the incorporation of the inpatient staff and primary care in the development of a discharge notification system, use of the level of patient activation to determine the postdischarge resources, and timing for follow-up. The evidence also suggested that a standard 4–7 day targeted follow-up call would measure the success of the discharge plan and allow for early adaptations. This clinical innovation resulted in a reduction in readmissions and was exported throughout the VHA.

continues to monitor the desired quality outcomes with data management systems and feedback to stakeholders. The CNL publishes or presents in order to disseminate the implementation of evidence into practice in local, regional, and national settings.

CNLs work as lateral integrators of care by removing silos and promoting teamwork across care settings (Begun, Torabeni, & White, 2006). The CNL mentors nursing staff, leads collaborative efforts between inpatient and specialty units to coordinate care, keeps a finger "on the pulse" of the primary care team, and works to improve operations with small tests of change. The case on the next page shows the role of the CNL as lateral integrator.

The CNL increases the safety and quality of patients' care by acting as a healthcare navigator, maximizing the use of information technology for population management at the microsystem level, and designing protocols with the default being the desired action rather than relying mainly on individuals. The CNL supports patients and staff through analysis of existing processes and assisting in changes that modify

Case Study

Care transition, responsibility for care, and patient autonomy are salient issues when patients are receiving both specialty and primary care services. Role confusion exists for both the healthcare team and the patient, placing the patient at risk for delays in care and unsatisfactory outcomes. The CNL in a urology specialty setting recognized this and designed a "nurses care across boundaries" program for patients in the urology surgical service. The urology care nurse developed a nurse transition note to convey both clinical and individual data to the registered nurse care manager (RNCM) in a primary care VHA facility. This note specifically provided information about the patient's clinical condition, the information the patient was given regarding contact with the urology team, and the clinical and self-care requirements of the unique patient. The CNL also set aside a call-in time for the RNCM to review concerns about patients shared by the urology and primary care teams. This program resulted in patient satisfaction, nurse satisfaction, and a reduction in readmission and urgent care visits in the posturology procedure period. The CNL addressed concerns with the RNCM when the patient called or came to an open access primary care appointment with an issue related to the urology procedure. The clinical concerns could then be addressed in the primary care clinic or through scheduling an outpatient appointment in the urology clinic, rather than through an urgent care visit or hospital admission. The CNL in the urology service acted as a mentor for the nurses in the cardiovascular service to develop a similar program. The CNL also was able to provide mentoring to the medical staff for the development of a similar note geared toward the provider group.

these practices to align with evidence, helping them become efficient and directing processes to support patients in disease management. Although the priority for process improvement is often with high-risk complex patients, the CNL also examines health promotion and disease prevention–oriented processes in this primary care setting. Because the CNL is an expert at process redesign using evidence and is also a skilled direct care provider, the CNL role involves mentoring and role modeling for nursing staff. Examples of where the CNL can role model and mentor staff to develop highly reliable approaches to care include the use of disease registries, information technology tools such as those reporting quantitative outcomes, and decision support systems. CNLs assist nursing staff in identifying patients who are highly complex, underpowered, and inefficient healthcare users, as well as underpowered patients who would benefit from prevention interventions. The evaluation of the CNL role can be measured by improved patient activation and biochemical, cost, efficiency, and other quantitative clinical outcomes. The success of the role of the CNL can also be gauged through measures geared to support of the practice of nursing such as reduced turnover, enhanced certification rates, and nurse satisfaction scores. In order for the CNL to maintain the ability to support clinical nursing, the CNL will lead the care for a group of patients. The CNL should provide direct care with a purpose beyond that of staff. Appropriate goals for CNLs in the role of direct care provision include participating in tests of change/process improvement evaluations, assessing processes to prepare for improvement, and mentoring or role modeling.

Jukkala, Greenwood, Ladner, and Hopkins (2010) describe the CNL role in a rural setting as geared to maximize wellness, health promotion, and risk reduction, and education programs by mentoring direct interaction with patients. The CNL in the outpatient setting has a substantial opportunity to improve many of the areas of care that are highly related to patient activation, such as weight management, tobacco and substance use, activity levels, medication management, and symptom recognition. The strengths of the CNL in ambulatory care are the skills in the use of clinical evidence regarding approaches, the use of data systems and systems redesign to implement evidence, and the power of the individual's adaptation of evidence as a care manager.

The CNL in the Long-Term Care Setting

There is a monumental role for the CNL in improving care and care processes for older Americans residing in long-term care (LTC) facilities. The CNL can work to improve clinical quality and respect for individual patients' preferences. The movement to improve quality of care in LTC facilities has been a slower process than quality improvement in the acute care setting. The Omnibus Budget Reconciliation Act of 1987 was the first national legislation to focus on quality outcomes in the LTC setting and to deliver sanctions for failure to achieve identified quality outcomes. The quality outcomes outlined in this act laid the foundation for the development of the national minimum data set (MDS) for documenting nursing care for public reporting of quality indicators (Weiner, Freiman, & Brown, 2007). This MDS clinical reporting system is one of the newer tools that will enable the CNL to measure outcomes. The MDS creates LTC population-based reports on quality for common clinical indicators. The trending of the clinical outcomes and the use of the specific data elements collected to create the outcome report provide the CNL with a data system for measurement.

The transition of the CNL role into the LTC setting lags behind the acute care setting, making the evidence of outcomes sparse. Recent improvement work in the LTC setting suggests that the CNL role may be exactly the nursing role needed in this setting. Rantz and colleagues (2012) reported that having a nursing leader with expert clinical skills to provide training and education, role modeling, and form clinical teams to use the MDS clinical data with process improvement cycles could create and sustain a meaningful improvement in clinical quality. The nurse in the role is described as a champion team builder, with a commitment to quality care. Nursing care given in LTC facilities is largely provided by nonnurse staff such as nursing assistants and licensed practical/vocational nurses. The clinical leadership in nursing and the development of strong clinical teams and clinical processes has been shown to have a larger effect on quality than staffing numbers or a staffing mix of developer/educator or director of nursing/supervisor (Rantz et al., 2004). Denham and colleagues (2008) documented the crucial role of communication and teamwork in providing a safe care environment. The CNL builds a clinical team of nurses and nonnursing staff using available resources, including gerontologists, gerontology APNs, mental health APNs; and wound, incontinence, and nursing safety specialists as they are available to be team members.

For example, one CNL in a facility recruited members of the rehabilitation staff, the dining room staff, and the nurses and nursing assistants to flow map the resources needed to mobilize resident patients to communal dining and to create an environment that facilitated increased nutrition and decreased dehydration while providing the therapy required by the resident patients in this transitional post-hospital setting (Hix, Mckeon, & Walters, 2009). The system analyst focused on the role of current nursing processes, the use of clinical evidence, and MDS data with the other professional and technical staff. In order to understand processes, CNLs provide hands-on nursing care and must have an intimate working knowledge of the effects of tests of change. In participating in change, the CNL is able to perceive areas for refinement before full analysis is completed.

Translating quality data from the MDS is crucial for the CNL in the LTC setting. Understanding the values of the data input, the power of the data to allow for change, and respect for the process is important to improving care, as well as financing the industry. Knowing how to "speak" MDS is a skill that many staff may not be fully versed in, even though they are providing daily care. The MDS assessment tool collects information about the type of care needed for an individual LTC resident and indicates actual or potential interdisciplinary team concerns that need to be addressed or monitored. For most, the process is complete at this step. The LTC CNL knows the purpose of the MDS is much broader than just completing an assessment and submitting for payment. The MDS data ultimately present outcomes known as quality indicators and measures, which are primarily based on actual nursing care.

The CNL can assist LTC facilities to make the transition to a newer model of delivery of care in the LTC setting that focuses on the creation of a "homelike setting." The focus of the CNL as a clinical nurse in the LTC setting is to balance patient centeredness and respect for human dignity with efficient and evidence-based processes. The CNL can examine and flow map to implement small tests of change, which can then become processes that balance the delivery of care with respect for the resident patient in their "home." The VHA Community Living Centers (CLC) are participating in the Advancing Excellence in America's Nursing Homes initiative to improve the goal of consistent assignment and clinical improvement in pain management. Consistent assignment reduces the number of caregivers who take care of an LTC resident during a month in order to enhance the provision of personnel preferences, reduce confusion and delirium, and promote early recognition in change in clinical status. The CNL leading the clinical microsystem team in these efforts will make tremendous contributions to the well-being of LTC resident patients.

Summary

- The examples in this chapter provide a general overview of how the CNL supports quality improvement and evidence implementation in a patient-centered manner to achieve population outcomes while respecting individual autonomy.
- In order to improve care at the bedside or within a nursing unit, it seems counterproductive to seek more education and then move away from direct patient care. The introduction of the CNL role within nursing reduces provides a solution to this challenge.

- Nurses choosing a career at the point of care have the opportunity to be academically educated with the skills needed to effect change.
- The ultimate goal of every nurse is to improve the care provided to all patients, either with help of a CNL or by becoming a CNL.

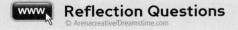

Reflection Questions

© Arenacreative/Dreamstime.com

1. What are the most important quality- and safety-related nursing-sensitive areas that could benefit from interventions to improve outcomes on your unit?
2. What processes did you use to determine which areas are the most important (e.g., volume, cost, potential for mortality or morbidity)?
3. How can the role of the CNL contribute to the improvement of outcomes in the areas identified as the most important?

Learning Activities

© Arenacreative/Dreamstime.com

1. Choose a nursing-sensitive issue to target for an improvement intervention. Develop a question to address a clinical concern and organize the evidence. Map out the current work flow processes related to the nursing care. Using the evidence (desired state) and the current workflow (as-is state), develop change ideas and implement plan-do-study-act (PDSA) cycles as tests of change. What process and or outcome indicators will be best suited for evaluation of the changes?
2. Consider a nursing quality or safety area of concern that occurs on an inpatient specialty care unit. Then develop a model for using the expertise of the CNL and the clinical nurse specialist to promote teamwork and achieve desired clinical outcomes while advocating for individual patient choice.

References

American College of Physicians. (n.d). Patient-centered medical home. Retrieved from http://www.acponline.org/running_practice/delivery_and_payment_models/pcmh/understanding/index.html

American Nurses Association. (2001). *Code of ethics for nurses with interpretive statements.* Silver Springs, MD. Author.

Begun, J. W., Torabeni, J., & White, K. D. (2006). Opportunities for improving patient care through lateral integration. The clinical nurse leaders. *Journal of Healthcare Management, 51*, 19–25.

Coleman, K., Austin, B. T., Brach, C., & Wagner, E. H. (2009). Evidence on the chronic care model in the new millennium. *Health Affairs, 28*(1), 75–85. doi: 10.1377/hlthaff.28.1.75

Dartmouth Institute for Clinical Microsystems. (n.d.) Home page. Retrieved from http://clinicalmicrosystem.org/materials/worbook

DeBoer, E. C. (2011). *Continuous renal replacement therapy for acute renal failure in the critically ill.* CNL Summit. Miami Marriott Biscayne Bay, Miami, FL.

Denham, C. R., Dingman, J., Foley, M. E., Ford, D., Martins, B., O'Regan, P., & Salamendra, A. (2008). Are you listening…are you really listening? *Journal of Patient Safety, 4*(3), 148–162.

Hix, C., Mckeon, L., & Walters, S. (2009). Clinical nurse leader impact on clinical microsystem outcomes. *Journal of Nursing Administration, 39,* 71–76.

Institute of Medicine. (2001). *Crossing the quality chasm: A new health system for the 21st century.* Washington, DC: National Academy Press.

Jukkala, A., Greenwood, R., Ladner, K., & Hopkins, L. (2010). The clinical nurse leaders and rural health. *Online Journal of Rural Nursing and Health Care, 10,* 38–44.

Kimball, B., Joynt, J., Cherner, D., & O'Neil, E. (2007). The quest for new innovative care delivery models. *Journal of Nursing Administration, 37*(9), 392–398.

Nelson, E. C., Batalden, P. B., Homa, K., Godfrey, M. M., Campbell, C., Headrick, L. A., … Wasson, J. H. (2003). Microsystems in healthcare: Part two, creating a rich environment. *Joint Commission on Quality and Safety, 29*(1), 5–15.

Rantz, M. J., Hicks, L., Grando, V., Petroski, G. F., Madsen, R. W., Mehr, D. R., … Mass, M. (2004). Nursing home quality, cost, staffing and staff mix. *Gerontologist, 44,* 24–38.

Rantz, M. J., Zwagarty-Stauffacher, M., Flesner, M., Hicks, L., Mehr, D., Russel, T., & Minner, D. (2012). Challenge of using quality improvement methods in nursing homes "needing improvement." *Journal of the American Medical Directors Association, 13,* 732–738.

Reid, K., & Dennison, P., (2011). The clinical nurse leader: Point-of-care safety clinician. *OJIN: The Online Journal of Issues in Nursing 16*(3), Manuscript 4. doi:10.3912/OJIN.Vol16No03Man04

Rusch, L., & Bakewell-Sachs, S. (2007). The CNL: A gateway to better care? *Nursing Management, 38*(4), 32, 34, 36–37.

Sherman, R., Clark, J., & Maloney, J. (2008). Developing the clinical nurse leader in the twelve bed hospital project: An education/service partnership. *Nurse Leader, 6*(3), 54–58.

Stanton, M. (2006). The health care quality challenge and the clinical nurse leader role (CNL). *Online Journal of Rural Nursing and Healthcare, 6.*

Wagner, E. H., Austin, B. T., Davis, C., Hindmarch, M., Schaefer, J., & Bonomi, A. (2001). Improving chronic illness care: Translating evidence into action. *Health Affairs, 20,* 64–78.

Weiner, J. M., Freiman, M. P., & Brown, D. (2007). *Nursing home care quality. Twenty years after the OMBA of 1987.* A Kaiser Foundation report. Retrieved from http://www.kff.org/medicare/upload/7717.pdf

CNLs Assigned to the 12-Bed Hospital Model

■ Donna Whitehead

WellStar Health System (WHS), located northwest of Atlanta, GA, embarked on a journey to place clinical nurse leaders (CNLs) on all acute care units in its five hospitals. WellStar granted scholarships to 40 baccalaureate (BSN) nurses. These nurses are currently enrolled at the University of West Georgia. CNL students were assigned to full-time, paid positions in acute care units during their immersion experience. The immersion experience allowed the CNL students to concentrate on implementing their newly acquired knowledge and skills to improve patient outcomes.

WHS is bringing the master's-prepared CNL to the bedside by implementing the 12-bed hospital model of care delivery. In the 12-bed hospital model, the CNLs' primary purpose will be to act as patient navigators and central contacts for communication working 5 days a week for continuity of care. The CNL will oversee the care of about 12 patients, allowing for adequate time for patient–CNL relationships to be built and critical situations addressed or prevented. The CNL will not be taking a patient load but serving the nursing team as role model and bedside leader.

WHS is where dreams of better healthcare come true. Now senior nursing leaders envision CNLs practicing on all inpatient units and expanding to the outpatient arena.

"patient navigators/central contacts"

CNL and Microsystem Assessment on a Trauma Unit

■ Tiffany Tscherne

Critical Thinking

The trauma program manager (TPM) is responsible for assessing the microsystem of the trauma patient to find out why poor outcomes have been obtained, and/or why evidence-based guidelines are not being adhered to. Through application of the chosen quality improvement model (plan-do-check-act [PDCA]), the how it can be corrected is created by the TPM as the CNL student in consultation with the trauma medical director or multidisciplinary trauma operations committee.

The microsystem assessment can be as simple as interviews, or as complex as work flow diagrams and retrospective analysis of charts and data from the trauma registry. Upon completion of the assessment through the CNL's clinical immersion experience, the CNL completed a new design for the corrections process and selected the outcome metrics, based on regulatory guidelines such as the American College of Surgeons or the state of Michigan, in concert with evidence-based practice.

Communication

In addition to email, the CNL student must master both business and clinical venues of communication. The CNL student in the TPM role is responsible for developing high-level reports to senior leadership utilizing the A3 and other standard formats. Identifying the route of communication with the direct-care level provider is necessary for program operations. So, familiarity with marketing tools throughout the hospital as well as the staff communication venues allows the TPM (CNL student) to share everything from "kudos" to classes to educational tools.

learn marketing tools
- pt
- agency (internal)

Assessment

The CNL student's assessment focused on identification of the primary trauma population for the area served by the hospital. In my case, falls in those over the age of 55, with orthopedic injury are my primary population of interest. The information on falls was obtained through chart reviews, usage trends, the Michigan Hospital Association MIDAS database, and the hospital's central data warehouse.

Why is this knowledge so important? It allows us to focus on our injury prevention activities to the community that we serve. While handing out bicycle helmets to children is a noble cause, it doesn't help the seniors who are falling due to poor knowledge of fall risks. Anticipating the risk allows us to decrease the high mortality rates that often follow falls in those considered to be in their golden years.

Assessment of the microsystem, especially when poor outcomes or regulatory standards are not being met, is a primary job role of the TPM. Whether through the 5 Ps, (patients/population, purpose, philosophy [mission], processes, and patterns), or a fishbone chart, the TPM utilizes tools to answer why this issue or outcome is occurring. This microsystem assessment when done correctly, will yield valuable information and data to improve fall reduction outcomes for the elder population.

Health Promotion, Risk Reduction, and Disease Prevention

Injury prevention activities are a mandate for a trauma center according to the American College of Surgeons. As discussed, after an assessment of the primary trauma risks to the community, the CNL student evaluates EBP to develop a plan that best addresses the risk. The CNL student develops the outcome matrix tool, gathers the relevant data from the trauma registry, and then reports the findings to the trauma operations committee. No change in outcomes? Back into the PDCA it goes!

So who is responsible for delivering the programming? The CNL serves as the primary creator and the educator as well by going out into the community to give lectures, provide health fairs, and to also serve on committees throughout the community. This level of community involvement lends the CNL expertise to shape policy for health promotion, risk reduction, and disease prevention.

Illness and Disease Management

The CNL student served as the case manager for the trauma patient throughout the care spectrum. Yes, the CNL student served as one of the primary authors of the process, but she will also be the de facto case manager for the trauma patient through daily rounding, participating in multidisciplinary care planning, and applying both EBP and regulatory guidelines in order to shape a positive patient outcome.

Information and Healthcare Technologies

In addition to being a clinical care force, the TPM is responsible for the trauma registry. The trauma registry serves as a clinical repository for trauma patient care data on a myriad of data points ranging from demographics to procedures and even comorbidities. The CNL student is responsible for the operations of the data collection, creating the data collection process, data integrity, and the management of the trauma registry.

Healthcare Systems and Policy

Writing policy, managing all aspects of trauma center operations including staff and budget, are part of the CNL student's role expectations. A CNL student managed a team of two or more and assumed responsibility for office operations. The CNL student is responsible for the trauma services budget, which can include not only paper clips, but on-call fees for physicians, and well as staff trauma training for an entire hospital.

The CNL student writes policy that affects not only trauma services, but the operations of the entire multidisciplinary team in regards to the trauma patient. Trauma policy must remain valid and applicable as the patient moves from the ED to diagnostic testing, to the inpatient realm, and upon discharge and transfer. Policies on trauma activations, transfer criteria, and even trauma education are crafted under the guidance of the CNL student.

Designer/Manager/Coordinator of Care

The CNL student bears the responsibility for the cornerstone of the trauma program for any hospital, of any size or designation: the process improvement/patient safety (PIPS) program. The PIPS program consists of daily activities, through trauma rounding and chart review, up to committee action by a physician peer review or the multidisciplinary operations committee. Whether a patient care failure or process failure, the issue moves through one of three levels of review, guided by the CNL student. The CNL student serves as the chief researcher, facilitator, and even outcomes manager for the issue in order to ensure loop closure.

CNS overlap?

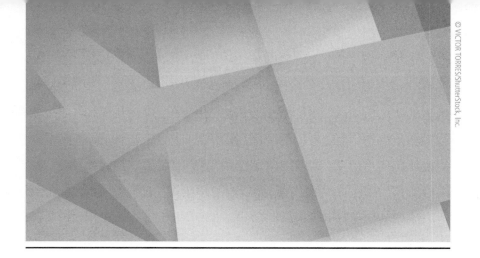

UNIT 5
Foundations for CNL Success

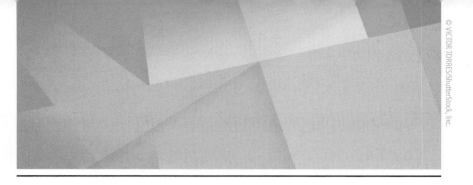

TWENTY-ONE

Creative and Meaningful Clinical Immersions

 Patricia L. Thomas, James L. Harris, and Linda Roussel

www Learning Objectives
© Arenacreative/Dreamstime.com

- Discuss why it is important for a clinical nurse leader to conduct a needs assessment and a gap analysis prior to beginning the clinical immersion experience.
- Discuss the importance of using business principles during the clinical immersion experience.
- Describe the role of nursing, clinical, and ancillary department leaders in the development of the clinical immersion experience.
- Discuss techniques and components to include when developing a portfolio of clinical experiences.
- Discuss the relevance of metrics for addressing needs and gaps during the immersion experience.

> There is only one thing stronger than all the armies in the world, and this is an idea whose time has come.
>
> **Victor Hugo**

Key Terms

Needs assessment	Gap analysis	Portfolio	
Business principles	Planning	Metrics	Collaboration

CNL Roles

Clinician	Outcomes manager	Coordinator of care
Information manager	Life-long learner	Team manager
Systems analyst/risk anticipator	Member of a profession	

CNL Professional Values

Accountability	Fiscal stewardship	Outcome measurement
Microsystem management	Quality improvement	
Evidence-based practice	Interdisciplinary teams	
Integrity	Quality patient care and safety	

CNL Core Competencies

Communication	Assessment
Environment of care management	
Membership in a profession	Team leadership
Design/management/coordination of care	
Information and healthcare technologies	

Introduction

An imperative for educating future generations is a philosophical and programmatic transformation that is aligned with the changing healthcare delivery system and reform legislation (Diefenbeck, Plowfield, & Herrman, 2006). Meaningful and innovative clinical immersions are imperative for clinical nurse leader (CNL) students to develop the skills to respond to the changing care environment. Immersions are the culmination of the academic and clinical experiences in a CNL program; their usefulness can be limited when faculty, clinical partners, and students do not mutually identify needs and create developmental opportunities within a microsystem. Clinical immersions for the CNL student should be based on identifying and assessing gaps and needs

> **Plans are nothing: planning is everything.**
>
> Dwight D. Eisenhower

within an organization that is focused on improving the health of a population of patients within a given microsystem. This critical point cannot be overstated. Without thoughtful planning that is detailed and deliberate, the clinical immersion experience can be misaligned and opportunities for successful launching into the CNL role can be missed.

Nelson, Batalden, and Godfrey (2007) identified the importance of discovering the microsystem by studying its "5 *Ps*"—purpose, patients, professionals, processes, and patterns—and the ways each of the parts interacts with one another. Even the smallest measurable details should be analyzed, and iterative work redesign and learning cycles should be developed that result in changing work processes and developing database and feedback systems at the microsystem level. Thus, gaps between the unit and organizational levels are closed, improvement in the usefulness of information occurs, and a management focus that corresponds with the real work is created. The unit of work is therefore aligned with the unit of analysis and unit of intervention (Nelson et al., 2007; Norman, 2007).

A meaningful clinical immersion is established when CNL students are able to integrate their course work into valued clinical work through the enactment of the CNL role. The clinical immersion experience is intended to provide the platform to support transformative learning, initially for the CNL student and the microsystem, and eventually for the organization. Transformative learning is the culmination of past experiences and perspectives, joined with new learning, to support resocialization. Resocialization involves critical reflection on past and present perspectives in an effort to understand the learner's essential self and thinking processes. Beliefs and old ways of thinking are examined, and critical reflection is triggered, leading to alternative ways of thinking and acting. Within a clinical immersion experience, students are encouraged and supported in changing their worldviews and roles, as well as in internalizing new ways of thinking, communicating, and behaving. They are supported by a precepted clinical immersion experience in a microsystem (Mezirow, 1997; Morris & Faulk, 2007). Fundamental to early outcomes, clinical partners and students need to question assumptions, beliefs, and values and consider multiple points of view while seeking to verify the rationale for the clinical immersion experience (Bouchard & Steel, 1980; Mezirow, 1997; Stanley, Holing, Burton, Harris, & Norman, 2007).

Because the CNL role is new, many CNL students and organizations struggle with developing an appropriate immersion experience. There are a limited number of CNL preceptors in a system. CNL faculty and nurse leaders are challenged to create structured immersions using CNL competencies and existing organizational roles. Their goal is to establish a tapestry of experiences that allows the novice CNL to use knowledge and skills that validate competence and that also addresses organizational needs within a microsystem.

Using Data and Resources to Identify Needs and Craft Meaningful Clinical Immersions

A variety of data and resources that correspond to the learning objectives of the CNL student are available for analysis at the microsystem level. Examples include balanced scorecards, quality markers, performance and target measures, satisfaction indices, and actions to reduce or eliminate inefficient practices. The identified microsystem gaps can be transformed into meaningful clinical immersion experiences and projects that develop CNL students, create additional examples of outcomes for their portfolio, and benefit the overall function of the unit. In examining unit data, CNL students can identify an area of interest to allow an innovative approach to issues that are easily recognized in the microsystem. **Table 21-1** provides examples of clinical project data and sources.

Selection and scoping of the clinical immersion is pivotal to success for both the CNL student and the organization that sponsors the immersion. The planning process, whereby the CNL student, the CNL faculty member, and the nurse leaders in the organization come together to craft a deliberate and detailed plan for success, is key. Outcome data can point the CNL student and faculty to areas that require change, but a critical success factor for the CNL is the ability to apply new tools and knowledge to "old problems." A potential pitfall for the clinical immersion experience is addressing a current situation with past problem-solving strategies, rather than engaging innovative and creative tools and tactics derived from evidence-based interventions found in the literature.

Table 21-1   Unit Clinical Project Data and Source

Type of Data	Source of Data/ Data Collection Method	Target Compliance Percentage	Actual Compliance Percentage
Troponin level returned to provider for review and action within 60 minutes of order	Acute coronary syndrome performance measure **Balanced scorecard**	100	90
Percentage of patients who received smoking cessation at least once during inpatient admission	Smoking cessation performance measure; inpatient **Inpatient education tracking**	80	50
Percentage of inpatients diagnosed with heart failure who received all five components of the discharge instructions	Heart failure discharge instructions; inpatient **Balanced scorecard**	100	15
Percentage of patient readmissions with heart failure within 30 days	Patient education on admission, during hospitalization, and telephone contact within 1 week of discharge **Balanced scorecard**	100	85
Percentage of skin assessment completion on admission and daily during hospitalization	Admission and daily skin documentation **Inpatient skin assessment form**	100	92
Percentage of overall patient satisfaction scores with admission and discharge processes	Patient satisfaction metrics **Press Ganey survey scores, patient satisfaction**	5*	4.2*

*Based on 5-point Likert scale where 1 = very poor and 5 = very good

The American Association of Colleges of Nurses' (AACN's) *White Paper on the Role of the Clinical Nurse Leader* (2007), the *CNL Job Analysis Study* (AACN, 2011), and strategic review of current organizational role competencies found in nursing and ancillary departments are key to the development of the clinical immersion experience. Often, no single person or department holds responsibility for measurement, leadership, and integration of practices. With support from CNL faculty and nurse leaders, the CNL student in an immersion experience has an opportunity to establish new relationships, new dialogue, new teams, and new ways to approach microsystem concerns. Detailed review and documentation of current process and practices and identification of points of coordination and competence can position the CNL students in their immersion environments to deal with complexities and organizational culture and norms. A thorough gap analysis is the starting point for their work. After identifying gaps, the CNL student can organize a clinical immersion project that meets the needs of the objectives in the clinical immersion course while simultaneously addressing important concerns in the organization. Linking a microsystem issue or concern to the planning of the immersion project then benefits both the student and the organization. Using the unit assessment tools provided in didactic courses offers the CNL a framework for analyzing opportunities in the microsystem. The assessment tool provides a springboard for specific problem identification, which leads to quality improvement methodologies, team engagement, and team leader opportunities, as well as specific measures and metrics to demonstrate outcomes. This also creates additional examples of outcomes for the CNL student's portfolio, benefits patient care delivery and patient outcomes, and ultimately creates a system transformation that builds a continuous improvement culture.

> **Start by doing what's necessary, then what's possible, and suddenly you are doing the impossible.**
>
> St. Francis of Assisi

When establishing a project status summary, attention needs to be placed on the process and patterns that the student observes in terms of collaboration with the interdisciplinary team members, inclusion of staff in quality improvement initiatives, relationships established with departments or project champions in the organization, and the responses of patients, family, and staff. Because CNLs are expected to serve as the team or project leader, insights are gained as students reflect on their interactions and leadership skills are expanded. CNL students can use tools from their didactic learning or incorporate the sponsoring organization's tools so that future replication and organizational learning can occur. For team and project leaders, leadership skills are requisite as projects and supporting structures and processes that then foster collaboration and redesign of care delivery within a given microsystem evolve (Cebel, Rebitzer, & Taylor, 2006; Porter-O'Grady, Clark, & Wiggins, 2010). **Figure 21-1** is an example format for a clinical summary project.

Applying the Business Model to CNL Clinical Immersions

The often uncontrollable issues in clinical settings can interfere with the development of innovative approaches to problem resolution and work redesign. Staff members find themselves performing multiple tasks, getting trapped in existent business models and processes that are ineffective and obsolete. Without insight, the CNL student's clinical immersion experiences may be less than meaningful and lack innovation that demonstrates the incorporation and integration of advances of new technologies and methods (Hwang & Christensen, 2008). This raises the question of how to use the elements of a business model to guide a CNL clinical immersion experience.

According to Hwang and Christensen (2008), all business models consist of three components: a value proposition, resources and processes, and a profit formula. The value proposition is the service (quality and safe patient care) that assists an individual in accomplishing desired goals and objectives. In order for the clinical

---

Figure 21-1   Clinical project status summary.

Summary of Project:

Problems Encountered:	*Actions Taken:*	*Milestone Achievements:*
1.	1.	1.
2.	2.	2.

Planned Activities and Milestones for Next Reporting Period:

---

immersion experience to be successful, resources must be dedicated, including expert and knowledgeable staff, engagement of academic partners, and the equipment necessary to provide care. Processes are identified to ensure activities and actions that result in desired outcomes are developed and initiated and are framed for data capture and future trending. The final component is the profit formula, where any organization determines the costs and benefits that can be sustained over time. Organizations can use this model as other services are envisioned and ultimately offered. The CNL student and the assigned preceptor can use this model as a road map in developing the clinical immersion experience.

The CNL student can work with clinicians and managers to develop a cost–benefit analysis in concert with course objectives. This project can continue throughout the entire clinical immersion. An example of a clinical immersion experience for a CNL student that incorporates each of the three components of the business model is illustrated in **Table 21-2**.

The Usefulness of Portfolios

The dynamic nature of the healthcare environment and the changing market with greater focus on value-based care requires educators to use innovative methods to measure learning outcomes. A professional portfolio is one such method. The portfolio is a summary and history of collected documents that showcases accomplishments and documents continuous improvement. It demonstrates how various elements of a professional's role functions are related, highlighting competence and the development of a role over time (Billings & Kowalski, 2008; Sherrod, 2005). Right from the beginning of their coursework in a CNL program, students should start collecting documents from assigned classroom activities and save examples of their writing and accomplishments. The examples become a tool kit that can be shared with prospective employers to demonstrate accomplishments shared on a resume. The examples become the vehicle to communicate to a prospective employer that academic knowledge has been translated into meaningful actions and interventions that can be used to improve a microsystem. Upon graduation, the portfolio is used to persuade an employer or supervisor that the CNL can enact AACN's CNL end-of-program competencies (AACN, 2006) and that the student has the experience to support what is claimed on his or her resume.

The portfolio presented at the fruition of a clinical immersion experience chronicles the process(es) and evidence used to successfully complete the capstone

Table 21-2   Clinical Immersion Project: Medical/Psychiatric Unit

Value Proposition	Resources and Processes	Profit Formula
Medical/psychiatric unit dedicated to comprehensive care for patients requiring acute and chronic medical and psychiatric interventions by an interdisciplinary team skilled in medical and psychiatric care	Unit design and construction, staff development, equipment purchase and staff training, and marketing strategies that include patient education materials	Cost–benefit analysis that includes all start-up costs and savings of a comprehensive unit that eliminates transfer of psychiatric patients with acute and chronic medical problems off a medical unit that historically required 1:1 sitters

project. The portfolio document for the clinical immersion includes a detailed plan that identifies the microsystem problem to be addressed, project objectives, deliverables, time lines, and data or metrics. Less evident to an untrained eye are the redesign efforts undertaken to improve clinical outcomes of care for the population of the microsystem and the leadership efforts required to guide an interdisciplinary team to success.

Aside from the information related to the CNL's education, licensure, work experience, and certifications, additional tips for creating effective portfolio designs include:

1. Creating a well designed cover;
2. Placing information behind tabs to organize the content;
3. Using colorful charts or graphics to demonstrate impact or outcomes achieved; and,
4. Include examples that illustrate cost savings and innovations (Elbow & Belanoff, 1997).

Performance Contracts

As CNLs graduate and accept positions, the performance contract is a common mechanism used to define the role expectations and markers of impact and success. The portfolio documentation serves as a quick reference to prospective employers about past performance—evidence that CNL performance has been demonstrated in the past and can be expected in the future. An example of a performance contract is shown in **Figure 21-2**.

Measurement of CNL Success

The challenge for the CNL student and those in practice is to design methods that measure impact and clinical outcomes that are sustainable. Nelson and colleagues (2007) stated that measurement is forward progress, and clinical leaders functioning within a microsystem must engage all staff to be innovative and creative and to participate in the improvement of healthcare delivery. Didactic coursework and clinical immersions must prepare the CNL student to understand and collaboratively develop measurement tools that are applicable to the practice environment. Within all microsystems are numerous data points waiting to be mined, analyzed, and displayed. Creating an area to display data as a "data board" allows the CNL to visually demonstrate each metric for the members of the microsystem to observe. This is a key role for the CNL. The data should represent the current value or target and the impacts over a period of time. This information can drive clinical and quality improvements and identify other improvement projects that are necessary to meet

Figure 21-2   Clinical nurse leader performance contract.

Rating Period: _____–_____

Name: _____   Unit Assigned: _____

Measure	Target	Comments from Quarterly Review
Infectious disease: Blood cultures collected before administration of first antibiotic	93%	
Immunizations: Patients received immunization during flu season (_____–_____)	90%	
Inpatient satisfaction: Evidence of satisfied inpatients during each stay	95% (6 months post-introduction of the CNL)	

_____/_____   _____
Clinical Nurse Leader/ Supervisor Signatures   Date

organizational goals, regulatory requirements, and specific microsystem improvements that ultimately enhance quality and delivery of care.

But how does the CNL identify appropriate metrics? A starting point is to review unit goals, the population served, and the services provided. For example, a CNL assigned to a long-term care area may focus on increasing residents' functional status by measuring involvement in daily activities offered by staff. The CNL assigned to an ambulatory surgery unit can measure the number of cancellations and the financial impacts incurred by each cancellation. This can be further measured and trended by service or product. The information can then be used by the project improvement team to develop strategies and tactics to improve efficiency. These are only two examples of the many projects CNLs can measure and have an impact on to enhance both financial and quality outcomes within a microsystem.

Summary

- CNL clinical experiences must be creatively developed, meaningful to the student, and add value for the organization.
- Multiple data and other resources are readily available for CNL students to access when developing a clinical immersion project.
- The business case for a CNL project must be supported by outcomes and evidence-based data.
- Portfolios of CNL projects can be of value to healthcare facilities for displaying quality outcomes and partnerships with academic affiliates, and to the CNL for applying for positions.
- A performance contact is a useful method for the CNL and the organization to track successes and identify opportunities for improvement.

WWW Reflection Questions
© Arenacreative/Dreamstime.com

1. What part of the clinical immersion project do you feel most prepared for? What part do you feel least prepared for?
2. What are the critical elements of a clinical immersion project?
3. What resources do you have to assist you in completing the clinical immersion?
4. What documents do you have that demonstrate your skills and accomplishments in the CNL role?

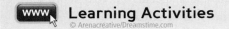

Learning Activities

1. Gather documents to create a professional portfolio. Consider how you will organize the information. Share your ideas and documents with a classmate and ask him or her to perform a peer review.
2. Form a group with two or three other students and brainstorm about assignments that have been completed that would be appropriate for inclusion in your portfolios.
3. Bring a project plan that you have completed for a past project to class. The project plan should include a time line with detailed action steps, contact persons/responsible parties, and deliverables. Describe how a project plan for your clinical immersion would be different from this previous project plan.

References

American Association of Colleges of Nursing. (2006, May). *End-of-program competencies & required clinical experiences for the clinical nurse leader*. Retrieved from http://apps.aacn .nche.edu/CNL/pdf/EndCompsgrid.pdf

American Association of Colleges of Nursing. (2007). *White paper on the role of the clinical nurse leader*. Retrieved from http://www.aacn.nche.edu/publications/white-papers/cnl

American Association of Colleges of Nursing. (2011). CNL job analysis study. Retrieved from http://www.aacn.nche.edu/cnl/publications-resources/job-analysis-study

Billings, D., & Kowalski, K. (2008). Developing your career as a nurse educator: The professional portfolio. *Journal of Continuing Education in Nursing, 39*(12), 532–533.

Bouchard, J., & Steel, M. (1980). Contract learning. *Canadian Nurse, 76*(1), 44–48.

Cebel, R., Rebitzer, J., & Taylor, R. (2006). Organizational fragmentation and care quality in the US health care system. *Journal of Economic Perspectives, 22,* 93–111.

Diefenbeck, C. A., Plowfield, L. A., & Herrman, J. W. (2006). Clinical immersion. A residency model for nursing education. *Nursing Education Perspectives, 27*(2), 72–79.

Elbow, P., & Belanoff, P. (1997). Reflections on an explosion: Portfolios in the 90's and beyond. In K. Yancey & I. Weiser (Eds.), *Situating portfolios: Four perspectives* (pp. 21–33). Logan, UT: Utah University Press.

Hwang, J., & Christensen, C. M. (2008). Technology: New technologies demand new business models. In *Futurescan: Healthcare trends and implications 2008–2013*. Chicago, IL: Health Administration Press.

Mezirow, J. (1997). Transformative learning: Theory to practice. *New Directions for Adult and Continuing Education, 74,* 5–12.

Morris, A. H., & Faulk, D. (2007). Perspective transformation: Enhancing the development of professionalism in the RN-to-BSN students. *Journal of Nursing Education, 46*(10), 445–461.

Nelson, E. C., Batalden, P. B., & Godfrey, M. M. (2007). *Quality by design. A clinical microsystems approach.* San Francisco, CA: Jossey-Bass.

Norman, L. (2007). Lecture, Vanderbilt University, Nashville, TN.

Porter-O'Grady, T., Clark, J. S., & Wiggins, M. (2010). The case for clinical nurse leaders: Guiding nursing practice into the 21st century. *Nurse Leader, 8,* 37–41.

Sherrod, D. (2005). The professional portfolio: A snapshot of your career. *Nursing Management, 36*(9), 74–75.

Stanley, J., Holing, J., Burton, D., Harris, J., & Norman, L. (2007). Implementing innovation through education practice partnerships. *Nursing Outlook, 55*(2), 67–73.

The Dedicated Education Unit: Innovative Model for Preparing Preceptors for CNL Clinical Experiences

Sherry Webb and Tommie Norris

Key terms: preceptor, dedicated education units, clinical teachers

Aim: To prepare preceptors for CNL clinical experiences

A new model nationwide for clinical education, the dedicated education unit (DEU), is a microsystem that is developed as an exemplar teaching–learning environment through the collaborative efforts of staff nurses, nursing administrators of the academic and practice partners, and nursing faculty. Students are educated in a positive clinical learning environment that maximizes student learning outcomes, uses proven teaching–learning strategies, and capitalizes on the expertise of both practice partner staff nurses and faculty.

The University of Tennessee Health's Science Center College of Nursing and its practice partner developed 6 DEUs for CNL clinical education over a 3-year period for its 2-year accelerated master's-entry CNL (Model C) program. Expert staff nurses, who were not CNLs, were selected by their nurse manager to serve as "clinical teachers" on the DEUs. In addition to prior hospital preceptor training, the clinical teachers, unit managers, and clinical unit educators were prepared for their roles during a 1-day workshop held at the College of Nursing. Participants received paid leave and were rewarded a certificate of completion, which could be used toward advancement on the agency's career ladder. Experienced faculty provided instruction for the workshop, which focused on the CNL role, quality and safety education for nurses (QSEN) competencies, adult learning principles, teaching–learning principles, and student evaluation. Because the preceptors were not practicing CNLs, a discussion of the AACN's CNL white paper and end-of-program outcomes was initiated, providing the opportunity to better understand experiences required in the clinical setting. Adult learning principles reinforced the individual learning needs influenced by prior life experiences. Students enrolled in the CNL program completed a "learning style inventory" and were asked to share their learning style with their clinical teacher to facilitate learning opportunities. Clinical teachers also completed the learning style inventory to better understand how best to provide instruction. Simulated clinical experiences provided experiences that included dealing with difficult conversations, summative versus formative evaluations, and recording anecdotal notes. Clinical teachers received ongoing support for their new role by working collaboratively with CNL faculty assigned to the DEU.

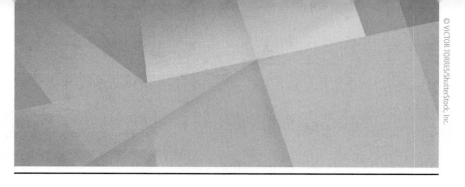

© VICTOR TORRES/ShutterStock, Inc.

TWENTY-TWO

Toward Achieving Desired Outcomes: The Clinical Nurse Leader's Transition to Practice

◼ Alice E. Avolio and Marjory D. Williams

 Learning Objectives
© Arenacreative/Dreamstime.com

- ◼ Describe the clinical nurse leader residency/transition to practice program
- ◼ Identify core elements included in a clinical nurse leader residency/transition to practice program, as well as the rationale and desired outcomes of such programs
- ◼ Describe clinical nurse leader residency/transition to practice program content

> **You first must be a believer if you would be an achiever.**
>
> **Anonymous**

Key Terms

CNL residency program	Outcomes	Evidence-based practice

CNL Roles

Outcomes manager	Clinician	Advocate
Information manager	Communicator	Educator
Life-long learner		

CNL Professional Values

Accountability	Integrity

CNL Core Competencies

Life-long learning	Communication	Innovation
Management	Education	Facilitation
Leadership		

Introduction

Healthcare organizations implementing the CNL role have varying levels of organizational knowledge and experience with the role. Many care facilities located in regional markets lack ready access to information and strategies related to CNL role implementation beyond the knowledge held by the novice CNL. While CNL education programs incorporate a robust clinical immersion, the specific circumstances of these immersions may fall short of adequately supporting the transition of a novice CNL to effective proficient practice as a generalist at the point of care.

The challenge of assuming a new role in a practice environment when the role lacks clear and broadly accepted standards of practice places a disproportionate burden on the novice CNL to successfully establish the role and integrate it into the organization. The organization may not have experienced CNLs to serve as preceptors/mentors, placing full responsibility for role definition and delineation within the microsystem of practice on the novice CNL. As distance learning options for CNL academic programs become more common, the nature of the academic–practice partnership may limit the CNL student's active engagement to the immersion component of their experience, making it all the more important to improve immersion experiences.

The development and implementation of a transition to practice program provides an organization with the opportunity for consolidation of a shared vision, understanding, and expectations regarding the CNL role among all organizational stakeholder groups. It provides specific strategies for embedding the role into a particular organization in a manner that is both meaningful to the organization and consistent with the academic preparation and intent of the CNL role. This chapter discusses frameworks for CNL transition to practice, identifies core elements and desired outcomes of CNL transition to practice programs, and provides examples of content elements included in a national healthcare delivery system's CNL transition to practice curriculum.

Defining a CNL Transition to Practice Program

Several terms are used to describe the professional development activities associated with the transition from being a student to becoming a provider of nursing care. These activities may be labeled a residency or a transition to practice program. For the purposes of this discussion, the two terms are considered equivalent; both refer to the initial practice period following completion of the academic program. While the value of registered nurse (RN) residency programs for new graduate nurses is well recognized, that value is primarily driven by the need to ensure that a novice nurse is sufficiently competent to provide safe care in an independent manner with sufficient self-assurance to support role satisfaction. The novice CNL, as a master's prepared advanced generalist, may not be viewed as a novice nurse upon entry into CNL practice and thus may not be afforded the same opportunity to develop sufficient proficiency of practice in the new role. A CNL transition to practice program provides a shared vision and set of expectations, acknowledges the new CNL as a novice in a new role, and provides a supportive structure within which the new CNL can transition to confident and effective practice at the point of care.

Core Elements of a CNL Transition to Practice Program

Five core elements of a CNL transition to practice program are identified and discussed in this section. The elements include (1) the framework; (2) curriculum development; (3) curriculum content, format, and learning activities; (4) program structure; and (5) evaluation framework.

Framework

In a recent review of the evidence behind nurse residency programs, Anderson, Hair, and Todero (2012) identified an opportunity for strengthening the link between theory and the design of these nursing educational efforts. This opportunity has implications related to evaluation of the effectiveness of individual programs, as well as knowledge building in the areas of organizational transformation and experiential–interactive learning. Framework-driven programs enhance the ability to measure the effectiveness of the CNL role in achieving positive organizational outcomes while promoting development of individual practice.

A suitable framework for CNL role transition should draw upon the theoretical frameworks that led to the initial vision for the role and guided its academic program development that underpin healthcare transformation and transformational leadership and that support clinical interprofessional learning and competency development. Although the focus of the role and the needs for transitioning to practice as an influential clinical leader at the point of care may be different than those of the new graduate nurse, the concepts are similar and applicable to the design, implementation, and evaluation of a CNL transition to practice program. Specific curricular components and experiential learning activities can be designed to focus on the components of the CNL role and the influence of the role on patterns of care and practice at the point of care.

The guiding framework provided by the American Association of Colleges of Nursing (AACN) in its white paper on the role of the CNL describes the components of the CNL role and expectations for practice as a generalist nurse (AACN, 2007). The AACN's *CNL Job Analysis Study* further identifies measureable competency elements derived from actual practice (AACN, 2012). Clinical microsystems provide a framework for the focus of CNL practice and are the locus of influence on healthcare delivery and organizational transformation (Nelson, Batalden, & Godfrey, 2007). As noted by Anderson and colleagues (2012), the guiding framework for transition to practice in the current healthcare delivery environment should support engagement in clinical learning environments characterized by interprofessional collaborative learning relationships and embed that learning to support high-quality, safe care and practice excellence.

An important consideration in the selection of a guiding framework for CNL transition to practice is the desired outcome of the transitional period. While measures of success for novice nurse residency programs are often focused on individual competency development to support independent safe practice and organizational retention of new nurses, the measures of successful CNL transition to practice are more focused on the ability of the CNL to influence patterns and processes reflecting microsystem performance and culture. The application of advanced knowledge and skill within the context of a microsystem of practice requires a framework that not only acknowledges the nature of the advanced generalist practice, but that also provides a vehicle for evaluating its impact within the context of organizational priorities and measures of performance. The ability to clearly communicate the framework guiding the CNL transition to practice provides opportunities for organizational learning and promotes the development of shared vision and expectations, as well as common language surrounding the nature of CNL practice and its significance to the organization.

A final consideration for a CNL transition to practice program is the opportunity to expand on the knowledge base across the multiple concept domains incorporated into the transition to practice focus. By drawing from and building upon past and current efforts, framework-driven CNL transition to practice program development and evaluation can contribute to knowledge regarding the CNL role, clinical microsystems, healthcare transformation, and interprofessional collaborative learning and practice.

Curriculum Development

Of particular importance to the development of curricular components for a CNL transition to practice program is selection of content and design. The curriculum should extend learning and development beyond the academic program and clinical immersion experience without duplicating academic course work. Significant attention should be given to linking practice to the foundations of training. This may be challenging for an organization that lacks experience with the CNL role or a clear understanding of the needs of a novice CNL, attesting to the importance of curricular development based on a well-defined and shared vision derived from a solid foundation.

Learning content that is specific to the organization or microsystem of practice should provide opportunities for the new CNL to use tools and apply knowledge from academic training to actual practice and role development. Selected content should reinforce CNL role components of particular significance to the organization and should promote consolidation of interprofessional relationships as the foundation for CNL influence on microsystem performance (Herbert, 2005; Scarvell & Stone, 2010). Exploiting opportunities to engage diverse partners and multiple stakeholders in shared ownership of successful transition of the new CNL supports organizational learning from curricular content.

The microsystem focus of the CNL role presents additional challenges and considerations for transition to practice curriculum development. The specific activities of a CNL are primarily driven by the needs of the microsystem within which their practice is based. General content about organizational priorities can be presented in a manner that allows the individual CNL to relate that knowledge to their microsystem. Content should include opportunities to identify organizational structures and resources that enhance the novice CNL's ability to solidify competency elements needed to influence microsystem practice and outcomes. Because a large portion of the CNL role is initially focused on embedding practice into the microsystem to promote the impact and influence of transformational clinical leadership (Moore & Leahy, 2012; Sherman, 2010), the ideal CNL transition to practice curriculum provides the vehicle for the novice CNL to begin this process.

Curriculum Content, Format, and Learning Activities

As noted previously, the concepts upon which transition of a novice CNL to proficient and meaningful practice is based are similar to the concepts of any sound transition to nursing practice program. Effective strategies identified by Anderson and colleagues (2012) include incorporation of trained preceptors, activities that build cohort relationships, time for exploring thoughtful approaches to commonly encountered challenges, and use of complex scenarios that engage practice teams. Additional strategies that warrant consideration consist of activities promoting reflective practice and professional socialization, as well as activities that promote interprofessional practice learning communities (Anderson et al., 2012; Scarvell

& Stone, 2010). Learning activities for the novice CNL expose stakeholders to the role and should be designed to reflect CNL practice, rather than simply represent projects in which CNLs participate. This is particularly important for organizations with minimal exposure to mature CNL practice. Learning activities should facilitate integration of CNL role components into a multidimensional point-of-care transformational clinical leadership practice.

The importance of preceptors to the success of the graduate RN is well described, and characteristics of preceptor support are predictors of novice nurse performance (Anderson et al., 2012). One challenge facing an organization may be the identification of appropriate preceptors if the role is new to the organization or the number of new CNLs exceeds the availability of seasoned CNLs. While the preceptor for a novice nurse is normally an expert nurse, the preceptor for a novice CNL does not necessarily need to be an expert CNL. The ideal preceptor must have sufficient understanding of the role and the expectations, have adequate professional development as a preceptor, and be in a position to facilitate the learning and competency development of the new CNL. Whenever possible, the novice CNL should be connected to an experienced CNL, either through a community of practice network or the establishment of a virtual mentor relationship that supports both the novice CNL and assists the on-site preceptor in providing appropriate guidance. Academic–practice partnerships are excellent resources for developing and supporting CNL preceptors.

Learning activities for a CNL transition to practice program are most easily identified from a guiding framework that designates critical skills and measures of success. Activities should be designed so that the novice CNL gains both competence and confidence within the context of their microsystem through active engagement in an interprofessional practice learning community. Activities that promote relationship building are key to the ability of the proficient CNL to influence patterns of practice as a transformational leader at the point of care. Opportunities to expose stakeholders to the CNL role promote the CNL's credibility as a leader and increase organizational knowledge about the potential impact of the role. Focused learning exercises during the transition to practice period can be employed to translate academic knowledge into practice and promote competency in core areas such as microsystem assessment, risk assessment, and continuous improvement methodologies. Participation in structured and strategic learning activities helps the novice CNL identify areas in which additional development may be required.

Two activities that have been identified as learning strategies (Anderson et al., 2012) but that have not been sufficiently evaluated in the practice environment, are worthy of consideration for inclusion in CNL transition to practice programs. Journaling is a form of reflective observation that can serve as a basis for CNL praxis, a method for promoting action that leads to change and transformation (Anderson et al., 2012). The second activity, establishing and maintaining a professional portfolio, provides a mechanism for tracking individual and microsystem development and supports dissemination of information related to outcomes and return on investment.

Program Structure

Considerations for the structure of a CNL transition to practice program include, but are not limited to, access, capacity, coordination, oversight, monitoring, and resources. Several dimensions of program structure may differ considerably from RN residency programs due to the nature of the novice, the expectations for practice, the number of novice CNLs at any given time, and the availability of local resources and expertise. As a master's prepared novice, the new CNL should not require the same degree of clinical oversight or program structure as a novice nurse. The microsystem of practice within the context of the organization is where competency development activities should occur to help the novice CNL embed his or her role and emerge as an influential clinical leader (Morrison & Symes, 2011). Online access to curricular components and self-paced self-study options may be more suitable than scheduled activities that divert the CNL's focus away from the microsystem. Ready access to a preceptor with regularly scheduled discussions rather than continuous oversight promotes independent problem solving and the development of key relationships with members of the microsystem's interprofessional team. Virtual access to experienced CNLs, especially those in similar microsystem environments, enhances the ability of the novice CNL to fully operationalize the role.

Evaluation Framework

Several levels of evaluation are indicated for a transition to practice program. Measures of program success may include the number of novice CNLs successfully completing the program, evaluation feedback from CNLs and preceptors, and indicators of satisfaction of key microsystem stakeholders with relevant components of CNL performance. Measures of successful transitions to practice focus on the impact of the CNL on the microsystem as evidenced by microsystem performance, patterns of practice and professional engagement of staff, and outcomes (Bender, Connelly, Glaser, & Brown, 2012; Harris, Tornabeni, & Walters, 2006; Hix, 2009; Sherman, 2009). Identifying measures and developing the evaluation framework prior to implementation of the CNL transition to practice program enhances the ability to establish sources of data and information and to demonstrate success.

CNL Transition to Practice Program Content

In 2011, the Veterans Health Administration (VHA) Office of Nursing Services (ONS) chartered a core team of CNL and education subject matter experts to develop and implement a CNL transition to practice program. The core team was tasked with refining a conceptual framework for the curriculum, leading the development of curricular components, designing a curriculum format, and formulating recommendations for the program structure of a 6-month transition to practice program. The core group recruited and engaged additional subject matter experts and practicing VHA CNLs in the development of curriculum content, learning activities, and evaluation strategies. Upon completion, the ONS CNL Implementation and Evaluation Service assumed responsibility for review, revision, testing, and full launch of a CNL transition to practice program. This section describes the evolution of this effort and provides examples of learning content and activities that can be adapted to address CNL transition to practice in any healthcare system.

Learning Domains, Modules, and Objectives

Five learning domains were identified as key to the transition of a novice CNL graduate into practice as a VHA CNL. The curriculum framework, illustrated in **Table 22-1**, is organized under domains of learning that represent critical components of the role, within which application and expansion of academic content would best facilitate the transition to effective practice. The five domains emerged from input provided by both CNLs and nursing leaders regarding identified learning needs of CNLs employed by the VHA during early role implementation. A core working group of CNL and education subject matter experts initially validated that the identified learning domains could serve as the guiding framework for content development and program evaluation for CNL transition to practice in any healthcare system.

Table 22-1 **The VHA ONS CNL Transition to Practice Curriculum Framework**

Learning Domain	Content Module	Learning Objectives
Role differentiation	ONS CNL strategic initiative and spread plan overview	1. Describe the ONS strategic vision for the CNL role. 2. Identify how the ONS vision is consistent with the AACN's CNL white paper. 3. Define individual CNL roles within the context of the ONS's vision. 4. Determine how the microsystem supports the organizational strategic plan.
	Establishing and sustaining interprofessional, collaborative relationships	1. Identify key collaborative relationships for the microsystem. 2. Understand the value of professional communication, leadership, and facilitation skills in establishing collaborative relationships. 3. Identify resources to help develop collaborative skills.
	Role differentiation	1. Be able to differentiate the CNL role from other nursing roles. 2. Describe how implementing the CNL role brings added value. 3. Identify resources to help differentiate the CNL role.
	Microsystems needs assessment and role establishment	1. Identify members of the team who will complete the clinical microsystem assessment. 2. Using the clinical microsystems workbook that is appropriate for your microsystem, begin an assessment, diagnosis, and treatment that focuses on patients, purpose, professionals, processes, and patterns ("5 *Ps*"). 3. Identify resources needed to complete the workbook.
	Owning your practice	1. Describe who you are as a professional. 2. Develop a professional portfolio. 3. Disseminate information about your CNL role. 4. Identify the elements of a culture of professional ownership.

Table 22-1   The VHA ONS CNL Transition to Practice Curriculum Framework (continued)

Learning Domain	Content Module	Learning Objectives
Clinical outcomes management	Care coordination	1. Describe transitions of care. 2. Identify a continuum of care collaborative team. 3. Describe elements of safe and effective handoffs. 4. Identify resources to facilitate seamless care transitions.
	Patient/family education	1. Outline the principles and expectations of patient- and family-centered care. 2. Identify the skills needed to achieve patient- and family-centered care outcomes through education. 3. Identify resources to support patient- and family-centered care.
	Staff education and learning environment	1. Identify competencies needed to achieve optimal outcomes in the microsystem. 2. Describe strategies for developing and maintaining competencies. 3. Identify resources to develop staff skills and create continuous learning environments.
	Products/technology	1. Identify the products and technologies that impact the microsystem. 2. Identify strategies to improve resource management. 3. Identify resources to support and optimize efficiency and effectiveness.
	Patient-driven care protocols	1. Identify opportunities to improve management of clinical outcomes. 2. Define processes and structures that impact clinical practice outcomes. 3. Identify resources available to achieve optimal outcomes.
	Health promotion and disease prevention (HPDP)	1. Describe how HPDP is integrated in all aspects of care across the care continuum. 2. Identify the performance measures related to the microsystem. 3. Identify HPDP internal and external resources related to the microsystem.

(continues)

Table 22-1 **The VHA ONS CNL Transition to Practice Curriculum Framework (continued)**

Learning Domain	Content Module	Learning Objectives
Care environment management	Team coordination	1. Identify the team structures within the microsystem. 2. Assess the communication pathways and patterns of team structures. 3. Identify resources that support team function.
	Accreditation readiness	1. Describe the accreditation processes for the microsystem. 2. Identify strategies to promote team ownership of readiness. 3. Identify accreditation resources.
	Performance improvement, safety, risk aversion	1. Describe the elements that contribute to risks in the microsystem. 2. Identify unique risks for obtaining optimal outcomes in the microsystem. 3. Describe risk anticipation strategies. 4. Identify resources to support performance safety and risk aversion.
	Change	1. Identify conceptual models and theories of change. 2. Identify a variety of strategies to approach and manage change. 3. Identify resources to support change management.
	Shared governance/ high-reliability organizations	1. Define shared governance. 2. Define "high-reliability organizations." 3. Identify strategies for leveraging microsystem governance structures. 4. Identify resources for supporting shared governance and the development of high-reliability organizations.
Data management	Data—general considerations	1. Identify sources of useful and appropriate data. 2. Describe elements of data collection strategies. 3. Describe considerations for protecting data.
	Data management	1. Identify available systems for organizing data. 2. Describe considerations related to ownership and accountability of data.

Table 22-1   The VHA ONS CNL Transition to Practice Curriculum Framework (continued)

Learning Domain	Content Module	Learning Objectives
	Data analysis/ interpretation	1. Describe strategies for analyzing and interpreting data. 2. Identify appropriate audience for different types of data reporting.
	Dissemination	1. Describe considerations when determining dissemination methods. 2. Identify suitable opportunities and venues for dissemination. 3. Identify levels of review and approval required for dissemination.
Using evidence to guide practice	Using the evidence-based practice (EBP) curriculum: transition to practice program	1. Define EBP. 2. Identify how EBP can improve patient safety and quality patient care.

Four to six learning content modules were developed within each of the five learning domains. Content was identified through facilitated brainstorming and concept consolidation, with the core working group of CNL and education subject matter experts. Within each content module, learning objectives were identified to guide CNL practice within a microsystem context. The core working group decided that a major focus of the learning objectives and corresponding learning content was to assist the new CNL in embedding his or her practice into the assigned microsystem in a manner meaningful for individual transition to practice as well as organizational priorities. A draft outline of learning domains, learning modules, and learning objectives was submitted for review and concurrence to a group of internal and external stakeholder groups prior to the development of learning content and activities. (See Table 22-1 for a listing of learning domains, content modules, and the learning objectives for each module.)

Learning Content and Activities

The knowledge and experience of practicing CNLs across the VHA system was used in the development of learning module content and activities related to the stated learning objectives. Members of the core working group coordinated authorship of an assigned group of modules that they had a special interest in or had access to content subject matter experts. Existing resources were researched, reviewed, and used to strengthen learning content. Learning activities were devised to both ground the new CNL in the assigned microsystem and to promote competency development in areas of practice crucial to the mission and strategic initiatives of the VHA. As illustration, **Table 22-2** describes learning activities for several learning objectives in the transition to practice curriculum.

Program Format

The development of a CNL transition to practice curriculum for a national healthcare delivery system required special consideration with respect to access, coordination, and resource impact. The core team decided early in the planning process that the program would be self-study based, self-paced, preceptor guided, virtually accessible, and would include regular opportunities for feedback and evaluation. This type of design supported the dissemination of a national curriculum that could be customized at the facility level and ensured sufficient flexibility for application across diverse organizations within the VHA system.

Content and evaluation materials were placed on a virtual national community of CNL practice. An invitation was sent to novice CNLs to register, with a preceptor, for the transition to practice program. Upon registration, CNLs and their identified preceptors were given full access to the curriculum materials. The CNLs were asked to complete Learning Domain I first, as this module formed the foundation for role differentiation and consolidation. Full access to the curriculum was also given to nursing leadership. Options for virtual distance mentoring relationships with experienced CNLs were facilitated. Beginning CNLs, preceptors, and experienced CNLs worked together in the virtual community of practice to connect, ask/share, collaborate, innovate, and consolidate practice networks.

Consideration should be given to the types of resources needed prior to implementing a CNL transition to practice program. Resources include CNL and preceptor's time, supportive infrastructures, and return on investment expectations. If a facility or microsystem has predetermined expectations for what the new CNL is supposed to accomplish, the ability of the new CNL to participate in the transition to practice learning activities may be limited. In these cases, it is important to evaluate whether expectations are consistent with the shared vision for the role, whether expectations involve proficiency that is developed through completion of transition to practice learning exercises, and if perception of the CNL role is consistent with the AACN's vision and intent.

Table 22-2   Examples of VHA ONS CNL Transition to Practice Curriculum Learning Objectives and Activities

Learning Objective	Learning Activity
Differentiate the CNL role from other nursing roles	1. Outline for yourself, and discuss with several staff nurses, how the CNL role compares to the staff nurse role in your microsystem. 2. Outline for yourself, and discuss with the nurse manager and/or assistant nurse manager, how the CNL role compares to the administrative management roles in your microsystem. 3. Identify any other nursing roles in your organization that might functionally partner or overlap with the CNL role and discuss with these individuals how you might establish collaborative practice.
Identify key collaborative relationships for the microsystem	1. Who are the members of the patient care delivery team for the microsystem and how can the CNL partner with each member and the team as a whole? 2. Specifically, how can the CNL partner with patients in this microsystem? 3. In the CNL role of lateral integrator, what collaborative relationships are key for this microsystem? 4. What opportunities for CNL collaboration with stakeholders external to this microsystem are essential to achieving optimum microsystem outcomes?
Identify resources for supporting shared governance and developing a high-reliability organization (HRO)	1. Ask staff nurses in your microsystem about their definition and understanding of nursing shared governance. 2. Identify the means of communication between microsystem staff nurses and facility committees. 3. Read the executive summary, introduction, and overview in *Becoming a High Reliability Organization: Operational Advice for Hospital Leaders* (available at http://psnet.ahrq.gov/resource.aspx?resourceID=7076) 4. Engage in a unit discussion about how to develop an HRO. 5. How does your microsystem and facility respond to errors? Create a root cause analysis (RCA) flow map showing how your microsystem responded. Are there gaps that can be remediated through a health failure mode event analysis (HFMEA)? Identify your facility's process for analyzing and reviewing system errors. Try to attend an interdisciplinary RCA meeting.

Preceptor Guide

Curriculum components for which preceptor engagement is required or may be sought by the CNL were highlighted in the VHA's preceptor guide. The preceptor guide includes general guidelines for precepting and links to additional resources available across the national system. Each preceptor was provided access to the full curriculum, with recommendations for application of content to organizational learning as well as to CNL development. Curricular components for which guided learning is most critical were identified for the preceptor, with examples of teaching styles and activities to enhance CNL competency development in those areas. Preceptors were provided access to other preceptors, as well as to national program and academic resources. Preceptors were asked to evaluate the novice CNL, the transition to practice curriculum, and the preceptor support components, and to provide indicators evidencing CNL successful transition to practice and microsystem influence.

Evaluation

Measures of success for the VHA's CNL transition to practice program included:

- Percentage of novice VHA CNLs who completed the transition to practice program within 6 months of appointment
- Average score on CNL feedback measures of accessibility, usability, and meaningfulness of curriculum; preceptor support; and access to national supportive resources
- Average score on preceptor feedback measures of accessibility, usability, and meaningfulness of curriculum and preceptor guide; application of knowledge to the practice of the novice CNL; and access to national supportive resources
- CNL retention in the role, retention in the system, and satisfaction

Measures of successful transition to practice (early influence on microsystem) included:

- Increased microsystem team knowledge about and satisfaction with the CNL role and CNL performance
- Improved microsystem patterns of communication and relationships
- Increased microsystem team engagement in continuous improvement and evidence-based practice activities

Summary

- A CNL transition to practice program provides a shared vision and set of expectations, acknowledges the new CNL as a novice in a new role, and provides a supportive structure within which the new CNL can transition to confident and effective practice at the point of care.
- The five core elements of a CNL transition to practice program are (1) the theoretical framework; (2) curriculum development; (3) curriculum content, format, and learning activities; (4) program structure; and (5) evaluation framework.
- The VHA's CNL transition to practice curriculum is organized under domains of learning that represent critical components of the CNL role within which application and expansion of academic content best facilitate transition to effective practice.
- The VHA's CNL transition to practice program is self-study based, self-paced, preceptor guided, virtually accessible, and includes regular opportunity for feedback and evaluation.

www. Reflection Questions
© Arenacreative/Dreamstime.com

1. What are the key elements of a guiding framework that best represents the outcomes you most desire from a transition to practice experience?
2. What are the key characteristics of learning activities that can best enhance a transition to practice experience?
3. What are important indicators or measures of a successful transition to practice for a novice CNL?

www. Learning Activities
© Arenacreative/Dreamstime.com

1. Obtain information from several healthcare systems about their approaches to supporting the transition of the novice CNL to practice. How well do these approaches reflect the core elements identified in this chapter? To what extent do these approaches address your expectations for a transition to practice experience?

2. Select one learning objective from the VHA's CNL transition to practice program framework and differentiate learning and competency development as a novice CNL from learning as a student in a CNL academic program.

References

American Association of Colleges of Nursing. (2007). *White paper on the role of the clinical nurse leader*. Retrieved from http://www.aacn.nche.edu/publications/white-papers/cnl

American Association of Colleges of Nursing. (2012). CNL job analysis study. Retrieved from http://www.aacn.nche.edu/cnl/publications-resources/job-analysis-study

Anderson, G., Hair, C., & Todero, C. (2012). Nurse residency programs: An evidence-based review of theory, process, and outcomes. *Journal of Professional Nursing, 28*(4), 203–212.

Bender, M., Connelly, C. D., Glaser, D., & Brown, C. (2012). Clinical nurse leader impact on microsystem care quality. *Nursing Research, 61*(5), 326–332.

Harris, J. L., Tornabeni, J., & Walters, S. E. (2006). The clinical nurse leader: A valued member of the healthcare team. *Journal of Nursing Administration, 36*(10), 446–449.

Herbert, C. P. (2005). Changing the culture: Interprofessional education for collaborative patient-centered practice in Canada. *Journal of Interprofessional Care, 19*(Supple. 1), 1–4.

Hix, C. (2009). Clinical nurse leader impact on clinical microsystems outcomes. *Journal of Nursing Administration, 39*(2), 71–76.

Moore, L.W., & Leahy, C. (2012). Implementing the new clinical nurse leader role while gleaning insights from the past. *Journal of Professional Nursing, 28*(3), 139–146.

Morrison, S. M., & Symes, L. (2011). An integrative review of expert nursing practice. *Journal of Nursing Scholarship, 43*(2), 163–170.

Nelson, E. C., Batalden, P. B., & Godfrey, M. M. (2007). *Quality by design: A clinical microsystems approach*. San Francisco, CA: Jossey-Bass.

Scarvell, J. M., & Stone, J. (2010). An interprofessional collaborative practice model for preparation of clinical educators. *Journal of Interprofessional Care, 24*(4), 386–400.

Sherman, R. O. (2009). The role of the clinical nurse leader in promoting a healthy work environment at the unit level. *Critical Care Nursing Quarterly, 32*(4), 264–271.

Sherman, R. O. (2010). Lessons in innovation: Role transition experiences of clinical nurse leaders. *Journal of Nursing Administration, 40*(12), 547–554.

Preceptors' Use of Portfolios for Career Advancement

Tommie Norris and Sherry Webb

Key terms: preceptor, dedicated education units, portfolios

Aim: To prepare preceptors on dedicated education units

Portfolios can be organized to showcase achievement of career advancement criteria. Preceptors working with CNL students assigned to dedicated education units (DEUs) were impressed by the portfolios prepared by their students. Faculty were interested in facilitating the development of the preceptors' portfolios as one way to express gratitude to the preceptors for sharing their expertise and role modeling professional nursing. Faculty worked with preceptors to develop portfolios that would demonstrate achievement of specialized skills and career advancement criteria established by the employer. In an informal survey, DEU preceptors reported that their portfolios helped them to feel prepared for their annual evaluations, impressed their supervisors, and provided evidence of meeting advancement criteria. Preceptors also reported that portfolios proved to be a great vehicle for retaining records of continuing education needed for certification renewal. All portfolios developed by preceptors contained an updated resume. Faculty provided a template that enabled preceptors to "click and insert" demographic information, work experience, education, and honors/awards. The portfolios were individualized and contained various sections such as evidence of achieving certification including basic CPR, advanced cardiac life support, and/or pediatric advanced life support. Continuing education (CE) hours earned in pursuit of life-long learning or as a requirement for employment (such as fire safety or HIPAA) were included. Membership in professional organizations and leadership positions was incorporated. Nurses returning to college to advance their education included transcripts of completed coursework, and many included examples of assignments such as quality improvement projects. Development of educational tools and patient pamphlets were included as examples of innovative practice. Of course, an agency always strives for patient satisfaction, and preceptors were encouraged to include "thank you" letters/notes from patients and peers providing evidence of patient-centered care or teamwork.

TWENTY-THREE

Clinical Nurse Leadership: Creating the Vision

■ Patricia L. Thomas and Linda Roussel

 Learning Objectives
© Arenacreative/Dreamstime.com

- ■ Define clinical nurse leadership
- ■ Identify the core skills necessary to lead change in a microsystem
- ■ Describe the impact of skillful leadership, giving examples of clinical nurse leaders in action

> **Leadership is an opportunity to serve. It is not a trumpet call to self-importance.**
>
> J. Donald Walters

Introduction

Clinical nurse leaders (CNLs) engage in clinical leadership. Clinical leadership is about clinicians informing the quality and safety of care through innovation and improvement—both in their organizational processes and in their individual care practices. Clinical leadership can be taken on by any direct provider of patient care, including doctors, nurses, allied health professionals, clinical pharmacists, and paramedics. Because CNLs have

Key Terms

Clinical leadership	Outcomes	Evidence-based practice

CNL Roles

Outcomes manager	Advocate	Communicator
Life-long learner		

CNL Professional Values

Accountability	Integrity

CNL Core Competencies

Life-long learning	Communication	Innovation
Education	Facilitating	Leadership
Collaboration		

advanced knowledge in quality improvement, measurement, systems, and change leadership strategies and actually deliver care, they are well positioned to evaluate its quality and guide its improvement. No matter where CNLs operate in the healthcare system, as clinical leaders they are able to critically appraise care processes with respect to outcomes. Not only do they ask: "Are we doing things right?," they also consider the more fundamental question, "Are we doing the right things?" Even more to the point they ask, "Should we be doing what we're doing?" Bleich (2012) notes in his discussion on leadership responses to the Institute of Medicine's (IOM's) report, *The Future of Nursing: Leading Change, Advancing Health* (IOM, 2010), that there are too few nurses at the table as models of accountable care and this, he asserts, is serious. "Nurse leaders must influence all nurses to give voice to and act on our unique roles as the singular health discipline who addresses both holistically and contextually" (Bleich, 2012, p. 184).

The American Association of Colleges of Nursing (AACN, 2007) posits that CNL education provides the graduate with the skill set necessary to assume horizontal leadership within the healthcare team. Horizontal organizations are described as having decentralized power and/or control, at least within specific departments, and support greater flow of communication and collaboration. In horizontal leadership a number of individuals can assume leadership of a team or teams in the attempt to achieve a common goal. Vertical leadership, in contrast, has one leader, often with centralized control. As a clinical leader in a horizontal organization, the CNL has the opportunity and responsibility of bringing individuals together, giving them a voice, and creating an environment that is safe for communication and feedback. As such, understanding and applying leadership theories are important aspects of the CNL role to demonstrate strong, effective clinical leadership (Woo, 2013).

> **Leadership is the capacity to translate vision into reality.**
>
> **Warren G. Bennis**

The Need for Clinical Leadership

There is need for a more programmatic, strategic approach to clinical leadership, because the U.S.'s ailing healthcare system is in urgent need of reform. Although many believe that the responsibilities of the clinician and the responsibilities of an administrator are completely separate, in reality, the distinction between clinical leadership and administrative leadership is often blurred. This chapter posits that while there are unique elements within each of these roles, there is far greater commonality than what is typically described in the literature. Beyond the scope of formal or informal leadership, bridging this false dichotomy with CNLs offers a transition point to support the transformation of care delivery across the continuum.

Porter-O'Grady (1997, 1999) proposed a new way of thinking about leadership, describing how the changing healthcare system necessitates new leadership characteristics and roles. He noted that knowledge of technology has changed the traditional hierarchy of leadership. That is, nursing knowledge rose vertically as the nurse moved up the chain of command. Historically, as the knowledge base increased, so did the demands and responsibilities that nurses experienced in their positions.

Leadership and the knowledge associated with it have shifted. The CNL has a burgeoning role as an information and outcomes manager. The CNL uses technology to lead as the lateral integrator.

The success of the U.S. healthcare system in treating infectious disease, the changing social and economic environment, modern lifestyles, and an aging population have dramatically shifted the burden of care from acute conditions to chronic disease. Chronic conditions such as some cancers, diabetes, cardiovascular disease, and asthma now account for some 80% of the total burden of disease (National Health Priority Action Council, 2006). CNLs are prepared and poised to assume leadership for coordinating care and collaborating with interdisciplinary teams necessary for management of chronic conditions. Clinical leadership brings this together for patients, stakeholders, and providers.

Clinical Leadership Behaviors

Clinicians can lead in many ways, both formal and informal, as part of their organizational position and/or through their collegial relationships. There are many ways to serve as a clinical leader, including:

- *Developing personal qualities:* qualities such as self-awareness, self-reflection, self-management, professionalism, and self-development
- *Working with others:* developing networks, building and maintaining relationships, team building, developing others, engaging with clients and consumers, and collaborating with other service providers
- *Improving services:* ensuring patient safety, critically evaluating, encouraging innovation, evaluating services, improving healthcare processes, and developing new services and roles
- *Managing services*: planning, managing resources, managing people, and managing performance
- *Setting direction*: identifying opportunities for change, applying knowledge and evidence, making decisions, and evaluating impact and outcomes

CNLs are well positioned to lead safety and quality improvement initiatives, and, at a practical level, this translates into a range of activities, including equipping themselves with the knowledge and skills to initiate and drive appropriate safety and quality activities at a professional and team level.

Additional tasks of CNLs include the following:

- Translating high-level organizational strategy into operational improvement activities
- Leading the development, implementation, and evaluation of quality and safety plans, systems, and activities, openly communicating and reporting safety and quality problems and adverse events and participating in developing solutions
- Adhering to policies and procedures for preventing, reporting, and disclosing adverse events, ensuring that care and services are delivered according to the best available evidence, health service protocols, and policies
- Ensuring that safety and quality risks are proactively identified and managed through effective systems, delegation of accountabilities, and properly trained and credentialed staff
- Developing a partnership approach with patients and their care givers in individual episodes of care as well as the prevention, treatment, and discussion of adverse events, leading a team approach to patient care, quality improvement, and problem solving, and ensuring that this adds to participants' organizational and professional status
- Fostering a culture that does not blame, but rather seeks to solve problems and learn from them, supporting staff in this process
- Empowering and holding staff accountable at all levels to be appropriately involved in monitoring and improving care and services
- Recognizing the importance of effective team communication in patient care, and supporting staff training and development in this area
- Improving systems to support and spread best practice individual patient care, modeling a professional, evidence-based approach to care delivery

Information Management, Technology, and Analysis

Healthcare information technology initiatives are more successful when a collaborative redesign approach is taken, in which clinicians are intimately involved in the entire change process. Clinical engagement is a well-documented determinant for the success of new initiatives (Boonstra & Broekhuis, 2010; Diamond, French, Gronkiewicz, & Borkgren, 2010; Yackanicz, Kerr, & Levick, 2010). A lack of clinical engagement is a commonly cited reason for failure (Westbrook et al., 2007). Garling (2008) notes that nonclinicians have limited opportunities to effect change in clinical practice. CNLs are well positioned to bridge the divide that often exists in organizations between those who understand clinical processes and those who understand information systems. The CNL has been educated to appreciate both equally and has the knowledge and language to narrow the space between what have historically been siloed decision-making bodies.

Change Paradigms

Clinical engagement is acknowledged as a critical success factor for change initiatives that involve patient care. However, clinicians and managers may have different change paradigms. Clinicians want progress but expect it to be delivered in the manner to which they are accustomed from experience with an emergent paradigm. In the context of organizational change, however, such a model is not practical. Organizational leaders place change in two categories: incremental change and revolutionary disruptive change. Both have value and purpose, but they have very different considerations. Incremental change is the change most people are comfortable with and anticipate. It is change that brings modest to moderate improvement, and it is typically supported by infrastructure changes and defining an aim or changing the focus of a group in response to clinical outcomes that did not meet a target.

Revolutionary or disruptive change, on the other hand, represents a radical shift in thinking, being, and doing—thus the disruption. CNLs, by virtue of their roles, are expected to lead change. Several change theories may guide their work, including appreciative inquiry, Lewin's theory, and Lippitt's theory of change. Each has unique advantages and disadvantages, but they hold in common systematic, defined, and prescriptive actions to support the change agent in managing resistance and promoting enthusiasm and engagement in the change process. A brief summary of each of these theories is offered, recognizing that many other change theories exist and could be used.

Appreciative Inquiry

Appreciative inquiry (AI) is about the coevolutionary search for the best in people, their organizations, and the relevant world around them (Cooperrider, 1990). At its center, AI focuses on the art and practice of asking questions that strengthen a system's capacity to apprehend, anticipate, and heighten positive potential. AI provides the mobilization of inquiry through the crafting of the "unconditional positive question," which may include any number of individuals from various disciplines. AI's intervention gives way to imagination and innovation rather than a negative, critical, or pessimistic trajectory. AI seeks to provide the opportunity to discover, dream, and create systems and designs that inspire and invigorate. Additionally, AI desires to develop a constructive union between the collective body and the entirety of what is being talked about through past and present capacities: successes, assets, untapped potentials, innovations, strengths, and opportunities. Benchmarks, high-impact moments, authentic values, traditions and rituals, strategic competencies, narratives, expressions of lived experiences, reflections on the corporate spirit, and insights into values are considerations. Taken as a whole, AI seeks to work from positive positions, reflecting that living systems have untapped potential and rich, in-depth inspiring accounts of affirmations. When the energy of this synergy is directed toward transformation, innovations that were never thought possible become real opportunities.

Hubbard (1998) defined AI as a paradigm of conscious evolution as considerations for realities of the new century. The paradigm purports a social construction of reality to its extreme, focusing on metaphor and story, relational ways of knowing, and language, thereby producing a type of generative theory, advancement in action research (Bushe & Pitman 1991), and a tribute to Maslow's vision of a positive social science (Chin, 1998; Curran, 1991; Westbrook et al., 2007). AI has also been considered a powerful second-generation organizational development practice (French & Bell, 1994; Porras, 1991), as well as a framework for participatory science (Harman, 1990). AI is an affirmative way to make changes, moving away from problem-based management and transforming strategic planning and survey methods to more integrative methods and approaches to quality management, measurement systems, and sociotechnical systems (White, 1996). AI is a theoretical approach to knowing and a conceptualization of change management that can be used as an approach to leadership and human development (Cooperrider, 1990).

Cooperrider's work on AI is seminal (1990). He describes four stages of AI: discovery, dream, design, and destiny. *Discovery* is the mobilization of an entire system of inquiry into the positive change core. The *dream* stage occurs when a transparent results-oriented vision is created through discovered potential and questions are posed that provide a higher purpose. *Design* happens when possibilities are realized of the ideal organization where people feel capable of expanding the positive core and making real new dreams and concepts. *Destiny* purports the strengthening of the positive capabilities and capacities of the whole system, building hope and momentum focused on a deeper purpose, and thereby creating processes for learning, adjustment, and improvisation.

Lewin's Change Model

The power of Lewin's work rests in his ability to build models that drew attention to the variables that need to be conceptualized and observed to explain change in human systems (Schein, 1999). The model of planned change and the process of change in human systems conceptualized in Lewin's planned change model created the foundation that allowed organizational thinking to evolve from a theory of planned change to a process of managed learning (Schein, 1999). Lewin's change model highlighted that human change, at both the individual and group levels, involves a psychological and dynamic process (Lewin, 1951). This process includes unlearning behaviors without the loss of ego identity and a relearning process that attempts to restructure thoughts, perceptions, feelings, and attitudes (Schein, 1999, p. 59).

Change, irrespective of the intervention used, requires energy to overcome system inertia. Lewin (1951) suggested that change occurs in a three-stage process at individual, group, or organizational levels. Lewin referred to the stages as unfreezing, change, and refreezing (Burnes, 2004; Marquis & Huston, 2006; Tomey, 2010). The *unfreezing* phase of the process requires an alteration of the positive and negative forces on an individual level that disrupts the social equilibrium enough to motivate a change. *Change* occurs when individuals are offered options by way of an attitude change or a role model. These efforts need to be coupled with a signal that the norms or culture will support the change. *Refreezing* occurs when the new behavior or attitude is incorporated into the existing relationships and a new stability in social support creates equilibrium (Burnes, 2004; Marquis & Huston, 2006).

The ability to unfreeze or learn new behaviors is dependent on an individual's ability to enter the learning or change process with the recognition that something is wrong or imperfect. This requires an admission of limitations and acceptance that effectiveness may be questioned and that parts of personal identity and self-esteem may be lost if a change occurs. Often, adapting poorly or not meeting expectations appears more desirable than risking failure or loss of self-esteem. This learning anxiety is a primary restraining force that leads to the maintenance of equilibrium by discounting information and resisting change (Schein, 1999, p. 60). The concept of a force-field equilibrium model, published by Lewin in 1951, described reasons, or forces, that support and encourage individuals to continue present behavior patterns compared to another set of forces that are trying to effect change (Burnes, 2004; Lewin, 1951; Tomey, 2010). Lewin's description of force fields provides a structure to examine human behavior based on the equilibrium supported by driving and restraining forces. For change to occur, force fields of driving (supportive behaviors) or restraining factors (real or perceived threats) need to be altered. By adding a driving force toward change, often a counterforce to maintain equilibrium will be introduced. This observation led to the insight that equilibrium can be more easily shifted if restraining forces are eliminated. Unfortunately, restraining forces are often personal psychological defenses or group norms embedded in organizational cultures (Schein, 1999).

Lippitt's Theory of Change

Lippitt's work has also been cited frequently as a useful change theory (Lippitt, Watson, & Westley, 1958). Lippitt's change theory provides a seven-step process that advances the work of Lewin, focusing on the person serving as the change agent. Lippitt purports that the key to successful change is having the right person be the voice of change, creating an empowering process. Having the right person as the voice of change and having support for the change further empowers the process. CNLs can be utilized as this change agent because they are not routinely part of the processes that create delays or barriers; rather they are observers of other nursing and interdisciplinary roles who recognize the need for process changes (Lippitt et al., 1958).

The seven stages of Lippitt's theory are as follows:

1. Diagnose the problem and include those who will be affected by a change
2. Assess motivation for the change and engage in small group discussions about the pros and cons of the change
3. Assess resources and the motivation of those who will need to make change
4. Choose elements that need change and develop and plan a time line to address the change
5. Choose those who will lead the change and manage the team dynamics and any conflicts that arise
6. Maintain the change and revise policies and procedures
7. Terminate the helping relationship

Each of the stages is moved through in a sequential manner and requires the involvement of members of a team or group for success. The stages emphasize that while there is an identified leader, many of the team members will contribute their knowledge and skill to the success of the team's work. If at any time the work of the group stalls, it is important to engage the project sponsor in discussion for recommendations on how to manage the obstacles (Lippitt et al., 1958).

Engagement, Teams, Satisfaction, and Outcomes

The key to achieving successful clinical outcomes is to develop a clinical engagement model where representative clinical leaders can have an empowered seat at the executive table to engage in strategic planning for initiatives that have an impact on care delivery. Subsequently, these clinical leaders can promote clinical engagement by driving awareness of change initiatives within their clinical communities. This clinical executive role can work to heal the divide between clinicians and management, facilitating successful change.

By including members of the interdisciplinary team in the creation of a change, the CNL emphasizes the shared goals, shared commitments, and shared successes in leveraging the strengths of the team members. As a facilitator of the team, the CNL manages the group dynamics, ensures participation of all team members, and fosters trust and respect. Major challenges in leading teams are to ensure that meetings start and end on time and that multiple means of gathering data (including observation of different processes) are built into the team interactions.

Several studies on the CNL have demonstrated increased patient satisfaction (Bender, Connelly, Glaser, & Brown, 2012; Hix, McKeon, & Walters, 2009), as well as staff satisfaction in qualitative examination (Hartranft, Garcia, & Adams, 2007). Additionally, studies on teams, staff satisfaction, and engagement demonstrate that healthy work environments are developed when strategies to enhance communication and promote interdependence of team members are established (Amos, Hu, & Herrick, 2005). Given this, the investment of CNL time in leading interdisciplinary teams could bring improved satisfaction and support healthier environments.

Contemporary Leadership Theories

Understanding contemporary leadership theories is foundational to the CNL assuming an effective leadership role. The following section offers a brief overview of principles of a variety of useful leadership theories. While no individual can embody every element of the tenets in a leadership theory, all nurses should ground their leadership in a particular leadership theory. It has been postulated that depending on the situation, nurses shift behaviors to address needs, underscoring flexibility that is principle based, embodied in a theory, and deliberate, rather than a function of personality.

Servant Leadership

Greenleaf (1977) describes servant-leaders as there to serve those they lead, implying that the employees are an end in themselves, rather than a means to an end (bottom line). Servant leadership can be an alternative to a command and control style, with a greater focus on how others can be served and their needs.

Greenleaf (1977) offers 10 principles of servant leadership: listening, empathy, healing, awareness, persuasion, conceptualization, foresight, stewardship, commitment to the growth of people, and building community.

Listening

Servant-leaders make a deep commitment to listening intently to others, seeking to identify and make clear the needs of the group. They are receptive to what is being said (and nonverbal cues of what is not being said). The servant-leader is self-aware, seeking to have a greater understanding of the connection of body, mind, and sprit communicated through self.

Empathy

The servant-leader accepts and recognizes the uniqueness of those he or she leads, assuming the good intentions of coworkers and accepting others for who they are.

Healing

Healing denotes a powerful force that transforms and integrates teams. This is considered one of the greatest strengths of the servant-leader. According to Greenleaf (1977), "There is something subtle communicated to one who is being served and led, if implicit in the compact between the servant-leader and led is the understanding that the search for wholeness is something that they have" (p. 345).

Awareness

Self-awareness is the cornerstone of the servant-leader's awareness of his or her own strengths and abilities to provide healing and a supportive environment. Developing inner security is paramount to the success of a servant-leader.

Persuasion

Persuasion is described as influence. The servant-leader focuses on persuading the process rather than using positional authority in making decisions. Rather than being coercive, the servant-leader seeks consensus. This is a distinguishing feature from a more traditional authoritarian model.

Conceptualization

Helping those they lead to see the big picture is particularly important to the servant-leader. The skill of looking at an issue (problem) from a conceptualizing view requires a focus beyond the day to day operations. This requires a balance between vision and real world thinking.

Foresight

Using these principles, the servant-leader helps others to understand lessons learned from past experiences, put into perspective the realities of the present, and consider implications of future decisions. This principle is grounded in self-knowledge, being intuitive, and trusting one's voice.

Stewardship

Transcending the self to consider the greater good of the organization defines stewardship. Being a good steward of the resources of time, humanity, and spirit requires dedication to all of the principles described.

Commitment to the Growth of People

Growing others means believing that the people the servant-leader serves have an intrinsic value beyond their "job worth" as workers. Servant-leaders are deeply committed to the personal, professional, and spiritual growth of those in the organization.

Building Community

Servant-leaders have a keen awareness that becoming a large institution may create feelings of loss for community and connectedness for those they serve. Servant-leaders, in building community, seek ways to bring people together for the good of individuals and the organization (Greenleaf, 1977).

Through their roles as strong, effective clinical leaders, CNLs can use servant-leader principles to enhance the effectiveness of patient outcomes through collaborative teams.

Transactional and Transformational Leadership

Transactional leadership is based on transactions or exchanges between the leader and the led where rewards and benefits are offered to subordinates if they fulfill agreements and contribute to the achievement of goals (Avolio & Bass, 2002; Bass, 1990). While transactional leaders tend to be caretakers, they often have little vision or few overtly shared values with followers (Avolio & Bass, 2002; Barker, Sullivan, & Emery, 2006). Transactional leaders focus on the completion of tasks or assignments and consider how to modify processes to incrementally improve and maintain the quality of performance, how to substitute one goal for another, and how to reduce resistance to a particular action and implement decisions (Avolio & Bass, 2002). The transactional leader strives to carry out decisions with little disruption or conversation (Klainberg & Dirschel, 2010). This can be effective for groups under stress, providing satisfaction through immediate solutions; however, long-term effectiveness is not often an outcome of transactional processes (Tomey, 2010). Transactional leadership is often displayed in healthcare organizations where immediate or unpredictable patient care needs necessitate immediate responses or actions. It is also congruent with traditional definitions of management that include goal setting, establishing priorities, developing an action plan, and delegating (Barker et al., 2006; Tomey, 2010).

As an extension of transactional leadership, transformational leadership includes a change or transformation of both the leader and the follower (Avolio & Bass, 2002; Barker et al., 2006, Tomey, 2010). Bass (1990) describes transformational leadership as a superior form of leadership that occurs when leaders act as agents of change influencing others through the change process. Transformational leaders expand the sphere of influence of their employees by increasing awareness and engagement of the aims and mission of the community of practice. Transformational leaders are instrumental in coaching employees to transcend their own self-interest thereby providing a means to think beyond what is their current reality.

Transformational leaders motivate followers to perform beyond normal expectations through a transformation of thoughts and attitudes and by enlisting vital support of the vision while striving for its fulfillment. Avolio and Bass (2002) and Tomey (2010) summarized the behaviors associated with transformational leadership, including attributed charisma (modeling behaviors), inspirational motivation (creating a vision for the future), intellectual stimulation (questioning assumptions and reframing problems from a new perspective), and individualized consideration (delegating work that attends to individual needs, abilities, and aspirations). Transformational leadership is a visionary leadership style that has a long-term focus. As a result, change focuses on the systems and culture of an organization. Transformational leaders act as agents of change for both the leader and the follower. They arouse strong positive emotion and influence the beliefs, behaviors, attitudes, and perceptions of others. Changes that occur using this leadership style have longer lasting effects because they change patterns of thinking, beliefs, and values through the interaction between the leaders and followers (Avolio & Bass, 2002; Bass, 1990; Tomey, 2010).

Transformational leadership has been defined as a superior form of leadership that occurs when leaders bring awareness to the shared or common desires of leaders and followers. This awareness, commitment, and acceptance of the purposes and mission of the group or organization are the motivating factors followers embrace as they look beyond self-interest and embrace change for the good of the group (Klainberg & Dirschel, 2010; Tomey, 2010). These goals are accomplished by using transformational leadership behaviors, including the aforementioned: attributed charisma or modeling behaviors that gain admiration and trust, inspirational motivation or the ability to envision and articulate a future, intellectual stimulation involving questioning assumptions and reframing problems from a new perspective, and individualized consideration by delegation and empowering groups while attending to individual needs, abilities, and aspirations (Klainberg & Dirschel, 2010; Marquis & Huston, 2006; Tomey, 2010). This contributes to increased satisfaction and meaningfulness in one's work (Tomey, 2010, Marquis & Huston, 2006).

The theory of transformational leadership suggests that people need a sense of mission that extends beyond transactions and interpersonal relationships (Avolio & Bass, 2002; Barker et al., 2006; Marquis & Huston, 2006; Tomey, 2010). This is especially true in the CNL role, where the commitment is made to remain at the point of care and service to lead efforts in improving quality and safety. Nurses often choose their profession as a means to display and convey a commitment to the greater good for humankind. Transformational leadership behaviors create unity, wholeness, and collective purpose though the use of a common vision and inspiration focused on a larger purpose that is fundamental to the CNL role (Barker et al., 2006; Tomey, 2010).

Microsystem Partnerships and Clinical Leadership

Team Science

Implied in clinical leadership at the point of care is the integration and collaboration between the CNL and all members of a team. The IOM (2003), in *Health Professions Education: A Bridge to Quality,* identified interprofessional collaboration and communication as needs of 21st-century healthcare delivery systems, and for the most part, the literature describes individual choices and individual professional development as cornerstones of this change imperative.

Depending on the care delivery system, organizational structures, and organizational cultures, CNLs can have a significant impact on teams, particularly interdisciplinary teams charged with improving clinical outcomes that have implications between departments or locations of care. Given the CNL's attention to evidence-based practice and commitment to safety and quality improvement, CNLs leading interdisciplinary teams within a microsystem can facilitate improved outcomes through team-determined metrics.

In *The Science of Improvement*, the Institute for Healthcare Improvement highlights characteristics of effective teams representing different kinds of expertise and leadership within the organization, within a system, holding technical expertise, and in day-to-day leadership (2011). Critical to the success of a team are a clinical leader with the authority to test and implement change, a technical expert who knows the subject of change intimately and understands the processes of care and quality improvement tools and strategies, and a day-to-day leader to drive and oversee the change project and facilitate changes in the system. CNLs are well positioned for each of these activities.

CNLs in Action

As clinical leaders, CNLs are action oriented, connecting mission and purpose to outcomes with impact. CNLs serve as leaders for the greater good of the microsystem. Collaborating with their interprofessional team, CNLs translate evidence into quality practice. They lead with heart and conviction. CNLs influence processes through deliberate, thoughtful inquiry, using such tools as AI, transformational leadership, and change strategies. They model positive communication strategies and relationship-based care. They are sensitive to the nuances at the intersection of the patient, system, and provider. Exemplars of outstanding leadership are peppered throughout this text, including reducing pressure ulcers and falls with harm, improving patients' abilities to self-manage their chronic illnesses, and improving lifestyles.

Conclusion

Clinical leadership is about CNLs informing the quality and safety of care through innovation and improvement—both in their organizational processes and in their individual care practices. It is based on the premise that because CNLs actually deliver care, they are well positioned to evaluate its quality and guide improvement. Clinical leadership can be taken on by any direct provider of patient care, including doctors, nurses, allied health professionals, clinical pharmacists, and paramedics.

Summary

- CNLs are in a key position to influence healthcare delivery models and outcomes.
- CNLs use a variety of leadership strategies to influence microsystems, resulting in positive outcomes.
- CNLs demonstrate a number of clinical leadership behaviors in the execution of their various role functions.
- CNLs consider a variety of change theories in leading innovation.
- CNLs engage stakeholders in understanding the improvement process.
- CNLs use improvement and team science to create interdisciplinary teams to foster greater coordination and collaboration.

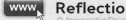 **Reflection Questions**
© Arenacreative/Dreamstime.com

1. Consider a typical day from your experiences as a CNL student, graduate, and then in the role. Identify at least one example in which you demonstrated clinical leadership. Were you intentional in your communication with others? How would you rate yourself? Would you respond differently now that you have had time to reflect on your actions, how individuals responded to you,

etc.? Then reflect on an interaction you observed in the last week in which leadership was critical to the outcome of decisions made during the interaction (meeting, task force, etc.). Were you able to recognize a particular leadership style? What constituted leadership in this example?

2. Assess your leadership style using any number of leadership appraisal tools. What are your areas of strength? What are the areas that need improvement? Share your assessment with your mentor as you develop an action plan for future growth.

www Learning Activities
© Arenacreative/Dreamstime.com

1. Consider a clinical situation on your unit where you have not been able to sustain a change. What elements of leadership were present? What elements of leadership were missing?
2. Examine the clinical indicators on your unit/microsystem. Select an indicator that could benefit from clinical leadership and propose how you would establish a team to address it. Who would be on the team? What tools would you use in planning the change? What evidence is available to support the change?
3. Consider a process that impacts your unit and the clinical outcomes that are possible. Is there clinical leadership of the initiative? An interdisciplinary team or task force responsible for the outcome? What do you attribute to the success or failure of this clinical intervention?
4. Describe the attributes of a clinical leader versus an administrative leader. What do they hold in common? What distinguishes them from one another?

   Using any number of self-appraisal leadership tools, assess your leadership abilities, developing an action plan to address areas that you would like to further develop. Have your mentor work with you to monitor your progress.

References

American Association of Colleges of Nursing. (2007). *White paper on the role of the clinical nurse leader*. Retrieved from http://www.aacn.nche.edu/publications/white-papers/cnl

Amos, M. A., Hu, J., & Herrick, C. A. (2005). The impact of team building on communication and job satisfaction of nursing staff. *Journal of Nurses Staff Development, 21*(1), 10–18.

Avolio, B., & Bass, B. (2002). *Developing potential across a full range of leadership: Cases on transactional and transformational leadership*. Mahwah, NJ: Lawrence Erlbaum Associates, Publishers.

Barker, A., Sullivan, D., & Emery, M. (2006). *Leadership competencies for clinical managers: The renaissance of transformational leadership*. Sudbury, MA: Jones and Bartlett.

Bass, B. (1990). *Bass & Stogdill's handbook of leadership: Theory, research, & managerial applications* (3rd ed). New York, NY: The Free Press.

Bender, M., Connelly, C. D., Glaser, D., & Brown, C. (2012). Clinical nurse leader impact on microsystem care quality. *Nursing Research, 61*(5), 326–332. doi: 10.1097/NNR .0b013e318265a5b6

Bleich, M. R. (2012). Leadership responses to the future of nursing: Leading change, advancing health IOM report. *Journal of Nursing Administration, 42*(4), 183–184. doi: 10.1097 /NNA.0b013e31824ccc6b

Boonstra, A., & Broekhuis, M. (2010). Barriers to the acceptance of electronic medical records by physicians from systematic review to taxonomy and interventions. *BMC Health Services Research, 10*, 231. doi: 10.1186/1472-6963-10-231

Burnes, B. (2004). Kurt Lewin and complexity theory: Back to the future? *Journal of Change Management, 4*(4), 309–325.

Bushe, G. R., & Pitman, T. (1991). Appreciative process: A method for transformational change. *Organization Development Practitioner, 23*(3), 1–4.

Chin, A. L. (1998, Spring). Future visions. *Journal of Organization and Change Management*.

Cooperrider, D. L. (1990) Positive image, positive action: The affirmative basis of organizing. In S. Srivastva & D. L. Cooperrider (Eds.), *Appreciative management and leadership* (pp. 91–125). San Francisco, CA: Jossey-Bass.

Curran, M. (1991). Appreciative inquiry: A third wave approach to OD. *Vision/Action, December*, 12–14.

Diamond, E., French, K., Gronkiewicz, C., & Borkgren, M. (2010). Electronic medical records: A practitioner's perspective on evaluation and implementation. *Chest, 138*(3), 716–723.

French, W., & Bell, C. (1994). *Organization development: Behavioral science interventions for organization improvement* (5th ed.). Englewood Cliffs, NJ: Prentice Hall.

Garling, P. (Ed.). (2008). Final report of the Special Commission of Enquiry. Acute care services in NSW public hospitals. Retrieved from http://www.lawlink.nsw.gov.au/lawlink/Corporate /ll_corporate.nsf/pages/attorney_generals_department_acsinquiry

Greenleaf, P. (1977). *Servant leadership: A journey into the nature of legitimate power and greatness*. Mahwah, NJ: Paulist Press.

Harman, W. W. (1990). Shifting Context for Executive Behavior: Signs of Change and Revaluation. In S. Srivastva, D. L. Cooperrider, & Associates (Eds.), *Appreciative management and leadership: The power of positive thought and action in organizations* (pp. 37–54). San Francisco, CA: Jossey-Bass, Inc.

Hartranft, S. R., Garcia, T., & Adams, N. (2007). Realizing the anticipated effects of the clinical nurse leader. *Journal of Nursing Administration, 37*(6), 261–263.

Hix, C., McKeon, L., & Walters, S. (2009). Clinical nurse leader impact on clinical microsystems outcomes. *Journal of Nursing Administration, 39*(2), 71–76.

Hubbard, B. M. (1998). *Conscious evolution: Awakening the power of our social potential.* Novato, CA: New World Library.

Institute for Healthcare Improvement. (2011, April 24). Science of improvement: Forming the team. Retrieved from http://www.ihi.org/knowledge/Pages/HowtoImprove/Science ofImprovementFormingtheTeam.aspx

Institute of Medicine. (2003). *Health professions education: A bridge to quality.* Washington, DC: National Academy Press.

Institute of Medicine. (2010). The future of nursing: Leading change, advancing health. Retrieved from http://www.iom.edu/Reports/2010/The-Future-of-Nursing-Leading-Change-Advancing -Health.aspx

Klainberg, M. K., & Dirschel, K. M. (2010). *Today's nursing leader: Managing, succeeding, excelling.* Sudbury, MA: Jones and Bartlett.

Lewin, K. (1951). *Field theory in social science: Selected theoretical papers.* K. Lewin & D. Cartwright (Eds.). Boston, MA: MIT Research Center for Group Dynamics; New York: Harper and Brothers Publishers.

Lippitt, R., Watson, J., & Westley, B. (1958). *The dynamics of planned change.* New York, NY: Harcourt, Brace and World.

Marquis, B., & Huston, C. J. (2006). *Leadership roles and management functions in nursing: Theory and application.* Philadelphia, PA: Lippincott Williams & Wilkins.

National Health Priority Action Council. (2006). *National Chronic Disease Strategy, Australian Government, Department of Health and Ageing, Canberra.* Retrieved from http://www.health .gov.au/internet/main/publishing.nsf/content/7E7E9140A3D3A3BCCA257140007AB32B /$File/stratal3.pdf

Porras, J. I. (1991). Organization development and transformation. *Annual Review of Psychology, 42,* 51–78.

Porter-O'Grady, T. (1997). Quantum mechanics and the future of healthcare leadership. *Journal of Nursing Administration, 27*(1), 15–20.

Porter-O'Grady, T. (1999). Quantum leadership: New roles for a new age. *Journal of Nursing Administration, 29*(10), 37–42.

Schein, E. (1999). Kurt Lewin's change theory in the field and in the classroom: Notes toward a model of managed learning. *Reflections: The SOL Journal, 1*(1), 59–74.

Tomey, A. (2010). *Guide to nursing management and leadership* (8th ed). Terre Haute, IN: Mosby-Elsevier.

Westbrook, I., Braithwaite, J., Georgiou, A., Ampt, A., Creswick, N., Coiera, E., & Iedema, R. (2007). Multimethod evaluation of information and communication technologies in health in the context of wicked problems and sociotechnical theory. *Journal of American Medical Information Association, 14*, 746 –755. doi:10.1197

White, T. W. (1996). Working in interesting times. *Vital Speeches of the Day, LXII*(15), 472–474.

Woo, T. (2013). Horizontal leadership. In C. King & G. O'Toole (Eds.). *Clinical nurse leader certification review*. New York, NY: Springer Publishing Company.

Yackanicz, L., Kerr, R., & Levick, D. (2010). Physician buy-in for EMRs. *Journal of Healthcare Information Management: Journal of Health Management, 24*(2), 41–44.

Suggested Readings

Centers for Medicare & Medicaid Services. (n.d.). The CMS innovation center. Retrieved from http://innovation.cms.gov/

Feldman, H. (Ed.). (2008). Nursing leadership: A concise encyclopedia. Retrieved from http://www.springerpub.com/samples/9780826102584_chapter.pdf

NHS Leadership Academy. (n.d.). Home page. Retrieved from http://www.leadershipacademy.nhs.uk/

Shirey, M. (2006). Authentic leaders creating healthy work environments for nursing practice. *American Journal of Critical Care, 15*, 256–267.

Valentine, S. (2002). Nursing leadership and the new nurse. Retrieved from http://juns.nursing.arizona.edu/articles/Fall%202002/Valentine.htm

Leading the Change in Insulin Delivery: Leading Groups/Moving Forward with Ideas Not in the Mainstream

Mary Harnish

Education of a CNL includes courses in quality improvement of microsystems and microsystem leadership. Our clinical facility/healthcare system challenged us as students to lead change projects identified by the clinical service directors and the chief nursing officer. These projects needed clinical leadership to be implemented. With years of experience in diabetes, I was selected to oversee implementing mainstream basal-bolus insulin as a hospital protocol.

I brought together a multidisciplinary team with key stakeholders including nursing staff, physicians, pharmacists, nutrition services, informatics, and administration. Clinical practice guidelines and literature reviews illuminated evidence-based practice (EBP) in this area, from which the team worked. The team met weekly, employing the Lean process to move this project forward.

Collaboration with nutrition services resulted in listing carbohydrate content of all foods on patient menus and on each meal ticket on the patients' food trays. The implementation of a standardized order set was accomplished by working with the pharmacy and information systems. The protocol was presented to the pharmacy and therapeutics, which, after reviewing the EBP literature, approved the protocol.

The biggest challenge was changing physician practice, especially the hospitalists group, who were responsible for the majority of insulin orders in the hospital. I presented the protocol and order sets to the hospitalists and residents and provided guidebooks on how to use the order sets.

Nursing staff education included a CD learning module and an instructional manual. I provided point-of-care education with multiple scenarios, color-coded dosing cards, and wall charts for reference material.

Months of work went into the challenge of changing clinical practice. Now, four years later, basal-bolus insulin is not the new way of ordering and administering subcutaneous insulin—it is the only way! Rates of severe hyperglycemia improved from a rate of 1.22% to 0.48%. Severe hypoglycemia with blood glucose < 50 mg/dL decreased from 1.5% to 0.48%.

The Need for Cross-Continuum Care

Elizabeth Triezenberg

The orthopedic program at Saint Mary's Health Care is a collaboration of a group of highly aligned surgeons not employed by St. Mary's Health Care. Prior to the implementation of the CNL role, there was limited communication between the office, surgeons, residents, and the staff nurses. Cross-continuum care was quickly identified as the root factor necessary for improving the orthopedic patient experience.

In order to define the cross-continuum, the CNL did a "gemba" walk of the orthopedic patient—starting in the outpatient surgeon's office and continuing through preadmission testing, surgical prep, surgery, recovery, inpatient unit, and returning to the office. Representatives from each of the areas were asked to participate in a short-term Lean project requiring weekly meetings.

The initial meeting was focused on identifying the experience of the patient undergoing a total joint replacement. It quickly became evident that the confusing, fractionated experience of the patient was a reflection of the team's knowledge of the system. Using Lean tools, the team decided to focus on preoperative patient education.

Structured weekly meetings were essential to the timely success of this work group. The group worked to identify, describe, and critique the patient experience. Barriers to care and communication were identified and addressed. Key information for each step of the system was defined and written into a preoperative patient education booklet, specific to our cross-continuum of care. The information the group felt was most important for the patient was summarized in a patient checklist in the front of the booklet.

The goal of the project was to improve the experience for the orthopedic patient by enhancing the cross-continuum of care. Once relationships were formed, the patient experience defined, and the patient preoperative booklet outlined, the group agreed to stop the weekly meetings. The remainder of the editing, marketing, and finalization of the book was done through small group meetings with email updates. The Lean team representatives were responsible for sharing the information with their departments and having the booklets available for reference. As a result of the Lean team's work, the conversations throughout the system have switched from "if the patients only knew _____" to patients stating "the book states _____ was going to happen." The established cross-continuum of orthopedic care has since created additional focus teams for short-term quality improvement projects.

Implementing Safe Insulin Infusion Dosing with a Computer Software Tool

Mary Harnish

Hyperglycemia in hospitalized patients increases infection rates, mortality, and length of stay (LOS). In turn, better glycemic control in hospitalized patients causes a decrease in LOS, infections rates, and mortality. Patients often require intravenous (IV) insulin infusion to maintain optimal glycemic control. Standardization of how IV insulin is titrated decreases blood glucose variability and maintains blood glucose in acceptable and preferred target ranges.

As a CNL for diabetes, I am a member of our hospital's diabetes operations team that works to improve glycemic care in our institution. A need to standardize titration of IV insulin was identified by this team. Various software tools were researched, and the team's clinical members made a choice.

In collaboration with a clinical nurse specialist, I implemented this new insulin titration software tool in the critical care unit. The rollout of this software tool challenged us with educating physicians, especially the intensivists, on use of this tool. Nursing staff were given hands-on training, along with "at-the-elbow" guidance during the initial few weeks of "going live" with the software.

After implementation of this software tool, critical care data on patients receiving insulin drips indicated a drop in the rate of hypoglycemia (blood glucose < 70 mg/dL) in patients on insulin drips from 2.1% to 0.5%. The rate of severe hypoglycemia (blood glucose < 50 mg/dL) decreased from 0.6% to 0.08%.

After the software tool proved useful in the critical care area, it became apparent that there was also a need for insulin drip standardization in step-down units. I assisted the cardiac step-down unit to go live with the software six months after the critical care unit. One year after initiating the use of the insulin titration software, all acuity adaptable units were trained and using the software.

The Implementation of the "Red Zone": An Evidence-Based Approach to Decreasing Medication Errors at The University of Alabama at Birmingham Hospital

Kristen Noles, Tina Fogel, Kathy Carter, Pamela Patterson, and Terri Johnson

Background

Healthcare workers are often interrupted during medication administration. Misdirection away from the task increases the risk of an error. Distractions and interruptions include anything that takes a caregiver's attention away from the current task. The distraction or interruption causes mental weariness, which leads to omissions, mental slips or lapses, and mistakes.

Aim

To describe how a CNL worked with a multidisciplinary team to address interruptions during medication stocking and retrieval.

Methods/Programs/Practices

A practice issue was submitted to the organization's shared governance structure, led by a CNL, called the nursing practice vongress (NPC), concerning medication administration interruptions and patient safety concerns. A multidisciplinary team was formed, including key stakeholders from nursing, pharmacy, ancillary staff, informatics, and medicine. A review of the current literature was completed and a best practice was identified. The team decided to test a time-out zone or "red zone" around the automated medication dispensing machines in both acute and intensive care units. This zone was created to prevent distractions and interruptions when medications were being dispensed, reviewed, and removed in this area. These red zones were established by using red mats and red signs as identifiers of the non-interruption zone. Education was provided to all members of the healthcare team, patients, and families. The expectation was established that when in the red zone, staff members would not answer phone calls, pages, or talk to others including family and staff. Results of the test in both units demonstrated a 50% reduction in medication errors. These results were significant enough to implement the red zone throughout the organization.

Outcome Data

"No interruption" zones around the automated medication dispensing machines were established in multiple care settings including outpatient clinics, acute care areas, operating rooms, intensive care units, and in the emergency department. Three months postimplementation, a decrease in the medication error rate was noted. Subsequent error rates continue to decline. Red zones currently are present around all automated medication dispensing machines throughout the organization. All disciplines acknowledge the importance of no interruptions in the red zone in an effort to prevent medication errors.

Conclusion

The CNL was integral in the identification of key stakeholders, review of the literature, educating staff, housewide implementation, and ongoing evaluation of the efficacy of the established no interruption zones. This has resulted in a sustainable change that has improved patient safety by decreasing medication errors across the organization.

Team Collaboration and Empowerment: Drug Shortages

Laura Bozeman

Medication shortage announcements are part of the daily routine within the Saint Joseph Mercy Health System. Duramorph (morphine), a medication used in spinal anesthesia, provides up to 24 hours of pain control. Shortages create dilemmas for postoperative pain management in cesarean section postoperative patients.

The labor and delivery (L&D) pain resource nurse (PRN), a staff nurse, attends monthly PRN meetings. In response to the Duramorph shortage, specialized pain management pharmacists submitted recommendations to the L&D PRN. Despite the recommendations, conflicting ideas arose from individual anesthesia providers,

L&D postanesthesia care unit nurses, and postpartum nurses. Postoperative cesarean patients did not receive adequate pain management, which contributed to growing concerns. The PRN consulted with the labor and delivery CNL.

The CNL organized a multidisciplinary team meeting, which included several pharmacists with various specialty backgrounds, the L&D and postpartum CNLs, the department head for obstetrics anesthesia, pain CNS, L&D staff nurse/PRN, and an obstetrics resident. The perinatal safety director was apprised via email. The collaborative 90-minute discussion concluded with a solid postoperative pain management plan to be implemented within one week.

The PRN was eager and willing to participate in the educational process. Empowering other staff members to contribute to educational endeavors is imperative for staff engagement. The department manager granted approval for the L&D PRN to be removed from staffing assignments to facilitate the educational sessions. Between the CNL and the PRN, 80 of 100 L&D nurses received the education within a 4-day period. The PRN shared information and managed questions in both the L&D and postpartum huddle discussions. Ongoing follow-up continued among the postpartum CNL, the labor and delivery CNL, and the PRN to assess effectiveness and patient satisfaction with the new regimen. Team collaboration and empowerment of front-line employees is necessary and effective when implementing practice changes.

Optimizing Patient Throughput at a Regional Hospital: Applying Lean Principles to Emergency Department Triage Methodology

Enna Edouard Trevathan and Sunny Rutter

Problem Statement

This community hospital has an 8-bed emergency department (ED) with an annual volume of 26,000 visits per year, three times the national average per-bed capacity. Arrival to triage time averaged 12 to 20 minutes with an additional 7 to 20 minutes per patient triage time, resulting in a bottleneck effect at the point of entry and therefore affecting the current rate of patients that are classified as left without being seen (LWBS).

Interventions

The team used principles and techniques of the Toyota Lean methodology in education and implemented the emergency severity index (ESI) Level 5 Version 4 for triage processes to reduce the redundancy in the nursing process and reduce patient wait times. All nursing staff received education and retraining on the ESI Level 5 triage process (national standard) and the facility's immediate bedding policy in the ED.

Implementation

- Implementation of a pilot process reducing turnaround time from arrival to triage
- Initiation of reduction in total time spent performing triage
- Planned annual revalidation of competencies at unit skills day
- Developed super users in all three shifts to support and sustain the adopted, newly developed policy
- Adoption of ESI Level 5 Version 4

Expected Outcome and Financial Impact

There was a reduction in arrival to triage times, triage process times, and LWBS 6 months to 1 year postimplementation. LWBS are now averaging 2.5% per month, with an average daily census of 72 patients per day or approximately 1.5 patients per day, above the national average of 2% and equating to an estimated 150 patients for the first quarter of the year. This is equal to an estimated loss of $197,700 using the current national average cost of an emergency visit of $1,318 (Agency for Healthcare Research and Quality, 2010; Machin, 2006). While not where the organization would like to be (below 2%), the current trends are moving in a positive direction.

References

Agency for Healthcare Research and Quality. (2010). Retrieved from http://www.ahrq.gov/health-care-information/topics/topic-emergency-room.html

Machin, S. R. (2006). *Expenses for a hospital emergency room visit, 2003*. Medical Expenditure Panel Survey, Statistical Brief #111, Agency for Healthcare Research and Quality. Retrieved from http://meps.ahrq.gov/mepsweb/data_files/publications/st111/stat111.pdf

Innovation in Nursing Quality Data Collection: Can an iPad Application Improve the Data Collection Process?

■ Enna Edouard Trevathan and Anita Girard

Problem Statement

The Institute of Medicine (IOM) estimates that more than 7,000 patients die each year in hospitals alone because of medication errors (Kohn, Corrigan, & Donaldson, 1999). Observations of the medication delivery process identified areas of improvement such as unit culture, delivery, and/or the auditing processes. There is a need for accurate data to drive process improvement projects in this large medical center.

Goal

To improve the quality and enhance the efficiency of medication safety data collection through the utilization of innovation and technology.

Implementation

The iPad technology provides an opportunity for an embedded system of data collection, ensuring decreased collection time and improved throughput while providing a fiscally sound solution that decreases the number of hours spent in data collection, data validation, and manual entry of data into California Nursing Outcomes Classification (CALNOC) spreadsheets for analysis and benchmarking with other Magnet facilities. Collaboration of the nursing quality team, business intelligence team, and the information technology team, with the support of nursing leadership, is imperative.

Expected Outcome and Financial Impact

The use of a secure iPad application allows timely data entry including all CALNOC medication naïve observation rules already embedded into the application software to ensure accuracy from the point of data collection to the completion of data interpretation at the microsystem level. There are 1,500 audits performed per quarter, or 6,000 audits per year. The current process involves 10 steps, with 6 of them involving moving the paper audit sheets from one location to the next. This intervention is in process and if successful, the iPad solution would decrease the steps to only 4 and would eliminate paper. The average registered nurse's wage is $60 per hour; by eliminating 30 minutes from the process, there would be a potential savings of $240,000 per year.

Reference

Kohn, L., Corrigan, J., & Donaldson, M. (Eds.). (1999). *To err is human.* Institute of Medicine. Committee on Quality of Health Care in America, Washington, DC: National Academies Press.

Index